NONPARAMETRIC STATISTICAL TESTS

Name (Test Statistic)	Purpose	Measurement Level*		Corresponding Index of Strength of Relationship
		IV	DV	
Chi-square goodness-of-fit test (χ^2)	To test the predicted value of a proportion for a population	—	N	—
Chi-square test of independence (χ^2)	To test the difference in proportions in 2+ independent groups	N	N	phi (2 × 2), Cramér's V
Fisher's exact test	To test the difference in proportions (2 × 2 table) when expected frequency for a cell < 5	N	N	phi
McNemar test (χ^2)	To test the difference in proportions for 2 related groups (2 × 2 design)	N	N	phi
Cochran's Q test (Q)	To test the difference in proportions for 3+ related groups	N	N	—
Mann-Whitney U-test (U)	To test the difference in the ranks of scores of 2 independent groups	N	O	Glass rank biserial correlation
Kruskal-Wallis test (H)	To test the difference in the ranks of scores of 3+ independent groups	N	O	Epsilon²
Wilcoxon signed ranks test (T or z)	To test the difference in the ranks of scores of 2 related groups	N	O	Matched pairs rank biserial correlation
Friedman test (χ^2)	To test the difference in the ranks of scores of 3+ related groups	N	O	Epsilon²
Spearman's rank order correlation (r_S)	To test the existence of a relationship/correlation between two variables	O	O	(r_S)
Kendall's tau (τ)	To test the existence of a relationship/correlation between two variables	O	O	(τ)

*Measurement level of the independent variable (IV) and dependent variable (DV): N = nominal, O = ordinal.

1

DATA
ANALYSIS &
STATISTICS
FOR NURSING RESEARCH

DATA ANALYSIS & STATISTICS

FOR NURSING RESEARCH

Denise F. Polit, PhD
Humanalysis, Inc.
Saratoga Springs, New York

Appleton & Lange
Stamford, Connecticut

Copyright © 1996 by Appleton & Lange
A Simon & Schuster Company

96 97 98 99 00 / 10 9 8 7 6 5 4 3 2 1

Prentice Hall International (UK) Limited, *London*
Prentice Hall of Australia Pty. Limited, *Sydney*
Prentice Hall Canada, Inc., *Toronto*
Prentice Hall Hispanoamericana, S.A., *Mexico*
Prentice Hall of India Private Limited, *New Delhi*
Prentice Hall of Japan, Inc., *Tokyo*
Simon & Schuster Asia Pte. Ltd., *Singapore*
Editora Prentice Hall do Brasil Ltda., *Rio de Janeiro*
Prentice Hall, *Upper Saddle River, New Jersey*

Library of Congress Catalog Card Number: 95-083509

ISBN 0-8385-6329-5

Acquisitions Editor: David P. Carroll
Editor-in-Chief, Nursing: Sally J. Barhydt
Production: Andover Publishing Services
Designer: Libby Schmitz

PRINTED IN THE UNITED STATES OF AMERICA

Contents

Preface

Few students in the health care professions enroll in a course on statistics because they have an inherent interest in *statistical theory* or *probability*. Typically, the primary reason for learning about statistics is because students want to (or are required to) better understand how to *analyze research data*. Yet, ironically, few statistics books teach readers much about the process of data analysis.

Data Analysis and Statistics for Nursing Research begins with the premise that learning about data analysis—how to do it and how to make sense of the results of others who have done it—is the ultimate goal of a statistics course in health care fields like nursing. Although this book *does* present statistical techniques, it does so within a broad data analytic framework. For example, each chapter tells students not only *how* to perform a statistical analysis, but *why* and *when* in the analysis process it should be done. Each chapter has a section on the *practical applications* of the material covered in the chapter—for example, under what types of situation would a researcher compute a *t*-test? Each chapter also includes a section on how to present statistical information in a research report.

Tables and figures are used throughout the text to enhance the presentation. The figures include computer printouts of the relevant statistical analyses, designed to help students learn how to read such printouts. Actual and fictitious research examples abound, to aid the students' understanding of research applications.

Data Analysis and Statistics for Nursing Research is designed as a textbook for a one-semester course on statistics and data analysis, primarily for nursing students. It covers descriptive statistics, bivariate inferential statistics, and many of the more commonly used multivariate statistics. It assumes virtually no prior knowledge of statistics, and advanced mathematical skills (e.g., calculus, matrix algebra) are not required. It is written in a nontechnical manner, and the emphasis is on understanding how to use and interpret statistics—not on how to calculate them. The textbook presents statistical concepts in an incremental fashion, introducing complex topics only after a firm foundation has been developed. It is hoped that the book will succeed in making a course on statistics less formidable than is often anticipated, and more practical than it often is.

Denise F. Polit

Acknowledgments

Although many individuals helped to make this book possible, I am primarily indebted to my editor, Dave Carroll, who not only suggested that I write it, but also provided unflagging moral support—during a period of considerable mutual turmoil—throughout the project. His friendship and loyalty can never be sufficiently repaid.

Many others, of course, made significant contributions. Dr. Susan L. Woods, who carefully reviewed the manuscript, provided numerous helpful suggestions and offered encouragement that saw me through to the last chapter. Hans Bos was an invaluable resource in the preparation of the *Applications Manual*. I am also indebted to Niels Buessem for his assistance, as well as to John Waggoner, Libby Schmitz, and to many others behind the scenes at Appleton & Lange.

Finally, deepest thanks to my husband Joe and my son Nate for their ongoing tolerance and strong support.

DATA
ANALYSIS &
STATISTICS
FOR NURSING RESEARCH

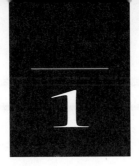

Introduction to Data Analysis

THE ANALYSIS OF RESEARCH DATA

A research investigation begins with a question to be answered. The researcher attempts to answer the question by collecting relevant information—typically, in nursing and in health fields, from human beings who serve as the participants in a study. In the context of a research investigation, the information usually is referred to as **data.** Data can be gathered in a number of different ways—by asking people questions, by observing and recording their behavior, or by taking biophysiologic measurements, to name the most typical methods. Whatever the method, the data serve as the foundation for addressing the research question.

Data in a research study can be of two basic types: qualitative or quantitative. **Qualitative data** consist of verbal, narrative pieces of information. For example, Box 1–1 presents some fictitious qualitative data provided by two people in response to the question, Have you felt sad or depressed at all lately, or have you generally been in good spirits? Here the data are narrative descriptions that summarize—and give details about—the respondents' emotional state.

Quantitative data consist of information that is in numerical form. Box 1–2 presents some quantitative data from two subjects responding to the question, Thinking about the past week, how depressed would you say you have been on a scale from 0 to 10, where 0 means "not at all" and 10 means "the most possible"? The subjects have provided a number indicating their degree of depression—9 for Subject 1, suggesting a high level of depression, and 0 for Subject 2, indicating no depression at all.

In a research study, the questions would be asked of many different people, who as a group constitute the research sample. The responses of the sample members would,

1-1

EXAMPLE OF QUALITATIVE DATA

Question

Have you felt sad or depressed at all lately, or have you generally been in good spirits?

Data (Subject 1)

Well, I've been in pretty rough shape lately, to tell you the truth. I mean, I haven't felt suicidal or anything like that, but I just can't seem to shake the blues. I just don't see anything to feel hopeful about in my future. I haven't really had anybody to talk to about my problems since my husband died last year.

Data (Subject 2)

I'm not at all depressed. I feel great! I love my new job. And I've lost 20 pounds and feel much healthier than I have in years. I can't remember any period of my life when I've been happier.

---

collectively, comprise the data for the study. By themselves, however, the data do not answer the research question. The data must be organized, synthesized, evaluated, and interpreted, through a process referred to as **data analysis.**

The analysis of qualitative data is a complex and labor-intensive process. Those interested in learning about methods of qualitative data analysis should consult references such as the books by Miles and Huberman (1994) or Wolcott (1993).

Quantitative data are almost always subjected to **statistical analysis.** This textbook is devoted to methods of analyzing data through statistics.

RESEARCH VARIABLES

In a scientific study, the concepts in which the researcher is interested are referred to as variables. A **variable** is something that varies or takes on different values. Height,

1-2

EXAMPLE OF QUANTITATIVE DATA

Question
Thinking about the past week, how depressed would you say you have been on a scale from 0 to 10, where 0 means "not at all" and 10 means "the most possible"?
Data (Subject 1)
9
Data (Subject 2)
0

weight, gender, blood pressure, and heart rate are all examples of characteristics that vary from one person to the next. (If they did not vary, they would be referred to as **constants**). Variation in our world is extensive, and it is this variation that is at the root of scientific inquiry. Researchers are interested in explaining and understanding variation: Why do some people smoke while others do not? Why do some people comply with a medical regimen while others fail to do so? Researchers collect data about those variables in which they are interested and examine relationships among them.

Independent and Dependent Variables

Variables can be characterized in several different ways that have implications for analyzing the data. One distinction concerns the role that the variable plays in an analysis—the distinction between independent and dependent variables. The **independent variable** is the hypothesized cause of, or influence on, the **dependent variable.** In the research question, "Does a low-cholesterol diet reduce the risk of heart disease?" the independent variable is the amount of cholesterol in a person's diet, and the dependent variable is heart disease. Cholesterol level is a variable, because people consume different amounts of it, and heart disease is a variable because not everyone has this disease. The research question is whether variation in the independent variable causes or influences variation in the dependent variable. Table 1–1 presents some examples of actual research questions from the nursing research literature, and indicates the independent variable and dependent variable of each.

Discrete and Continuous Variables

Another distinction that has relevance for statistical analysis concerns discrete and continuous variables. A **discrete variable** is one that has a finite number of values between any two points. For example, if people were asked how many times they had ever been hospitalized, they might answer 0, 1, 2, 3, or more times. The variable for number of times hospitalized is discrete, because a number such as 1.5 is not a meaningful value: between the values 1 and 3, the only possible value is 2. A **continuous variable** is one that, at least in theory, can assume an infinite number of values between any two points. Weight is an example of a continuous variable. Between 1 and 2 pounds, there is an unlimited number of possible values: 1.01, 1.245, 1.379, and so on.

LEVELS OF MEASUREMENT

In a quantitative study, the researcher must have a method of measuring the research variables. That is, for every variable, there must be a method of assigning a numerical value. **Measurement** involves the assignment of numbers to qualities of objects to designate the quantity of the attribute, according to a set of rules. No attribute *inherently* has a numerical value. Human beings invent the rules to quantitatively measure abstract concepts.

TABLE 1–1. EXAMPLES OF INDEPENDENT AND DEPENDENT VARIABLES

Research Question	Independent Variable	Dependent Variable
Is facilitated tucking effective in reducing crying in preterm neonates in response to heelsticks? (Corff, Seideman, Venkataraman, Lutes, & Yates, 1995)	Facilitated tucking vs. no facilitated tucking	Amount of crying
Are prodromal symptoms in suspected acute myocardial infarction (AMI) related to a final diagnosis of AMI? (Hofgren, Karlson, & Herlitz, 1995)	Presence vs. absence of prodromal symptoms	Final diagnosis of AMI vs. other diagnosis
What is the effect of ovarian hormone cessation and supplementation on the body weight of rats? (Bond, Heitkemper, & Jarrett, 1994)	Ovarian hormone status	Body weight
Do coronary angioplasty patients have more symptoms of psychologic stress than coronary artery bypass patients 1 month after treatment? (White & Frasure-Smith, 1995)	Type of treatment	Symptoms of psychologic stress
What is the effect of attendance at a long-term exercise program on the physical functioning of older adults? (Topp & Stevenson, 1994)	Attendance vs. non-attendance at exercise program	Physical functioning

For some variables, measurement is straightforward. There are widely accepted rules for measuring such variables as height, weight, and blood pressure, for example. For other variables, the researcher must often develop new rules of measurement. Sometimes the rules are complex—for example, when the researcher is measuring psychological concepts such as stress, coping, health beliefs, and so on, complex rules are generally required. In other cases, the rules simply involve the assignment of an arbitrary numerical **code**—for example, when the researcher designates a code of 1 for females and a code of 2 for males, for the variable gender.

Thus, there are different types of measurement rules. The most widely used system for describing these differences concerns the **level of measurement** of a variable. There are four different levels of measurement commonly used in nursing and health research: nominal, ordinal, interval, and ratio. This classification system is important because the type of analysis that the researcher can undertake depends on the level of measurement of the research variables.

Nominal Measurement

Nominal measurement, the lowest form of measurement, involves using numbers simply as labels to classify attributes into different categories. (In fact, variables measured on the nominal scale are sometimes referred to as **categorical variables.**) A wide variety of characteristics can be measured on a nominal scale: a person's gender, marital status, blood type, and religion, for instance. Some examples of nominal-level variables and their codes are shown in Box 1–3. In nominal measurement, the numbers are completely arbitrary and have no inherent quantitative meaning; it would be just as appropriate to code males as 1 and females as 2 as vice versa. Because the numbers are arbitrary, they cannot be treated mathematically. For example, it would not be meaningful to compute the average gender of a sample, although it would make sense to compute the percentage of males and females.

Ordinal Measurement

Ordinal measurement involves the use of numbers to designate ordering on an attribute. Ordinal measurement allows the researchers to classify subjects *and* to indicate their relative standing on some dimension of interest. The numbers are no longer arbitrary, but rather convey information about the *amount* of some attribute. Some examples are presented in Box 1–4. The codes for educational attainment, for instance, indicate incremental amounts of schooling, from high school diploma (code 1) to a graduate degree (code 4). Ordinal measurement does not, however, tell us anything about the distance between categories. The difference between having a graduate degree and a college degree is not equivalent to the difference between having a college degree and some college education, but the ordinal codes provide no clue about the relative magnitude of the differences. As with nominal-level measures,

1-3

EXAMPLES OF NOMINAL-LEVEL VARIABLES

VARIABLE	VARIABLE CODE			
Gender	1 = Female	2 = Male		
Marital Status	1 = Single	2 = Married	3 = Divorced	4 = Other
Group	1 = Experimental	2 = Control		
Blood Type	1 = Type A	2 = Type B	3 = Type AB	4 = Type O

1-4

EXAMPLES OF ORDINAL-LEVEL VARIABLES

VARIABLE	VARIABLE CODE	
Educational Attainment	1 = High school diploma	3 = College degree
	2 = Some college	4 = Graduate degree
Academic Rank	1 = Instructor, lecturer	3 = Associate professor
	2 = Assistant professor	4 = Full professor
Socioeconomic Status	1 = High	4 = Lower middle
	2 = Upper middle	5 = Low
	3 = Middle	

it is not generally meaningful to compute an average with variables measured on an ordinal scale.

Interval Measurement

Interval measurement involves assigning numbers that indicate both the ordering on an attribute, and the distance between different amounts of the attribute. Temperature on the Fahrenheit scale is an example of interval-level measurement. Equal distances on the Fahrenheit scale represent equal differences in temperature. That is, the difference between 100°F and 101°F is equivalent to the difference between 101°F and 102°F. Thus, interval-level measures provide information about not only rank ordering but also about the magnitude of difference between different values on the scale. When a variable is measured on the interval scale, there are a great many analytic possibilities. For example, it is perfectly reasonable to compute an average for interval-level variables (e.g., the average body temperature of a sample of patients).

Ratio Measurement

Ratio measurements combine the features of interval-level measurements with one additional characteristic: the presence of a natural, meaningful zero point. Because of this feature, variables measured on the ratio scale provide information about the absolute amount of the property being measured. If we were measuring the amount of pain medication administered to a patient, 0 milligrams would be a perfectly legitimate value, indicating the total absence of pain medication. Interval measures, by contrast, do not have a rational zero point. A temperature of 0°F does not indicate the total absence of heat. Because ratio-level measures have an absolute zero, all mathematical operations are possible. It is possible to add, subtract, multiply, and divide the values on a ratio scale. Thus, it is possible to say that 80 inches is twice as long as 40 inches (inches are on a ratio scale), although it is not meaningful to say that 80°F is twice as hot as 40°F (degrees Fahrenheit are on an interval scale).

Considerations in Using Measurement Scales

Researchers need to be aware of the measurement levels of their variables when they are collecting and analyzing data. The four types of measurement scale can be thought of as a hierarchy, with nominal measures at the bottom of the hierarchy and ratio measures at the pinnacle. Researchers generally strive to have variables measured on the highest level of measurement possible. There are three advantages to using higher levels of measurement: greater analytic flexibility, availability of more powerful statistical techniques, and a greater amount of information than at lower levels.

As we move from ratio measures to interval, ordinal, and nominal measures, there is a successive loss of information. We can demonstrate this information loss with a fictitious example. Table 1–2 presents data on the amount of sodium intake for six people,

TABLE 1–2. FICTITIOUS DATA SHOWING FOUR MEASUREMENT LEVELS FOR DAILY AMOUNT OF SODIUM INTAKE

Subject	Ratio (mg)	Interval	Ordinal	Nominal 1 = low 2 = high
Nathan	4000	1500	3	1
Chad	7500	5000	6	2
Travis	2500	0	1	1
Justin	3500	1000	2	1
Ryan	6000	3500	5	2
Tom	5500	3000	4	2

measured on the four measurement scales. The first column of data shows the actual amount of sodium consumed in milligrams. These ratio measures give us complete information regarding the absolute amount of sodium each subject consumed, and the absolute differences between subjects. The next column shows interval measures that represent the amount of sodium over a specified criterion, which in this case we have set at 2500 mg. Travis has a value of 0 (2500 − 2500), while Chad has a value of 5000 (7500 − 2500) on this measure. These interval measures provide no clue about the absolute amount of sodium consumed, although the distances between the values are still meaningful. For example, the difference in sodium consumption between Justin and Tom is the same as the difference between Tom and Chad (i.e., 2000 mg). In the next column, the data have been converted to an ordinal measure by rank ordering the subjects with regard to sodium intake. Travis is ranked first because his sodium intake was lowest, Justin is ranked second, and so forth. These measures no longer tell us how much more sodium was consumed by one person than the next. The amount separating Travis and Justin might be 1 mg or 5000 mg. Finally, the last column presents nominal-level measures, wherein the subjects are simply classified as being low or high on sodium intake, using 5000 mg or greater as the cutoff value for the "high" category. Within each category, there is no information regarding who consumed more sodium than whom: Nathan, Travis, and Justin are considered equivalent with regard to their sodium intake.

Thus, it generally is preferable to use the highest possible level of measurement so that the fullest information available can be exploited. Exceptions sometimes arise,[1] but this general rule should be kept in mind in making analytic and measurement decisions.

For the most part, the measurement level of variables is fairly easy to determine. However, there is some controversy regarding the level of many measures of psychosocial attributes (e.g., scales that measure stress, cognitive ability, self-esteem, attitudes,

---

[1]For example, for some health-related variables there may be cutoff values that designate important clinical categories, such as the distinction between low-birth-weight and normal-birth-weight infants. In some analyses, therefore, it may be more appropriate to use this nominal-level categorization than to use actual birthweights, which are ratio measures.

and so on). Such scales typically have been treated in statistical analyses as interval-level measures, but some people argue that they are really ordinal measures. Although many psychosocial scales do yield measures that are, strictly speaking, ordinal, some methodological studies have suggested that treating them as interval measures is not likely to introduce major distortions if the scales approximate interval characteristics.

One further distinction between types of measures is sometimes important. The measurement scales can be categorized into two basic groups. Variables measured on the nominal level are sometimes referred to as **qualitative variables** because the numbers associated with the variables convey no quantitative information. By contrast, variables measured on the ordinal, interval, or ratio scale—all of which convey information about the *amount* of an attribute—are referred to as **quantitative variables.**

THE USES OF DATA ANALYSIS

Once the research variables have been measured, the resulting quantitative data can be analyzed in a variety of ways, and the analyses can serve many different purposes. The purposes can be categorized and illustrated along three different dimensions, as discussed in the next sections.

Analyses for Description versus Inference

One of the most basic distinctions in statistical analysis is the difference between descriptive statistics and inferential statistics.

Descriptive Statistics. All researchers want, at a minimum, to describe their data in a convenient and informative manner. Figure 1–1 presents an array of data that is sometimes referred to as a **data matrix.** The rows in this table correspond to 25 different research subjects, and the columns correspond to different research variables. Looking at the numbers in this table, it is clearly impossible to make any sense of the data. **Descriptive statistics,** which are used by researchers to describe and summarize data, help to make data readily comprehensible.

A wide variety of descriptive statistics is available to researchers. Averages and percentages are examples of descriptive statistics. Through descriptive statistics, we would be able to ask and answer the following questions with regard to the data in Figure 1–1[2]:

1. What percent of the sample is male?
2. What is the average age of the subjects in the sample?
3. What is the age range of subjects in the sample?
4. Are men, on average, older than women?
5. Is there a relationship between age and number of years of schooling?

---

[2]In this table, column 3 contains data on gender, columns 4 and 5 contain data on age, and columns 6 and 7 contain data on years of schooling.

```
0113512031276122111321113016716131221111   1112133211563413121
0224114114133122122132541448815122112231121223412131876121122
0315210041255211221132321131781728112111212232121231111 5121211
0423916121231212312316761212131212312312312312311423123141212122
0516112123131210209121232123129912313181212191231231214321121
0613117121231291821231231231231231413121423214132123 912381200112
0724013121231817311213123191213121219121212313121912121122112
0824412132121191212122221222221213121151213121211112131210123
0915018212312311111211121211199991212   1212312123121111112111
1014314121233331211121231212  19999  121212222121121231221211
1122918222212232123123111219111212131212432114312123211121122
1212917411413312212213254144881512211223112122341213187612129
1323315041255211221132321131781728112111212232121231114212111
1424512221231212312316222212131212312123121231423123141211118
1515111123131210208121212312121112313181212111231231214322212
1614112212312221821231231231231413121423214132123111238120222
1723418121231113311213123121213121219121212313121912121121111
1822812132121191212122221222221213112131213121211112131210121
1915210212312311111211121211199991212111123121231211112122
2013715121233331211121231212112222121212122221211212312223322
2112516031276122111321113016716131221111221112133211563413122
2224911111413312212213254122121512211223112122341213187612111
2313212041255211221132321131781728112111212232121231111121221
2423814121231212312313421212131212312123121231423123141211222
2514113123131210209121232123121112313121212131231231214321122
```

FIGURE 1–1.   A MATRIX OF DATA FOR 25 SUBJECTS

As these illustrative questions suggest, descriptive statistics allow researchers to *describe* (questions 1 through 3); to *compare* (question 4), and to *determine a relationship* (question 5). Descriptive statistics can involve a single variable at a time (e.g., question 1 involves the variable gender) or two variables simultaneously (for example, question 4 involves the variables gender and age). Descriptive statistics generally are straightforward computationally.

Descriptive statistics can be communicated in three ways: in a narrative fashion, in a graph, or in a table. Narratively, we could describe a sample as being 50% white, 40% African-American, and 10% Hispanic. We could display this same information graphically, as shown in Figure 1–2. A table could be used to summarize the percentage distribution of the sample in terms of race/ethnicity, gender, and other characteristics. Throughout this book, we offer suggestions for when graphs or tables can be used effectively to supplement a narrative presentation.

Inferential Statistics. Researchers typically derive their data by obtaining measurements from a **sample,** that is, from a relatively small group of people with characteristics that are relevant to the research question. However, researchers are almost always interested in answering research questions about a **population**—the entire group of people with the relevant characteristics—rather than about the particular individuals comprising the sample.

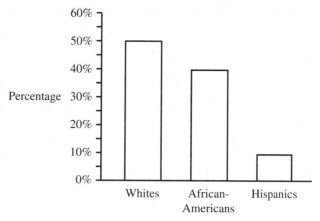

Racial/Ethnic Distribution of Sample

FIGURE 1–2.   GRAPHIC PRESENTATION OF DESCRIPTIVE STATISTICS

When researchers use data from a sample to make inferences or draw conclusions about a population, they use **inferential statistics.** Inferential statistics use the laws of probability to help researchers draw conclusions about population characteristics, based on information from samples. Most researchers use statistics based on samples to address questions about a population, and thus inferential statistics are widely used in research.

Inferential statistics are sometimes used to draw conclusions about a single population value. For example, a researcher might want to know the average birth weight of infants born with AIDS. Without data from all babies born with AIDS, the researcher would estimate the value based on data from a sample of AIDS babies. Inferential statistics would allow the researcher to infer how accurate the estimate was.

More frequently, inferential statistics are used to draw conclusions about the relationships between variables in the population. A **relationship** is a bond or association between variables. For example, the researcher might want to determine whether the average birth weight of AIDS babies is *lower than* the birth weight of other babies. The relationship in question concerns birth weight (the dependent variable) in relation to the infants' AIDS status (the independent variable).

Inferential statistics about relationships can be used to address three separate questions:

1. *Existence.* Is there a relationship between variable X and variable Y in the population?
2. *Magnitude.* How strong is the relationship between variable X and variable Y in the population?
3. *Nature.* What type of relationship exists between variable X and variable Y in the population?

Sometimes a single statistic can be computed to address all three of these questions, but often separate statistics are needed for different questions. Statistics for all three types of question are described in this book.

Univariate, Bivariate, and Multivariate Statistics

Another dimension along which statistical methods can be described concerns the number of variables in the analysis. **Univariate statistics** involve one variable at a time. Examples include the percentage of men and women in the sample, or the average heart rate of the sample members. **Bivariate statistics** involve two variables examined simultaneously. If the researcher compared the average heart rate of men versus women, bivariate statistical procedures would be used. When three or more variables are included in the same analysis, **multivariate statistics** are needed. For example, a researcher might use gender, weight, and amount of exercise (three independent variables) to better understand variations in heart rate (the dependent variable). Although multivariate statistics are computationally formidable, the widespread availability of computers has made these complex statistical procedures accessible to growing numbers of researchers.

Analyses for Different Purposes

A third dimension for characterizing quantitative analysis concerns the role that the analysis plays in the research process. Statistical analysis is typically used for many more purposes than simply to answer the researcher's substantive questions. (Indeed, even qualitative researchers sometimes use quantitative analyses for some purposes.) Here are a few examples of different purposes for using statistical analysis:

1. *Data Cleaning.* Typically, one of the first things that a researcher does with a data set (we are assuming that the researcher is using a computer for data analysis) is to determine if the data are "clean". Before the more substantive analyses can begin, the researcher must have confidence that the numbers and codes entered in the computer file are accurate. For example, if the researcher used descriptive statistics to determine the gender of the sample and found that 55% had a code of 1 (female), 44% had a code of 2 (male), and 1% had a code of 3 (not a valid code), then a correction to the file would need to be made.

2. *Sample Description.* Researchers almost always want to learn the main characteristics of their sample. Even though the research question may have nothing to do with the background characteristics of the subjects, researchers generally compute descriptive statistics that summarize the sample's main attributes (e.g., age, gender, race/ethnicity, marital status, and so on).

3. *Assessment of Bias.* Researchers often perform statistical analyses to determine if there might be systematic biases that need to be taken into consideration in interpreting the results of the substantive analyses. For example, in a study that

recruited subjects on a voluntary basis, the researcher might want to compare the background characteristics of people who agreed to participate in the study with those of people who declined, to determine the nature and magnitude of any differences.

4. *Evaluation of Measuring Tools.* In many studies, the researcher undertakes analyses designed to examine whether the measuring instruments used to collect the data are reliable and valid. In studies that are primarily methodologic in nature (for example, a study to develop and refine a new tool to measure stress), this type of analysis often constitutes the central focus of the investigation.

5. *Evaluation of the Need for Transformations.* Data that are gathered by the researcher often need to be transformed or altered before the substantive analyses can proceed, and the use of descriptive statistics comes to the researcher's assistance. As but one example, researchers usually have to make decisions about how to handle missing values. The term **missing values** refers to the absence of information for a specific variable for some of the subjects, as a result of errors, refusals, misunderstandings, and so on. Through descriptive statistics, the researcher can examine the extent of missing data for all the research variables, can evaluate whether the data are missing at random, and can make decisions on how best to handle the problem. This sometimes involves replacing the missing values with some other, legitimate values through a data transformation.

6. *Addressing Research Questions.* Finally, statistical analyses are used to directly address the substantive research questions. In some cases, descriptive statistics can be used for this purpose, but most researchers apply inferential statistics for establishing the extent to which their results are likely to be reliable for the population of interest.

THE DATA ANALYSIS PLAN

In most studies, the researcher does not move directly from the collection of the data to the substantive analyses of those data. As the preceding list of purposes suggests, there are many preliminary analyses that researchers typically undertake with their **data set** (i.e., the total collection of data for all sample members). The prudent researcher endeavors to develop a realistic **data analysis plan** that guides progress toward the goal of answering the research questions and interpreting the results.

Figure 1–3 presents a flow chart that depicts what the flow of tasks might look like in progressing from data collection to the attainment of the final results. Not all of these steps are necessary in all studies, and in some cases the ordering of the steps might be different. The figure is intended not as an explicit guide, but rather to show that careful planning of analytic activities is critical. Throughout this textbook we describe statistical techniques that are appropriate for many of the steps in this flow of analytic activity.

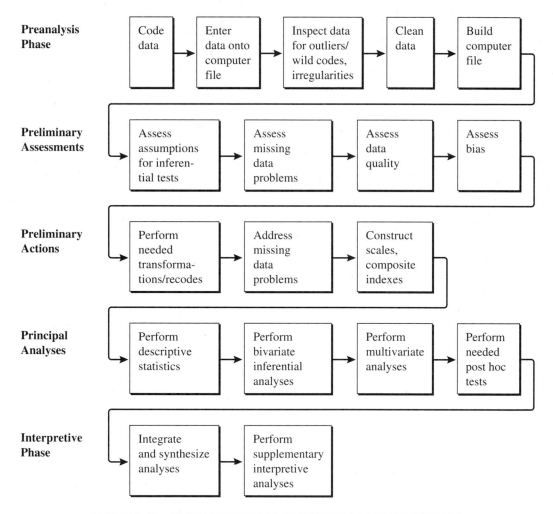

FIGURE 1–3.   FLOW OF TASKS IN ANALYZING QUANTITATIVE DATA

RESEARCH EXAMPLE

Nurse researchers typically measure their research variables on several different measurement levels. Here we describe the measurement levels used in a study that appeared in a recently published study.

> Kollef (1995) conducted a study that was designed to identify predictors of mortality for patients in intensive care units (ICUs). The dependent variable in this study was a nominal-level variable: survival versus nonsurvival.

Data on dozens of potential predictor variables (that is, independent variables) were collected from medical records, flow sheets, and various patient reports in a sample of 277 ICU patients. The independent variables were measured at every level of measurement. Nominal-level variables included the following: patient gender (male/female), smoking status (smoker/nonsmoker), private health insurance (yes/no), admission from a chronic health care facility (yes/no), presence of immunosuppression (yes/no), occurrence of an iatrogenic event (yes/no), need for acute dialysis (yes/no), and type of nutritional support (parenteral/enteral). An example of an ordinal-level variable was a five-point lifestyle score, designating the following categories of increased dependency: 0 = employed; 1 = independent and ambulatory; 2 = restricted activities; 3 = housebound; and 4 = bed/chairbound. An example of an interval-level variable was the patient's score on a widely used mortality prediction instrument, the Acute Physiology and Chronic Health Evaluation (APACHE) scale. Finally, there were a number of ratio-level variables, including the patient's age, pack years of cigarette smoking, and admission albumin level.

Kollef also used an index known as the Organ System Failure Index (OSFI), which involves counting the number of dysfunctional organ systems. Although scores on the OSFI could be considered ratio-level, Kollef found that this index proved to be an especially powerful predictor when dichotomized as a nominal-level variable that contrasted three or more organ system failures versus two or fewer. The dichotomized OSFI variable was an important predictor of mortality in the medical, surgical, and cardiothoracic ICU.

SUMMARY

Quantitative data are pieces of information that are in numerical form. Researchers who collect quantitative data to answer their research questions almost always subject their data to **statistical analysis.**

In a quantitative study, the research must develop a method of measuring the concepts of interest, which are referred to as **variables.** The researcher typically measures both an **independent variable** (the presumed cause, influence, or antecedent) and a **dependent variable** (the presumed effect). Some variables are **discrete** (take on a finite number of values), while others are **continuous** (capable of assuming an infinite number of values between two points).

Measurement involves assigning numbers to qualities of objects to designate quantitative information, according to a set of rules. The four **levels of measurement** for research variables are **nominal, ordinal, interval,** and **ratio.** Variables measured on the nominal scale are sometimes referred to as **qualitative variables,** while those measured on the ordinal, interval, or ratio scale are referred to as **quantitative variables.** The measurement level often determines the type of analysis that is appropriate.

Statistical analysis can be described according to different dimensions. One dimension concerns the distinction between **descriptive statistics,** which are used to summarize and describe quantitative information, and **inferential statistics,** which are used to make inferences about **population** values based on information from a **sample.** The second dimension concerns the number of variables in the analysis (**univariate, bivariate,** and **multivariate statistics**). The third dimension concerns the role the analysis plays in the research process (e.g., data cleaning, sample description, assessment of bias, etc.). Given the many uses and types of statistical analysis, the prudent researcher develops a **data analysis plan** to guide the analytic activities.

EXERCISES

The following exercises cover concepts presented in this chapter. Exercises indicated with a dagger (†) can be checked against answers appearing in Appendix A. Additionally, Chapter 1 of the accompanying *Applications Manual* offers supplementary exercises, some of which require analysis of the data set on diskette.

† 1. For each of the following, indicate which is a variable and which is a constant:
   a. The number of minutes in an hour
   b. Patients' diastolic blood pressure
   c. Pi (π)—e.g., for finding the circumference of a circle
   d. College students' level of depression

† 2. For each of the following research questions, identify the independent variable and the dependent variable:
   a. Does a person's age affect psychosocial adjustment following a burn injury?
   b. How do physically handicapped children differ from nonhandicapped children with respect to health self-concepts?
   c. Do patients who administer their own pain medication have lower pain ratings than patients whose pain medication is administered by nurses?
   d. Is the intracranial pressure of comatose patients affected by the presence of conversing visitors?
   e. How does a bonnet compare to a stockinette in preventing heat loss in newborns?

† 3. For each of the variables listed below, indicate which is discrete and which is continuous:
   a. Number of beds in a hospital
   b. Height in inches
   c. Number of pregnancies a woman has had
   d. Amount of time spent sleeping
   e. Body temperature measured in Fahrenheit degrees
   f. Self-esteem as measured on a 10-question scale
   g. Annual income

† 4. For each of the variables listed below, indicate whether the measure is nominal, ordinal, interval, or ratio:
   a. Degrees on the Celsius scale
   b. Students' class rank

c. Number of cigarettes smoked per day
d. Scores on an intelligence test
e. Religious preference
f. Military rank (private, sergeant, etc.)
g. Type of delivery (vaginal versus cesarean)
h. White blood cell count

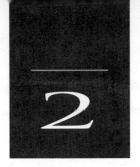

Univariate Statistics: Tabulating and Displaying Data

Researchers use a variety of descriptive statistics to describe data from a research sample. (Descriptive indexes computed for a population are referred to as **parameters;** descriptive indexes for a sample are **statistics**.) This chapter presents methods of organizing and displaying research data through univariate statistics.

FREQUENCY DISTRIBUTIONS

When researchers begin to analyze their data, they rarely attempt to make sense of the mass of numerical information without first imposing some order. A simple listing of the **raw data** (the actual numerical values before any analysis or transformation) rarely conveys much information about the research variables, unless the sample is very small. Take, for example, the data listed in Table 2–1, which represent fictitious heart rate values for 100 patients. It is difficult to understand these data simply by looking at the numbers; we cannot readily see what the highest and lowest values are, nor whether, overall, the heart rate for the sample as a whole is high or low.

Ungrouped Frequency Distributions for Quantitative Variables

One of the first things that researchers typically do with data is to construct frequency distributions. A **frequency distribution** is a systematic arrangement of data values—usually from lowest to highest[1]—together with a count of how many times each value

---

[1]Some statistics books suggest an ordering from highest to lowest. However, the standard procedure for most computer programs (i.e., the **default**) is to order the values from lowest to highest, and we have therefore used this ordering method.

TABLE 2–1. FICTITIOUS DATA ON HEART RATE FOR 100 PATIENTS

60	65	63	57	64	65	56	64	71	67
70	72	68	64	62	66	59	67	61	66
56	69	67	73	68	63	69	70	72	68
60	66	61	60	65	67	74	66	65	66
65	72	66	58	62	60	73	64	59	72
65	68	61	59	68	71	75	65	63	70
75	59	66	69	61	70	58	62	66	63
74	69	68	57	63	65	71	67	62	66
55	70	69	62	66	67	62	72	64	68
66	58	64	66	63	69	71	64	67	57

was observed in the data set. Table 2–2 presents a frequency distribution for the heart rate data. Now we can tell at a glance that the lowest value is 55, that the highest value is 75, and that the value with the highest frequency (12 patients) is 66.

Researchers constructing a frequency distribution manually list the obtained values (the Xs) in a column in the desired order, and then keep a tally next to each value for each occurrence of that value. In Table 2–2, the tallies are shown in the second column, using the familiar system of four vertical bars and then a slash for the fifth case. The tallies can then be totaled, yielding the frequency (f), the count of the number of cases for each value.

In constructing a frequency distribution, the researcher must make sure that the list of score values is mutually exclusive and collectively exhaustive. The sum of the frequencies *must* equal the number of cases in the sample. We can express this with some notation that will appear throughout this textbook:

$$\Sigma f = N$$

where Σ = the sum of
$\quad f$ = the frequencies
$\quad N$ = the sample size

This equation simply states that the sum of (symbolized by the Greek letter sigma, Σ) the frequencies (f) of score values equals the total number (N) of sample members.

A frequency count of data values usually communicates little information in and of itself. In Table 2–2, the fact that five patients had a heart rate of 70 is not very informative without knowing how many patients there were in total, or how many patients had lower or higher heart rates. Because of this fact, frequency distributions almost always show not only **absolute frequencies** (i.e., the count of cases), but also **relative frequencies,** which indicate the percentage of times a given value

TABLE 2–2. FREQUENCY DISTRIBUTION OF HEART RATE SCORES

Score (X)	Tallies	Frequency (f)	Percentage (%)
55	I	1	1.0
56	II	2	2.0
57	III	3	3.0
58	III	3	3.0
59	IIII	4	4.0
60	IIII	4	4.0
61	IIII	4	4.0
62	NN I	6	6.0
63	NN I	6	6.0
64	NN II	7	7.0
65	NN III	8	8.0
66	NN NN II	12	12.0
67	NN II	7	7.0
68	NN II	7	7.0
69	NN I	6	6.0
70	NN	5	5.0
71	IIII	4	4.0
72	NN	5	5.0
73	II	2	2.0
74	II	2	2.0
75	II	2	2.0
		$N = 100 = \Sigma f$	$100.0 = \Sigma\%$

occurs. The third column of Table 2–2 indicates that 5.0% of the sample had a heart rate of 70. Percentages are useful descriptive statistics that appear in the majority of research reports. A percentage can be calculated easily, using the following simple formula:

$$\% = (f \div N) \times 100$$

That is, the percentage for a given value is the frequency for that value, divided by the number of subjects, times 100. Since the sum of all the frequencies should equal the total sample size, the sum of all percentages should equal 100% (i.e., $\Sigma\% = 100\%$).

Another commonly used descriptive statistic is the **cumulative relative frequency,** which presents information about the percentages for the given score value, combined with percentages for all those values that preceded it in the distribution. To illustrate, the heart rate data have been analyzed on a computer, using the Statistical

HARTRATE

Value Label	Value	Frequency	Percent	Valid Percent	Cum Percent
	55	1	1.0	1.0	1.0
	56	2	2.0	2.0	3.0
	57	3	3.0	3.0	6.0
	58	3	3.0	3.0	9.0
	59	4	4.0	4.0	13.0
	60	4	4.0	4.0	17.0
	61	4	4.0	4.0	21.0
	62	6	6.0	6.0	27.0
	63	6	6.0	6.0	33.0
	64	7	7.0	7.0	40.0
	65	8	8.0	8.0	48.0
	66	12	12.0	12.0	60.0
	67	7	7.0	7.0	67.0
	68	7	7.0	7.0	74.0
	69	6	6.0	6.0	80.0
	70	5	5.0	5.0	85.0
	71	4	4.0	4.0	89.0
	72	5	5.0	5.0	94.0
	73	2	2.0	2.0	96.0
	74	2	2.0	2.0	98.0
	75	2	2.0	2.0	100.0
	Total	100	100.0	100.0	

FIGURE 2-1. COMPUTER PRINTOUT OF A FREQUENCY DISTRIBUTION

Package for the Social Sciences (SPSS), and the resulting computer printout is presented in Figure 2–1.[2] Cumulative relative frequencies are shown in the last column, under the heading **Cum Percent.** The advantage of these statistics is that they allow you to see at a glance the percentage of cases that are equal to or less than a specified score value. For example, Figure 2–1 shows that 85.0% of the patients had heart rates of 70 or lower.

Note that in Figure 2–1 there is a column headed **Valid Percent.** The values in this column are, in this example, identical to the values in the preceding column (headed **Percent),** because there are no missing data; heart rate information is available for all 100 fictitious patients. However, in actual studies, it is common to have missing data. The percentages in the column **Valid Percent** are computed after removing any missing cases. Thus, if heart rate information was missing for 10 sample members, the valid percentage for the value of 55 would be 1.1% ($(1 \div 90) \times 100$) rather than 1.0%.

---

[2]The printouts shown in this textbook were all produced through SPSS/PS+ on a personal computer. The SPSS/PC command that produced the printout in Figure 2–1 is as follows:

FREQUENCIES VARIABLES=HARTRATE.

Grouped Frequency Distributions

The values in the heart rate example ranged from a low of 55 to a high of 75, for a total of 21 different values. For some variables, the range of values is much greater. For example, in a sample of 100 infants, it would be possible to obtain 100 different values for the variable birth weight measured in grams. An ordinary frequency table to examine the birth weight data would not be very informative, because each value would have a frequency of 1. When a variable has many possible values, researchers often construct a **grouped frequency distribution.** Such a distribution involves grouping together values into sets, called **class intervals,** and then tabulating the frequencies of cases within the class intervals. For example, for infants' birth weights, we might establish the following class intervals:

- 1001-1500 grams
- 1501-2000 grams
- 2001-2500 grams
- 2501-3000 grams
- 3001-3500 grams
- 3501-4000 grams

In grouping together data values, it is important to strike a balance between insufficient detail resulting when too few groups are used in the frequency distribution, and problems of comprehensibility when too many groups are used. For example, if infants' birth weights were grouped in clusters of 10 grams (e.g., 1001 to 1010, 1011 to 1020, and so on), there would likely be dozens of groups. On the other hand, for most purposes it would likely be inadequate to cluster the birth weight data into only two groups (e.g., 1001 to 2500 grams and 2501 to 4000 grams). As a rule of thumb, a good balance can usually be achieved using between 5 and 15 class intervals.

Once you have a general idea about the desired number of intervals, you need to determine the size of the interval. By subtracting the lowest data value in the data set from the highest data value and then dividing by the desired number of groups, an approximate interval size can be determined. However, you must also strive for intervals that arc psychologically appealing. Interval sizes of 2, 3, and multiples of 5 (e.g., 10, 50, 100) usually work best. All class interval sizes in a grouped frequency distribution should be the same.

Given that the heart rate data resulted in a total of 21 different values, it might be useful to construct a grouped frequency distribution with these data. By clustering three values per class interval, for example, we would arrive at seven intervals. The printout for this grouped frequency distribution is presented in Figure 2–2.[3] This distribution results in a display of information that is easier to digest than the original ungrouped frequency

---

[3]The SPSS/PC commands for producing the frequency distribution in Figure 2–2 are as follows:

    RECODE HARTRATE (55 THRU 57=1) (58 THRU 60=2) (61 THRU 63=3) (64 THRU 66=4)
       (67 THRU 69=5) (70 THRU 72=6) (73 THRU 75=7).
    FREQUENCIES VARIABLE=HARTRATE.

HARTRATE

Value Label	Value	Frequency	Percent	Valid Percent	Cum Percent
55-57 BPM	1	6	6.0	6.0	6.0
58-60 BPM	2	11	11.0	11.0	17.0
61-63 BPM	3	16	16.0	16.0	33.0
64-66 BPM	4	27	27.0	27.0	60.0
67-69 BPM	5	20	20.0	20.0	80.0
70-72 BPM	6	14	14.0	14.0	94.0
73-75 BPM	7	6	6.0	6.0	100.0
		-------	-------	-------	
	Total	100	100.0	100.0	

Valid cases   100   Missing cases   0

FIGURE 2–2.   COMPUTER PRINTOUT OF A GROUPED FREQUENCY DISTRIBUTION

distribution. We can readily see, for example, that there were relatively few cases at either the low end or high end of the distribution, and that there is a substantial clustering of values in the 64 to 66 interval. On the other hand, there is also an information loss; for example, we cannot determine from this distribution what percentage of cases is 70 or below, as we could with the original ungrouped distribution. Decisions on whether to use an ungrouped or grouped distribution depend, in part, on the researcher's reason for constructing the distribution. Some examples are presented later in this chapter.

Frequency Distributions for Qualitative Variables

When a variable is qualitative (i.e., measured on the nominal scale), a frequency distribution can also be constructed. As with quantitative variables, the variable categories are listed in the first column, followed by frequencies and/or relative frequencies in succeeding columns. A fictitious example of a frequency distribution for the nominal variable marital status is shown in Table 2–3.

With qualitative variables, it is usually not meaningful to display cumulative relative frequencies because there is no natural ordering of the categories along any dimension. In Table 2–3, for example, the ordering of the categories could be changed without affecting the information (e.g., the category "Single, Never Married" could come first). Several strategies can be used to order the categories. The most common are ascending or descending order of the frequencies, and alphabetical order of the categories. We ordered the categories in Table 2–3 in descending order of frequency.

TABLE 2–3. FREQUENCY DISTRIBUTION OF A QUALITATIVE VARIABLE: PATIENTS' MARITAL STATUS

	Frequency (f)	Percentage (%)
Married	124	49.6
Single, Never Married	55	22.0
Divorced/Separated	49	19.6
Widowed	22	8.8
	250	100.0

GRAPHIC DISPLAYS OF FREQUENCY DISTRIBUTIONS

Frequency distributions can be presented either in tabular form, as in Tables 2–2 and 2–3, or graphically. Graphs have the advantage of being able to communicate a lot of information quickly.

Bar Graphs and Pie Charts

When the variable of interest is measured on a nominal scale (and sometimes when it is measured on an ordinal scale with a limited number of values), researchers can construct a **bar graph** to display frequency information. An example of a bar graph for the marital status data from Table 2–3 is presented in Figure 2–3. As with other types of frequency distribution graphs, a bar graph consists of two dimensions: a horizontal dimension (sometimes referred to as the **X axis** or **abscissa**) and a vertical dimension (sometimes called the **Y axis** or **ordinate**). In a bar graph, the categories are typically listed along the horizontal X axis, and the frequencies or percentages are displayed along the vertical Y axis. The bars above each category are drawn to the height that indicates the frequency or relative frequency for that category. In a bar graph, the bars for adjacent categories should be drawn not touching each other; each bar width and the distance between bars should be equal. If frequencies are listed along the ordinate, researchers sometimes indicate percentages above the bars, as shown in Figure 2–3.

Sometimes bar graphs are used to display frequencies for several related variables simultaneously. For example, suppose a researcher administered a questionnaire to a sample of nurses and one question asked respondents to indicate how satisfied (very satisfied, satisfied, dissatisfied, very dissatisfied) they were with various aspects of their job (salary, benefits, schedule, and job security). A bar graph might profitably be used to display the percentage of nurses who said they were very satisfied with each of these four aspects of their job, as shown in Figure 2–4.

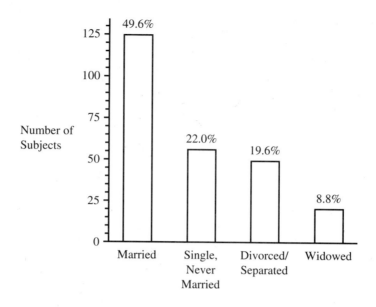

Marital Status of Subjects ($N = 250$)

FIGURE 2–3.   EXAMPLE OF A BAR GRAPH FOR A NOMINAL-LEVEL VARIABLE

An alternative to a bar graph is a **pie chart** (sometimes called a **circle graph**), which is a circle divided into pie-shaped wedges corresponding to the relevant percentages. Figure 2–5 presents a pie chart for the marital status data. All the pieces of the pie must add up to 100%. The pie wedges are generally ordered from highest to lowest frequency, with the largest segment beginning at "12 o'clock."

Histograms

Frequency information for interval-level and ratio-level variables can be displayed in a **histogram,** which is a graphic display similar to a bar graph. However, in a histogram the bars touch one another because adjacent values do not represent distinct categories, but rather contiguous scores on an ordered dimension.

An example of a histogram is shown in Figure 2–6, which is a graphic presentation of the heart rate data from Table 2–2. The data values are normally indicated on the X axis, arranged from lowest to highest, and the frequencies (or relative frequencies) are presented on the Y axis. The numbering on this vertical axis normally begins with 0, or 0%. The height of each bar corresponds to the frequency (or percentage) of cases with the specified score value. Note that the line of the X axis is broken, a convention that is sometimes used to designate a gap between 0 and the first number shown on the scale.

A histogram can also be constructed from a grouped frequency distribution. As with a tabular frequency display, it is advantageous to group score values when the

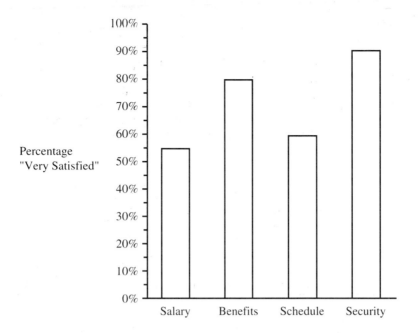

**Nurses' Satisfaction with Various Aspects
of Their Jobs ($N = 300$)**

FIGURE 2–4.   EXAMPLE OF A BAR GRAPH FOR SEVERAL RELATED VARIABLES

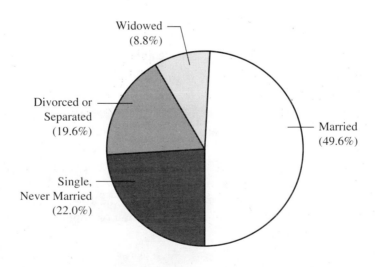

Marital Status of Subjects ($N = 250$)

FIGURE 2–5.   EXAMPLE OF A PIE CHART FOR A NOMINAL-LEVEL VARIABLE

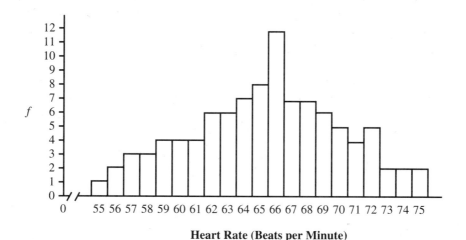

FIGURE 2–6.   EXAMPLE OF A HISTOGRAM: HEART RATE DATA

range between the highest and lowest scores is great. Most histograms display no more than about 20 bars (in Figure 2–6, there are 21). When the scores are grouped, the values shown on the horizontal axis are usually the midpoints of the score intervals.

Computer programs can be instructed to produce histograms; in most cases frequencies are presented along the horizontal dimension in computer printouts. To illustrate, Figure 2–7 presents a histogram of the grouped heart rate data.[4] In this printout, the computer listed the midpoint of the class interval—that is, 56 is the midpoint of the interval from 55 to 57, and so forth. This histogram corresponds to the information presented in Figure 2–2. Computer-generated histograms are useful for examining data, but may not be adequate for direct publication in research reports.

Frequency Polygons

Another method of displaying interval-level and ratio-level data is with a **frequency polygon.** A frequency polygon uses the same *X* axis and *Y* axis as for histograms, but instead of vertical bars, a dot is used above each score value to designate the appropriate frequency. The dots are then connected by a solid line. The heart rate data from Table 2–2 are displayed in a frequency polygon in Figure 2–8.

Frequency polygons show one score value below the lowest obtained value and one score value above the highest obtained value on the horizontal axis, so that the line

---

[4]The SPSS/PC command that produced the printout in Figure 2–7 is as follows:

    FREQUENCIES VARIABLES = HARTRATE
      /HISTOGRAM = MIN (54.5) MAX (75.5) INCREMENT (3).

HARTRATE

```
  Count    Midpoint
     6       56.00  |XXXXXXXXXX
    11       59.00  |XXXXXXXXXXXXXXXXX
    16       62.00  |XXXXXXXXXXXXXXXXXXXXXXXXXXX
    27       65.00  |XXXXXXXXXXXXXXXXXXXXXXXXXXXXXXXXXXXXXXXXXXXXXXX
    20       68.00  |XXXXXXXXXXXXXXXXXXXXXXXXXXXXXXXXXXX
    14       71.00  |XXXXXXXXXXXXXXXXXXXXXXXX
     6       74.00  |XXXXXXXXXX
                    I....+....I....+....I....+....I....+....I....+....I
                    0         6        12        18        24        30
                              Histogram frequency

Valid cases      100      Missing cases      0
```

FIGURE 2–7.   COMPUTER PRINTOUT OF A GROUPED FREQUENCY HISTOGRAM

connecting the dots can be brought down to the axis to show a frequency of 0 for these two values. An exception occurs if a higher or lower value is not possible. For example, if we were graphing a frequency distribution for number of correct answers on a 15-question test of knowledge about AIDS, a score of 16 would be impossible. In such a situation, a vertical *dotted* line would be drawn from the point designating the frequency for a score of 15 down to the X axis.

There are no strict rules regarding whether a histogram or a frequency polygon should be used to display data. By convention, histograms are usually the preferred method of displaying data for discrete variables, while frequency polygons are more

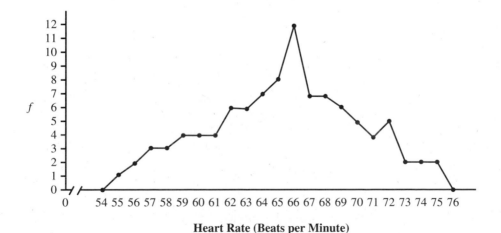

Heart Rate (Beats per Minute)

FIGURE 2–8.   EXAMPLE OF A FREQUENCY POLYGON: HEART RATE DATA

likely to be used with continuous variables. From a visual perspective, a frequency polygon is more likely than a histogram to emphasize the shape of an entire distribution, and does a better job of highlighting the notion of a continuum.

General Issues in Graphic Displays

Graphic displays of frequency distributions can communicate a lot of information at a glance, but graphs can be constructed in such a way that the information is misleading or ineffective. One issue concerns the grouping of values in a grouped distribution. If the heart rate data were clustered into three class intervals, for example (50 to 59, 60 to 69, and 70 to 79), the resulting histogram or frequency polygon would not be especially informative.

Another issue concerns the height and width of the display. The American Psychological Association (1983) has published guidelines for preparing research reports that are used by many nursing research journals. These guidelines suggest that the height of a graph (i.e., the height at the highest frequency) should be about two-thirds the width of the X axis.

SHAPES OF DISTRIBUTIONS

Distributions of quantitative variables can be described in terms of a number of features, many of which are related to the distributions' physical appearance or shape when presented graphically. The shape of a distribution is most readily discernible when the data values are arrayed in a frequency polygon.

Modality

The **modality** of a distribution concerns how many peaks or high points there are. A distribution with a single high peak—that is, a single value with a high frequency—is referred to as a **unimodal distribution.** The distribution of heart rate data (Figure 2–8) is unimodal, with a single peak at the value of 66.

Some distributions have two or more peaks, and these are referred to as **multimodal distributions.** (When there are exactly two peaks, the distribution is called **bimodal.**) Figure 2–9 presents six distributions (A through F), with different shapes. In this figure, the distributions labeled A, E, and F are unimodal, while B, C, and D are multimodal. Distributions B and D have two peaks and thus can also be described as bimodal.

Symmetry and Skewness

Another aspect of a distribution's shape concerns symmetry. A distribution can be described as **symmetric** if the distribution could be split down the middle to form two halves that are mirror images of one another. In Figure 2–9, distributions A through C are symmetric, while D through F are not.

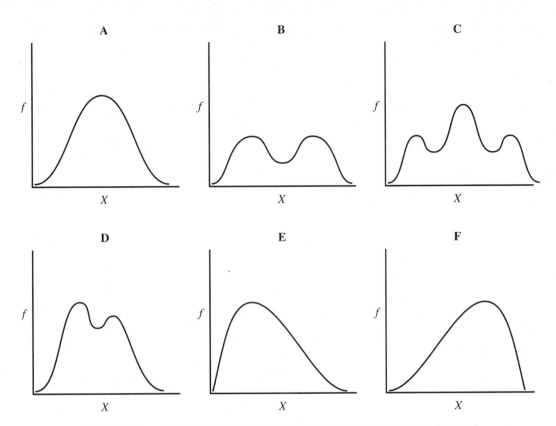

FIGURE 2–9.   EXAMPLES OF DISTRIBUTIONS WITH DIFFERENT SHAPES

With actual data collected in a study, the distributions are rarely as perfectly symmetric as those shown in Figure 2–9. For example, the distribution of heart rate values in Figure 2–8 is roughly symmetric, and we would likely characterize the data as symmetrically distributed. Minor departures from perfect symmetry are generally ignored when describing the shapes of actual data distributions.

The peaks of **asymmetric distributions** are off center, with a bulk of scores clustering at one end, and a tail trailing off at the other end. Such distributions are often described as being **skewed,** and they can be characterized in terms of the direction of the skew. When the longer tail trails off to the right, as shown in D and E of Figure 2–9, the distribution is said to be **positively skewed.** An example of an attribute that is positively skewed is annual income in the United States; most people have low or moderate incomes and would cluster at the left side, while the relatively small numbers in upper income brackets would be distributed in the tail. When a skewed distribution has a long tail pointing to the left (Figure 2–9, F), it is described as **negatively skewed.** As an actual example, if we drew a frequency polygon for people's age at death, we would construct a negatively skewed distribution; most people would be at the far right side of the distribution, with relatively few people dying at a young age.

It should be noted that skewness and modality are independent aspects of a distribution's shape. As Figure 2–9 shows, a distribution can be multimodal and skewed (D), or multimodal and symmetric (B and C)—as well as unimodal and skewed (E and F), or unimodal and symmetric (A).

Statisticians have developed methods of quantifying a distribution's degree of skewness. These indexes are almost never reported in research reports, but they can be useful for determining whether statistical tests that are described later in this book are appropriate. A statistical index for skewness is routinely calculated by most statistical computer programs in conjunction with frequency distributions. The index has a value of 0 for a perfectly symmetric distribution, a positive value if there is a positive skew, and a negative value if there is a negative skew. For the heart rate data (Figure 2–8), the skewness index is $-.109$, indicating a modest negative skew.

Kurtosis

A third aspect of a distribution's shape concerns how pointed or flat its peak is, which is referred to as the distribution's **kurtosis.** Two distributions with different peakedness are superimposed on one another in Figure 2–10. Distribution A in this figure is more peaked, and would be described as being **leptokurtic** (from the Greek word *lepto,* which means thin). Distribution B is flatter, and would be described as **platykurtic** (from the Greek word *platy,* which means flat).

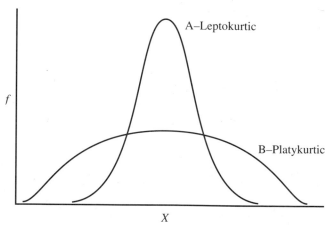

FIGURE 2–10.   EXAMPLE OF DISTRIBUTIONS WITH DIFFERENT KURTOSES

Verbal descriptors typically are used to describe the peakedness of a distribution. For example, we might say that distribution A in Figure 2–9 is symmetric, unimodal, and neither playtkurtic nor leptokurtic. As with skewness, there is a statistical index of kurtosis that is usually computed when computer programs are instructed to produce a frequency distribution. For the index of kurtosis, a value of 0 indicates a shape that is neither flat nor pointed, as might be the case for Figure 2–9 (A). Positive values on the kurtosis statistic indicate greater peakedness, while negative values indicate greater flatness. For the heart rate data displayed in Figure 2–8, the kurtosis index is −.541, indicating a platykurtic distribution.

The Normal Distribution

A distribution that has special importance in statistical analysis is the normal distribution (also known as the bell-shaped curve or normal curve). A **normal distribution** is one that is unimodal, symmetric, and not too peaked or flat. Figure 2–9 (A) illustrates a distribution that is normal. The normal distribution was given its name by the French mathematician Quetelet who, in the early nineteenth century, noted that many human attributes—such as height, weight, intelligence, and so on—appeared to be distributed according to this shape. That is, most people are in the middle range with respect to say, height, with the number of people tapering off at either extreme: there are few adults who are under 4 feet tall, and similarly few who are over 7 feet tall. Much more will be said about the normal distribution in subsequent chapters.

Because of the importance of normal distributions in statistical analysis, some computer programs (such as SPSS) have a special subcommand associated with the frequency distribution command that allows researchers to examine the extent to which their data approximate a normal distribution. Figure 2–11 presents a computer printout of a histogram for the heart rate data.[5] The bars are drawn to correspond to the percentage of cases at each score value; the dots superimposed on the histogram indicate what the distribution would look like if the data were normally distributed. This information indicates, for example, that with normally distributed data, only about 8% of the cases (rather than 12% of the cases) would have had a heart rate of 66. However, the heart rate distribution is not markedly nonnormal.

RESEARCH APPLICATIONS OF FREQUENCY DISTRIBUTIONS

Readers who have some experience reading research reports in professional journals may have noticed that most journal articles do not present frequency distributions in ei-

---

[5]The SPSS/PC command that produced the printout in Figure 2–11 is as follows:

```
FREQUENCIES VARIABLES=HARTRATE
    /HISTOGRAM=MIN (54.5) MAX (75.5) INCREMENT (1) PERCENT NORMAL.
```

HARTRATE

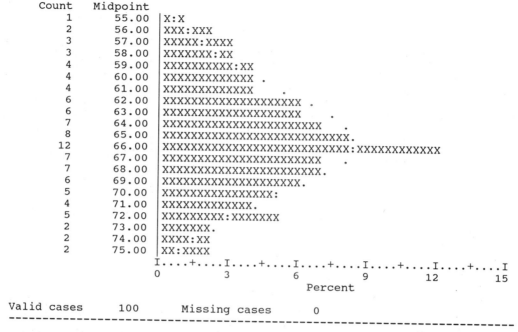

```
    Count   Midpoint
        1     55.00  |X:X
        2     56.00  |XXX:XXX
        3     57.00  |XXXXX:XXXX
        3     58.00  |XXXXXXX:XX
        4     59.00  |XXXXXXXXX:XX
        4     60.00  |XXXXXXXXXXXX .
        4     61.00  |XXXXXXXXXXXX     .
        6     62.00  |XXXXXXXXXXXXXXXXXX .
        6     63.00  |XXXXXXXXXXXXXXXXXX      .
        7     64.00  |XXXXXXXXXXXXXXXXXXXXXX    .
        8     65.00  |XXXXXXXXXXXXXXXXXXXXXXXXX.
       12     66.00  |XXXXXXXXXXXXXXXXXXXXXXXXX:XXXXXXXXXXX
        7     67.00  |XXXXXXXXXXXXXXXXXXXXXX    .
        7     68.00  |XXXXXXXXXXXXXXXXXXXXXXX.
        6     69.00  |XXXXXXXXXXXXXXXXXXXX.
        5     70.00  |XXXXXXXXXXXXXXX:
        4     71.00  |XXXXXXXXXXXX.
        5     72.00  |XXXXXXXXX:XXXXXXX
        2     73.00  |XXXXXXX.
        2     74.00  |XXXX:XX
        2     75.00  |XX:XXXX
                      I....+....I....+....I....+....I....+....I....+....I
                      0         3         6         9        12        15
                                            Percent
```

Valid cases   100   Missing cases   0

FIGURE 2–11. COMPUTER PRINTOUT OF A HISTOGRAM WITH NORMAL DISTRIBUTION SUPERIMPOSED

ther tabular or graphic form. This does not mean, however, that frequency distributions are unimportant in data analysis. This section examines some of the main reasons for constructing frequency distributions, and offers suggestions regarding the display of frequency distribution information in reports.

The Uses of Frequency Distributions

There are many reasons for constructing frequency distributions. A few of the major uses of frequency distributions within a research context are described here.

1. *Becoming Familiar with the Data Set.* Most researchers routinely begin their data analysis by running the **marginals** (instructing a computer program to construct frequency distributions) on all or most variables in their data set. Researchers want to make sense of their data, and a good place to begin is to inspect the data after they have been organized in frequency distributions. The first inspection normally involves tabular rather than graphic displays, as in Figure 2–1. Of course, in the process of inspecting the data, researchers may actually be addressing some of the research questions. For example, a researcher might be interested in determining

the extent to which people use vitamin supplements. A frequency distribution of responses to a question on the use of vitamin supplements would directly answer this
question.

2. *Cleaning the Data.* Data that have been input onto some medium for subsequent
computer analysis typically contain some errors, because data entry is an error-
prone activity. One aspect of data cleaning involves a search for **outliers**—that is,
values that lie outside the normal range of values for other cases. Outliers can be
found by inspecting the values in a frequency distribution, with special scrutiny of
the highest and lowest values. For some continuous variables, outliers are legitimate. For example, a question about sample members' annual income might yield
responses primarily in the $10,000 to $100,000 range, but a response of $5 million
would not be impossible. In many cases, however, outliers indicate an error in data
entry that needs to be corrected, as when the frequency distribution reveals a **wild
code**—that is, a code that is impossible. For example, Figure 2–12 presents a
computer-generated frequency distribution for responses to the question, "Have
you had a mammogram performed in the past 12 months?" In this example, only
the codes 1 (YES) and 2 (NO) represent legitimate responses to the question. The
codes 3 and 5 are wild codes resulting from data entry errors. In this situation, the
researcher would need to identify the four cases with the improper codes (three
cases coded 3 plus one case coded 5), determine the correct codes, and then make
the appropriate corrections. If the data cleaning is extensive, a whole new set of
marginals should be run to ascertain that the problems have been corrected
as intended.

3. *Inspecting the Data for Missing Values.* Researchers strive for what is referred to as
a **rectangular matrix** of data—data for all sample members for all key variables.

- -

MAMOGRAM   MAMMOGRAM IN PAST YEAR?

Value Label	Value	Frequency	Percent	Valid Percent	Cum Percent
YES	1	23	23.0	23.2	23.2
NO	2	72	72.0	72.7	96.0
	3	3	3.0	3.0	99.0
	5	1	1.0	1.0	100.0
	9	1	1.0	Missing	
	Total	100	100.0	100.0	

Valid cases   99   Missing cases   1

- -

**FIGURE 2–12. COMPUTER PRINTOUT OF A FREQUENCY DISTRIBUTION WITH WILD
CODES AND MISSING DATA**

This ideal is seldom achieved, and so researchers typically must make decisions about how to handle missing data. The first step is to determine the extent of the problem by examining frequency distributions on a variable-by-variable basis. In Figure 2–12, we see that only one case (1% of the sample) had a missing values code (code 9) on the mammogram question.

Another step might be to examine the cumulative extent of missing values. If 5% of the cases have missing values for variable X and 5% have missing values for variable Y, there could be missing data for anywhere between 5% and 10% of the sample on these variables, depending on how much overlap there is. In statistical software packages, it is possible to construct flags to identify how many variables are missing for each sample member.[6] Once a flag variable is constructed, a frequency distribution can be computed for the flag; this would show how many cases had no missing values, one missing value, and so on.

4. *Testing Assumptions for Statistical Tests.* As we discuss in subsequent chapters, many of the most widely used inferential statistics are based on a number of assumptions. In statistics, an **assumption** is a condition that is presumed to be true and, when violated, can lead to misleading or invalid results. Many inferential statistics assume that variables in the analysis (usually the dependent variables) are normally distributed. Frequency distributions provide researchers with information on whether the key research variables conform to this assumption. For example, the researcher can see whether the data are severely skewed. When the variables are not normally distributed, the researcher has to chose between three options: (1) select a statistical test that does not assume a normal distribution; (2) ignore the violation of the assumption—an option that is attractive if the deviation from normality is modest; or (3) transform the variable. Various transformations can be applied to alter the distributional qualities of a variable. For example, a logarithmic transformation tends to normalize a distribution. Annual income is an example of a variable that is often severely skewed and lends itself to a logarithmic transformation. Once a transformation has been performed,[7] the transformed data rather than the raw data are used in subsequent analyses. Dixon and Massey (1969) and Ferketich and Verran (1994) provide additional guidance regarding the use of transformations for changing the characteristics of a distribution.

5. *Obtaining Information about Sample Characteristics.* Frequency distributions are widely used to provide researchers with descriptive information about the back-

---

[6]As an example using SPSS/PC, suppose we had 10 variables (VAR1 through VAR10), all of which had a missing values code of 9. We could create a flag called MISSFLAG that would count the number of variables with a missing values code with the following command:

COUNT MISSFLAG = VAR1 TO VAR10 (9).

[7]For example, in SPSS/PC the command to create a logarithmically transformed income variable would be:

COMPUTE LOGINC = LN (INCOME).

where INCOME is the name of the original variable and LOGINC is the name of the logarithmically transformed variable.

ground characteristics of their sample members. This information is often of great importance in interpreting the results and drawing conclusions about the generalizability of the findings. For example, if a frequency distribution revealed that 80% of a research sample were college graduates, the researcher would need to be careful about generalizing the findings to less well-educated people.

6. *Directly Answering Research Questions.* Although researchers typically use inferential statistics to address their research questions, descriptive statistics are sometimes used to summarize substantive information in a study. For example, DiIorio, van Lier, and Manteuffel (1994) examined the methods that clinicians recommend most often for relieving nausea and vomiting in pregnant women. They presented a table that showed the absolute and relative frequency of 34 relief measures used by 130 clinicians, according to whether the nausea was mild, moderate, or severe.

Although the construction of frequency distributions is a routine part of data analysis in quantitative studies, frequency distributions are sometimes used by qualitative researchers as well. For example, qualitative researchers often analyze information about the background characteristics of their sample members. They may also use what Becker (1970) has called quasi-statistics. **Quasi-statistics** involve the tabulation of the frequency with which certain themes or coding categories exist in qualitative data.

The Presentation of Frequency Information in Research Reports

Most research reports that appear in professional journals include at least one table or figure, and typically they include several. Nevertheless, univariate frequency distributions are not often presented in research reports, in large part because tables and figures are expensive and take a lot of space and are thus reserved for presenting more complex information. Take, for example, the marital status information shown in Table 2–3 and in graphic form in Figures 2–3 and 2–5. This information could be more efficiently reported directly in the text of the report:

Nearly half (49.6%) of the sample was married, while 22.0% had never been married, 19.6% were divorced or separated, and 8.8% were widowed.

The publication guidelines of the American Psychological Association (1983) advise that tables should not be used for simple data presentations (e.g., one column by five or fewer rows, or two columns by two rows).

Frequency information is most likely to be presented in a table or figure when there are several related variables being reported simultaneously. One of the most frequent uses of tables for presenting frequency information involves the background characteristics of research subjects. For example, Tumulty, Jernigan, and Kohut (1994) studied the relationship between the work environment and job satisfaction of hospital staff nurses. A table in their report, reproduced here as Table 2–4, included three frequency distributions for key background variables. This method of presentation is efficient, because it provides readers with a quick summary of important sample characteristics.

**TABLE 2–4. EXAMPLE OF FREQUENCY
DISTRIBUTIONS OF SAMPLE CHARACTERISTICS**

Characteristics	N	%
*Clinical Specialty (N = 120)**		
Critical care	56	47
Medical/surgical	41	34
Maternal child	19	16
Other	4	3
Employment Status (N = 138)		
Full-time	79	57
Part-time	32	23
Weekend or Baylor plan	27	20
Professional education level (N = 136)		
Associate degree	34	25
Diploma	37	27
Bachelor's degree	53	39
Master's degree	12	9

*Does not include managers

*Adapted from Tumulty, Jernigan, & Kohut, 1994. Originally part
of Table 3 in their report, titled **Respondent Characteristics**.*

Researchers are most likely to present *substantive* frequency information in tables or graphs when there are several variables that have the same codes or score values, so that an entire matrix of frequency information can be presented simultaneously. For example, O'Brien (1993) studied self-esteem and coping in multiple sclerosis patients. Her report included a table (shown here as Table 2–5) that presented the distribution of the frequency with which the research subjects experienced various types of dysfunction. Note that if the researcher had gathered information on only one type of dysfunction, it would have been inefficient to report this in a table, but with multiple types the table presents a wealth of information in a compact format.

Another situation in which researchers can profitably display frequency distribution information in a table or graph is when there are data for the same variable measured at multiple points in time. For example, Bruce and Grove (1994) studied the effects of a coronary artery risk evaluation (C.A.R.E.) program, and displayed the percentage of subjects classified in high, moderate, and low risk groups before the program began and then 6 months later. Their bar graph is shown here as Figure 2–13.

In summary, frequency information is often presented in the text of a research report—typically as relative frequencies—rather than in graphs or tables. However, when multiple variables or multiple data collection points can be presented simultaneously, a graphic or tabular presentation of frequency distributions can be highly efficient. Despite the fact that graphs require considerable space, they do have an arresting

TABLE 2–5. EXAMPLE OF FREQUENCY DISTRIBUTIONS FOR MULTIPLE VARIABLES

Dysfunction	Never %	Occasionally %	Usually %	Always %
Vision	27.7	57.4	5.9	8.9
Speech	58.4	37.6	—	4.0
Coordination	9.9	40.6	23.8	25.7
Walking	3.8	14.9	14.9	67.3
Bladder function	19.8	30.7	21.8	27.7
Bowel function	33.7	44.3	11.9	12.9
Transferring	32.7	37.6	13.9	15.8

Originally Table 1 in O'Brien's (1993) report, titled **Selected Dysfunction of Subjects with Multiple Sclerosis (N = 101).**

quality that captures the readers' attention. If graphs are used to emphasize or clarify important pieces of information, they can be very effective.

Tips on Preparing Tables and Graphs for Frequency Distributions

Although frequency distributions are not often presented in tabular or graphic form in research reports, we can offer a few tips regarding the display of distributions. Some of these tips also apply to tables and graphs of other types of statistical information that we discuss in subsequent chapters.

- When percentage information is being presented, it is generally not necessary (or desirable) to report the percentages to two or more decimal places. For example, a calculated percentage of 10.092% usually would be reported as either 10.1% or 10%.

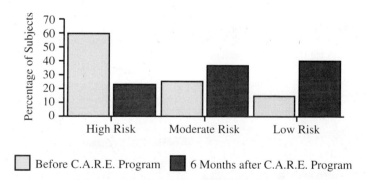

Before C.A.R.E. Program   6 Months after C.A.R.E. Program

FIGURE 2–13.   EXAMPLE OF A BAR GRAPH AT TWO TIME PERIODS

Originally Figure 2 in Bruce & Grove's (1994) report, titled **Percentage of Subjects in Each Cardiovascular Risk Category Before and After Treatment**

- In reporting percentages, the level of precision should be consistent throughout any specific table or figure. Thus, if the percentages in a distribution were 10.1%, 25%, and 64.9%, they should be reported either as 10%, 25%, and 65% *or* 10.1%, 25.0%, and 64.9%.
- A reader should be able to interpret graphs and tables without being forced to refer to the text. Thus, there should be a good, clear title and well-labeled headings (in a table) or axes (in a graph). With frequency information, the table should generally include information on the total number of cases on which the frequencies were based.
- Occasionally, there is a substantive reason for showing how much missing information there was. For example, if we were asking people about whether they used illegal drugs, it might be important to indicate what percentage of respondents refused to answer the question. In most cases, however, missing information is not presented, and only valid percentages are shown. For example, in Table 2–4, the percentages for the three background characteristics were based on slightly different numbers for each one because of missing data.

RESEARCH EXAMPLE

Almost all research reports include some information on frequencies or relative frequencies. Here we describe a recently published study that used frequency information extensively.

Gray, Rayome, and Anson (1995) undertook a descriptive study to determine the incidence and characteristics of urinary incontinence among patients with urologic complications caused by spinal injury and managed by clean intermittent catheterization (CIC). A sample of 150 spinal injured patients who had been discharged from a rehabilitation hospital on CIC were questioned about their experiences in the year following their injuries. The data were analyzed through descriptive statistics.

The investigators presented a wealth of descriptive information, primarily in the text of the report. For example, the findings indicated that only 54% of those patients who performed CIC experienced any incontinent episodes. Of those with any incontinence, 53% reported only episodic incontinence with minimal or moderate leakage. This information was noted in the text and also displayed in bar graphs.

The investigators found that the use of containment devices was the mostly commonly used coping strategy among those who experienced incontinence. Twenty-nine percent of the incontinent patients leaked sufficiently small volumes that no containment device was necessary. However nearly half (48%) of the 62 incontinent subjects regularly used a condom with a leg bag or a diaper-type device. Pharmacotherapy was the most commonly cited method for preventing leaking, mentioned by 69% of the incontinent patients. The study also revealed that 85% of the sample experienced one or more symptomatic urinary tract infections, and 42% had at least one febrile urinary infection since the commencement of the CIC program.

SUMMARY

A **frequency distribution** is a simple but effective method of imposing order on raw data. A frequency distribution arranges the data values in a systematic sequence (often from lowest to highest), with a count of the number of times each value was obtained. The sum of all the frequencies must equal the sample size (i.e., $\Sigma f = N$). In a frequency distribution, the information can be presented as **absolute frequencies** (the counts), **relative frequencies** (the percentage of cases with a given value), and **cumulative relative frequencies** (cumulative percentages for a given value plus all the values that preceded it). When there are more than 20 or so data values, it may be preferable to construct a **grouped frequency distribution,** which involves grouping values together into **class intervals.**

Frequency distribution information can be presented in graphs as well as in tables. Graphs generally involve plotting the score values on a horizontal axis (the X **axis** or **abscissa**) and frequencies or percentages on the vertical axis (the Y **axis** or **ordinate**). Nominal (and some ordinal data) are often displayed in **bar charts** or **pie charts,** while interval and ratio data are usually presented in **histograms** or **frequency polygons.**

Data can be described in terms of the shape of the frequency distribution. One aspect of shape is **modality;** if there is one peak or high value, the distribution is **unimodal,** but if there are two or more peaks it is **multimodal.** Another aspect of shape concerns symmetry; a **symmetric distribution** is one in which the two halves are mirror images of one another. A **skewed distribution** is asymmetric, with the peak pulled off center and one tail longer than the other. A **negative skew** occurs when the long tail is pointing to the left, and a **positive skew** occurs when the long tail points to the right. A third aspect of a distribution's shape is **kurtosis;** distributions with sharp, thin peaks are **leptokurtic,** while those with smooth, flat peaks are **platykurtic.** A special distribution that is important in statistics is known as the **normal distribution** (bell-shaped curve), which is unimodal and symmetric.

EXERCISES

The following exercises cover concepts presented in this chapter. Exercises indicated with a dagger (†) can be checked against answers appearing in Appendix A. Additionally, Chapter 2 of the accompanying *Applications Manual* offers supplementary exercises, including ones that require analysis of a data set on diskette.

† 1. The following data represent the number of times that a sample of residents in a nursing home who were aged 80 or older fell during a 12-month period.

0	3	4	1	0	2	0	1	2	0
1	0	0	1	2	5	0	1	0	1
0	2	1	0	1	1	3	2	1	0
1	3	1	1	0	4	6	1	0	1

Construct a frequency distribution for this set of data, showing the absolute frequencies, relative frequencies, and cumulative relative frequencies.

† 2. Using information from the frequency distribution for Exercise 1, answer the following: (a) What percentage of the nursing home residents had at least one fall?

(b) What number of falls was the most frequent in this sample? (c) What number of falls was the least frequent in this sample? (d) What percentage of residents had two or fewer falls? (e) What is the total size of the sample? (f) Are there any outliers in this data set?

† 3. Would it be advantageous to group the data in Exercise 1 before constructing a frequency distribution? Why or why not?

4. Draw a frequency histogram for the data shown in Exercise 1. Now superimpose a frequency polygon on the histogram. Using a ruler, measure the height and width of your graphs. Is the height about two-thirds of the width?

† 5. Describe the shape of the frequency distribution drawn in Exercise 4 in terms of modality and skewness. Is the number of falls normally distributed?

† 6. If you were going to display data on nurses' clinical specialty (Table 2–4) graphically, would you construct a bar graph, histogram, or frequency polygon? Construct such a graph.

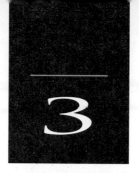

Univariate Statistics: Central Tendency and Variability

A distribution of data values for quantitative variables can be described in terms of three independent characteristics: the shape of the distribution, central tendency, and variability. Chapter 2 discussed various aspects of a distribution's shape. This chapter examines descriptive statistics that are indexes of central tendency and variability.

CENTRAL TENDENCY

One of the reasons that entire frequency distributions typically are not presented in research reports is that, for quantitative variables, there is a more convenient and succinct way of summarizing a distribution of scores: by reporting one or more indexes of central tendency. **Central tendency** refers to the general location of a "typical" data value—in other words, the data value around which other scores tend to cluster. Because a value is more likely to be typical if it is in the middle of a distribution than if it is an extreme value, the term *central* tendency has come to be used for this class of descriptive statistics.

In lay terms, the word *average* usually is used in connection with central tendency. For example, with regard to the heart rate data that were used to illustrate many concepts in Chapter 2, we could convey more useful information by reporting the research sample's average heart rate than by reporting what percentage of cases had a heart rate of 55, 56, 57, and so on. Researchers usually do not use the term average, because there are three alternative types of average: the mode, the median, and the mean. Each of these descriptive statistics can be used to describe the central tendency of an entire set of data values.

The Mode

The **mode** is the numerical value in a distribution that occurs most frequently. Take, for example, the following set of values:

20   21   21   22   22   22   22   23   23   24

We can readily see that the mode is 22, because this score occurred four times—a higher frequency than for any other value. If we constructed a frequency polygon for these 10 numbers, the highest peak in the graph would occur at the modal value of 22. In the heart rate example, we can tell from Figure 2–8 that the mode is 66; 12 people in the sample had a heart rate of 66 bpm, and no other heart rate value occurred more frequently.

Although the mode is very easy to determine, it has a number of drawbacks as an index of central tendency. One problem is that there may be two or more modes in a single distribution—that is, the distribution might be multimodal. The following example illustrates a bimodal distribution:

20   20   20   21   22   23   24   25   25   25

Here both 20 and 25 are the most frequently occurring numbers and both would be considered the modes. In this example, it is impossible to characterize the distribution with a single numerical value using the mode as the index of central tendency.

Another limitation is that the mode tends to be a fairly unstable index of central tendency. By unstable, we mean that the values of modes tend to fluctuate considerably from one sample to another drawn from the same population. Given its instability, it is difficult to attach much theoretical importance to the mode.

Because the mode has these shortcomings as an index of central tendency, it is not used extensively in research, except when the researcher is interested in describing typical (modal) values for nominal-level variables. For example, using the frequency distribution information from the study by Tumulty, Jernigan, and Kohut (1994) presented in Table 2–4, we could characterize the research subjects as follows: "The typical (modal) subject was a full-time nurse, had a clinical specialty in critical care, and had earned a bachelor's degree."

The Median

A second descriptive statistic used to indicate central tendency is the median. The **median** (sometimes abbreviated as **Mdn**) is the point in the distribution of data values that divides the distribution into two equal halves. In other words, the median is the score value corresponding to the 50th **percentile:** 50% of the score values lie above the median, and the other 50% lie below the median. As an example, the median of the following set of values is 25:

21   22   22   23   24   26   26   27   28   29

The point that has 50% above it and 50% below it is halfway between 24 and 26. Even though no subject had a score of 25, the value of 25 is the median because it splits the distribution exactly into two equal halves.

The method of computing the median depends on two factors: (1) whether there is an odd or an even number of data values, and (2) whether there are two or more cases with the same value near the median point. Each situation is illustrated here:

1. *An even number of cases with no duplicate values near the middle of the distribution.* In this situation, exemplified in the preceding example with 10 cases, the computation is straightforward. After the values are ordered from lowest to highest, the median is the arithmetic average between the two middle scores—i.e., $(24 + 26)/2 = 25$. This is illustrated in Figure 3–1 (A).

2. *An odd number of cases with no duplicates near the middle of the distribution.* In this situation, the median is simply the middle score. Take the following nine data values, for example:

   22   23   23   24   25   26   27   27   28

   In this example, which is presented graphically as Figure 3–1 (B), the median is the value in the middle, or 25. Some readers may have noticed that, in this example, it cannot be said that 50% of the cases are above and below 25: four out of nine cases (44.4%) are above the value of 25 and four out of nine cases (44.4%) are below it. However, the number 25 can be thought of as the midpoint of an interval extending between the values of 24.5 and 25.5. These are sometimes referred to as the **real limits** of a number. Thus, to find the median in this example, we would use the midpoint between the number's real limits, or $(24.5 + 25.5)/2 = 25.0$.

3. *Duplication of scores near the middle of the distribution.* Suppose, now, that we had the following distribution of 10 scores, with duplications of the middle score of 25:

   23   23   24   25   25   25   26   26   27   28

   In this situation, there are three cases with exactly 25, three cases below it, and four cases above it. The point that divides the distribution in half lies between the second and third values of 25. If, as just described, a score of 25 can be conceptualized as a value between 24.5 and 25.5, the median for this distribution must lie somewhere between these limits, such that exactly 50% of the distribution would

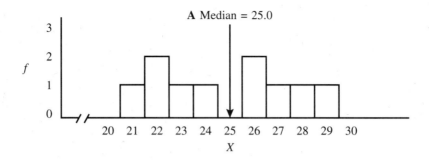

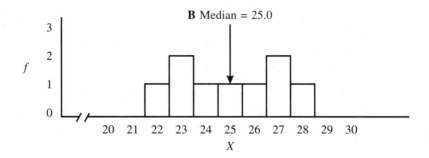

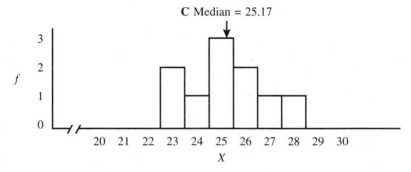

FIGURE 3–1. CALCULATION OF THE MEDIAN IN THREE CONDITIONS

be above and below it. Since two of the three values of 25 fall in the first half of the distribution, and the remaining value falls in the second half of the distribution, the median is the point at two-thirds the distance between the real limits of the number 25:

$$24.5 + .67 = 25.17$$

Thus, the median for these 10 numbers is 25.17, as shown in Figure 3–1 (C). This situation, with duplicate values near the middle of a distribution, is the most common of the three discussed here.[1]

The median, then, is an index of the average *location* or position in a distribution of numbers. Because of this fact, the median is insensitive to the distribution's actual numerical values. Suppose, for example, we changed the last number in the previous example:

23   23   24   25   25   25   26   26   27   128

Although the tenth value in the distribution has been changed from 28 to 128, the median is still 25.17—this remains the point that divides the distribution into two equal halves. Because of this characteristic, the median is often the most useful index of central tendency when a distribution is highly skewed and one wants to find a "typical" value.

The Mean

The most commonly used index of central tendency is the **mean,** which is the term used in statistics for the arithmetic average. The equation for calculating the mean is as follows:

$$\overline{X} = \frac{\Sigma X}{N}$$

where $\overline{X}$ = the mean
Σ = the sum of
X = each individual data value
N = number of cases

That is, the mean (often symbolized either as $\overline{X}$—pronounced "X bar"—or **M**) is computed by summing each individual score (ΣX), and then dividing by the total number of cases (N).

---

[1]Computers are almost always used to determine the median of a variable. However, for interested readers, the formula for calculating the median for ungrouped data is as follows:

$$\text{Median} = L + \frac{(N)(.50) - n_L}{n_w}$$

where L = lower real limit of the value at the median
N = total number of scores in the distribution
n_L = number of cases with scores less than L
n_w = number of cases with scores with the same value as the median

As an example, let us take the original set of 10 scores whose median was 25.17:

$$\overline{X} = \frac{23 + 23 + 24 + 25 + 25 + 25 + 26 + 26 + 27 + 28}{10} = 25.2$$

The value of the mean, unlike the median, is affected by every score in the distribution. Thus, although the median remained unchanged at 25.17 when we changed the tenth value in the distribution from 28 to 128, the mean would change markedly:

$$\overline{X} = \frac{23 + 23 + 24 + 25 + 25 + 25 + 26 + 26 + 27 + 128}{10} = 35.2$$

The mean has an interesting property that underscores why it is a good index of central tendency: *The sum of the deviations of scores from their mean is always equal to zero*. That is, if the mean is subtracted from every score in the distribution, the sum of these differences invariably is zero. As an example, consider the following numbers, which have a mean of 5.0: 9, 7, 5, 3, and 1. Now, if we subtract the mean from each score, we would obtain five **deviation scores:**

Score	Mean		Deviation Score
9	− 5	=	4
7	− 5	=	2
5	− 5	=	0
3	− 5	=	−2
1	− 5	=	−4

When the deviation scores are added, we obtain the sum of 0. It is this property of the mean—the fact that it balances the deviations above it and below it—that qualifies the mean as an important index of central tendency.

Comparison of the Mode, the Median, and the Mean

In a normal distribution for a quantitative variable, the mode, the median, and the mean have the same value, as illustrated in Figure 3–2. Most distributions of real data, however, are rarely perfectly normal, and thus the values of the three indexes of central tendency are typically not exactly the same. When this is the case, the researcher must decide which of the three indexes to report.

The mean is generally the preferred index of central tendency for variables measured on an interval or ratio scale, and is by far the most widely reported descriptive statistic for quantitative variables. The mean has a number of desirable features, including the fact that it takes each and every score into account. It is also the most stable index of central tendency, and it therefore yields the most reliable estimate of the central ten-

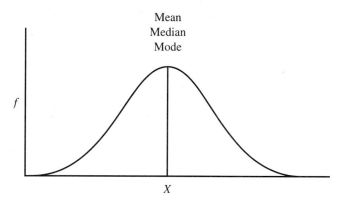

FIGURE 3–2. THE MEAN, MEDIAN, AND MODE IN A NORMAL DISTRIBUTION

dency of the population. Many of the inferential statistics that are described later in this book are based upon the mean.

While in many situations the mean's ability to capture every score value is an advantage, there are situations in which this feature is a disadvantage, at least for descriptive purposes. Suppose, for example, we collected data on the annual income of 10 research subjects and obtained the following:

$17,000
$20,000
$20,000
$20,000
$22,000
$24,000
$25,000
$26,000
$30,000
$200,000

In this example, the mode is $20,000, the median is $23,000, and the mean is $40,400. Despite the fact that 90% of the subjects had annual incomes of less than $40,000, the mean is greater than this figure. Extreme scores can exert a powerful influence on the mean and result in a misleading picture of the distribution of values. Thus, when the primary aim of summarizing a distribution is to describe what a typical value is, the median may be preferred. In this example, the value of $23,000 (the median) does a much better job of communicating the financial circumstances of the sample than does the mean. In general, the median is a better descriptive index when the data are highly skewed or when there are extreme, but valid, outliers. The median

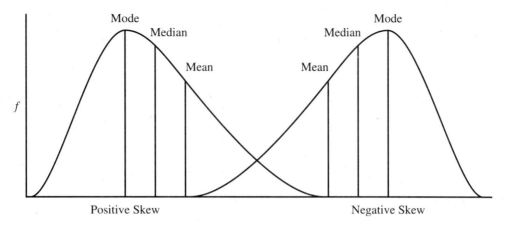

FIGURE 3–3. THE MEAN, MEDIAN, AND MODE IN SKEWED DISTRIBUTIONS

is also generally preferred for ordinal-level variables that cannot reasonably be viewed as approaching interval-level measurement.

Figure 3–3 illustrates that in skewed distributions the values of the mode, the median, and the mean are different. The mean is always pulled in the direction of the long tail—that is, in the direction of the scores at the extreme. Thus, for variables that are positively skewed (like income), the mean is higher than the mode or the median; for negatively skewed variables (like age at death), the mean is lower.

In distributions that are close to being normal, researchers usually report only the mean. However, when the distribution is asymmetrical, researchers sometimes report two or more indicators of central tendency, because each communicates new information about the distribution of values.

VARIABILITY

In addition to a distribution's shape and central tendency, another important characteristic is its variability. **Variability** refers to how spread out or dispersed the scores in a distribution are—in other words how similar or different the sample members are from one another with respect to the variable of interest.

Two distributions with identical means and similar shapes (e.g., both symmetrical or both positively skewed) could nevertheless differ considerably in terms of variability. Consider, for example, the two distributions presented in Figure 3–4. This figure presents body weight data for two hypothetical samples, both of which have means of 150 pounds. Clearly, the two samples differ considerably with respect to weight. In sample A, there is considerable intersubject diversity with respect to weight: some subjects weigh as little as 100 pounds, while others weigh up to 200 pounds. In sample B, by

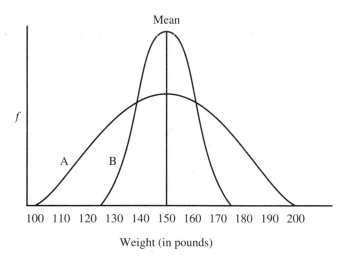

FIGURE 3–4. TWO DISTRIBUTIONS WITH DIFFERENT VARIABILITY

contrast, there are few subjects at either extreme: the weights cluster more tightly around the mean of 150.

We can provide verbal descriptors of the variability of a sample on a given attribute. We can say, for example, that sample A is **heterogeneous** with regard to weight, while sample B is **homogeneous** with regard to weight. These verbal descriptors, however, are not very precise and may be open to subjective interpretations. Therefore, statisticians have developed quantitative indexes that express the extent to which scores on quantitative variables[2] deviate from one another in a distribution. The three most widely used measures of variability are the range, the semiquartile range, and the standard deviation.

The Range

The **range** is the simplest measure of variability. It is the difference between the highest score and the lowest score in the distribution. In the example shown in Figure 3–4, the range for sample A is approximately 100 (200 − 100 = 100), while the range for sample B is about 50 (175 − 125 = 50). In a research report, the range is often shown as the minimum and maximum value, without the subtracted difference score.

The range provides a quick summary of a distribution's variability, and is easy to compute. The range also provides useful information about a distribution when there are outliers or extreme values. For example, a researcher might well want to know that the

---

[2]There are no widely used indexes of variability for variables measured on a nominal scale, although the range can be used as an indicator of the number of categories.

range of values for annual income is (to use the example presented previously) from $17,000 to $200,000 (i.e., a range of $183,000).

However, as an index of variability, the range has several drawbacks. Because the range is based on only two values, it can be highly unstable. For example, in another sample of 10 people, the annual incomes might range from $20,000 to $30,000 (a range of only $10,000). Another problem is that the range tends to increase with sample size; the larger the sample, the greater the likelihood that an extreme value will be obtained. It is more likely, for example, that a sample of 1000 people would include a millionaire than a sample of 10 people. Because of these limitations, the range is rarely used as the only descriptive index of a distribution's variability.

Semiquartile Range

As previously described, the median is the score at the 50th percentile—the point below which 50% of the cases fall. Percentiles can be computed at any point in a distribution. A familiar use concerns test scores; for example, a score of 700 on the Scholastic Assessment Test (SAT) might place a student at the 95th percentile, indicating that 95% of the students taking the test obtained a lower score.

The **semiquartile range** (sometimes referred to as the **semiinterquartile range**) is an index of variability that is calculated on the basis of quartiles. The lower quartile (Q_1) is the point below which 25% of the scores lie, while the upper quartile (Q_3) is the point below which 75% of the scores lie. The semiquartile range (*SQR*) is half the distance between these two values, or:

$$SQR = \frac{Q_3 - Q_1}{2}$$

Thus, the *SQR* indicates *half* the range of scores within which the middle 50% of the score values lie. In Figure 3–4, sample A would have an *SQR* of about 20, while sample B would have an *SQR* in the vicinity of 10.

Because the *SQR* is based on middle-range cases rather than extremes, it is more stable than the range. However, in practice the *SQR* is rarely used because it is not amenable to further analysis and because it is less useful than the range as a pure descriptor of the distribution. The semiquartile range is most likely to be used in conjunction with the median.

The Standard Deviation and the Variance

The most widely used index of variability is the **standard deviation** (often abbreviated as **SD** or **s**). Like the mean, the *SD* takes into consideration every score in the distribution, not just those at the extreme (like the range) or at a fixed point in the distribution (like the *SQR*).

Variability refers to differences among scores, and thus an index of variability necessarily captures quantitatively the degree to which scores are different from one another. In the range and *SQR,* this notion of differences is indicated by a minus sign, which represents the difference between two score values. The standard deviation is also based on differences—in this case, differences between each and every score and the value of the mean. Thus, the first step in calculating a standard deviation is to calculate deviation scores. The formula for a deviation score (often symbolized as x) is:

$$x = X - \overline{X}$$

For example, if a person weighed 200 and the average weight of the sample were 150, that person's deviation score would be 50.

Indexes of central tendency are useful because they offer a *single numerical value* that describes the "average" score in a distribution. Researchers also want as an index of variability a single number that describes the "average" amount of dispersion. This might lead you to surmise that a good indicator of variability could be obtained by summing the deviation scores and dividing by the number of cases to obtain an average deviation. However, as we have already seen, the sum of the deviation scores about a mean is *always* equal to 0, or:

$$\Sigma x = 0$$

The standard deviation addresses this problem by squaring the deviation scores before summing them and dividing by the number of cases. Then, to return to the original unit of measurement, the square root is taken. The formula[3] for the *SD* is:

$$SD = \sqrt{\frac{\Sigma x^2}{N - 1}}$$

An example of the computation of a standard deviation is presented in Table 3–1. The first column presents the weights of 10 subjects. At the bottom of this first column, the mean weight is computed to be 150.0 pounds. In the second column, a deviation score for each subject is calculated by subtracting the mean of 150.0 from each original weight value. In the third column, each deviation score is squared, and the sum of these squared deviation scores (Σx^2) is calculated to be 6000. At the bottom of the table, the

---

[3]There is some discrepancy among statistics textbooks as to whether the denominator of the standard deviation formula should be N or $N - 1$ (as shown here). There is generally agreement that N is appropriate for computing the *SD* of a population value. Knapp (1970) indicates that N should also be used in the denominator when computing an *SD* purely as a descriptive index of variability; the denominator should be $N - 1$ when calculating an *SD* as part of an inferential test— i.e., to estimate the population *SD*. Computer programs that compute the *SD* (such as SPSS) usually use $N - 1$ in the denominator. The discrepancy between the two computations is usually negligible, unless the sample is very small.

TABLE 3–1. EXAMPLE OF THE COMPUTATION OF A STANDARD DEVIATION

X	$x = X - \bar{X}$	$x^2 = (X - \bar{X})^2$
110	−40	1600
120	−30	900
130	−20	400
140	−10	100
150	0	0
150	0	0
160	10	100
170	20	400
180	30	900
190	40	1600
$\Sigma X = 1500$	$\Sigma x = 0$	$\Sigma x^2 = 6000$

$\bar{X} = 1500/10$

$\bar{X} = 150.0$

$$SD = \sqrt{\frac{6000}{9}} = \sqrt{666.67} = 25.820$$

SD is computed; 6000 is divided by 9 (the number of cases minus 1), and then the square root is taken. The value of the standard deviation of the weights for the 10 subjects is 25.820 (or, rounding to one decimal place, 25.8).

What does the number 25.8 represent? While it is easy for most students to understand that the average weight in this example is 150.0, it is less easy to understand what is meant by the fact that the standard deviation is 25.8. There are several ways to explain the concept of the *SD*.

The *SD* of 25.8 signifies the "average" deviation from the mean. The mean indicates the best single point in the distribution for summarizing a set of values, but the *SD* tells us how much, on the average, the values deviate from that mean. In essence, the *SD* communicates how wrong, on average, the mean is as an overall summary of the distribution of scores. The smaller the *SD,* the better is the mean as the summary of a typical score. To take an extreme case, if all 10 subjects in our example weighed 150 pounds, the *SD* would be 0, and the mean of 150.0 would communicate perfectly accurate information about all the subjects' weights. At the other extreme, suppose the first five subjects weighed 100 and the last five subjects weighed 200. In this case, the mean would still be 150.0, but the *SD* would be 52.7. In this situation, the mean of 150.0 contains a lot of "error" as a single descriptor of the 10 weights.

An *SD* is often easier to interpret when put in a comparative context. For example, looking back at Figure 3–4, both distributions A and B had a mean of 150, but sample A would have an *SD* of about 20, while sample B would have an *SD* of about 10. The *SD* index communicates clearly that sample B is considerably more homogeneous than sample A.

Another way in which the *SD* can be interpreted concerns the evaluation of any single score in a distribution. In our example of 10 subjects' weights, the *SD* was 25.8. This actually represents a good "standard" of variability against which individual weights can be compared. Subjects with weights that are greater than 1 *SD* away from the mean (i.e., less than 124.2 pounds or more than 175.8 pounds) have weights that are farther away from the mean than the average. Conversely, weights between 124.2 and 175.8 pounds are closer to the mean than the average.

When data values are normally distributed, the standard deviation can be used in an even more precise way to evaluate individual values. In a normal distribution, there are approximately 3 *SD*s above the mean, and 3 *SD*s below it, as shown in Figure 3–5. This figure shows a distribution of scores with a mean of 500 and an *SD* of 100, which is similar to the distribution of scores for the SAT or the Graduate Record Examination (GRE). When data are normally distributed, a fixed percentage of cases fall between the mean and distances from the mean, as measured in standard deviation units. Sixty-eight percent of the cases fall within 1 *SD* of the mean: 34% above the mean and 34% below it. In the example shown in Figure 3–5, nearly 7 out of every 10 people obtained a score between 400 and 600. A full 95% of the cases fall within 2 *SD*s of the mean. Only a very small percentage of cases (about 2.5% at each end of the distribution) are more than 2

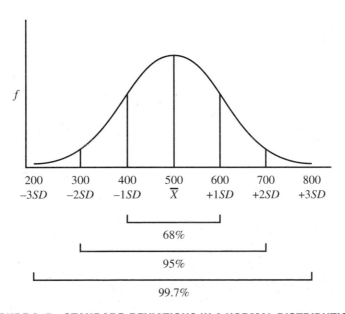

FIGURE 3–5. STANDARD DEVIATIONS IN A NORMAL DISTRIBUTION

SDs away from the mean. With this information, it is easy to interpret any individual score. A person with a score of 600, for example, obtained a higher score than 84% of the sample (i.e., 50% below the mean and 34% between the mean and 1 SD above it).

The SD is often reported in research reports in conjunction with the mean, and is the most widely used descriptive index of variability. However, another index of variability, called the variance, plays an important role in inferential statistics. The **variance** is simply the value of the standard deviation before the square root is taken; that is:

$$Var = \frac{\Sigma x^2}{N - 1} = SD^2$$

In the example worked out in Table 3–1, the variance is 666.67 (6000 ÷ 9), which is the same as 25.820^2. Because the variance is not in the same measurement units as the original data (in this example, the variance is in pounds squared), the variance is rarely used as a descriptive statistic.

STANDARD SCORES

Means and SDs are sometimes used to compute standard scores. **Standard scores** are scores that are expressed in terms of their relative distance from the mean. Researchers most often use standard scores to make their data more interpretable or amenable to comparisons. For example, SAT scores are actually standard scores—they do not represent the number of questions a person answered correctly on the test. By standardizing SAT scores, comparisons can be made between those taking the test at one time and those tested at a different time. As another example, suppose we were measuring children's behavior problems on a standard instrument such as the Behavior Problem Index (BPI), an index that quantifies the number of behavior problems a child has, as reported by a parent or a teacher. Since children's behavior is age-sensitive, it might be problematic to use the raw BPI scores in a study if the sample included children spanning several years. In such a situation, we could age-standardize the scores by computing standard scores within age groups in the sample.

A standard score (sometimes symbolized as **Z**)[4] is easy to compute once the raw score mean and standard deviation have been calculated. The formula is:

$$Z = \frac{X - \overline{X}}{SD}$$

That is, for each person, the deviation score (the raw score minus the mean) is divided by the standard deviation to yield a standard score. This converts all raw scores to SD

---

[4] A standard score in a normal distribution is, by convention, referred to as a z **score.** We use Z rather than z for a standard score when the distributional properties are unknown.

units—a raw score that is 1 *SD* above the mean would become a standard score of +1.0; a raw score 2 *SD*s below the mean would become a standard score of −2.0; and a score directly at the mean would be a standard score of 0.0. The mean of a distribution of standard scores is necessarily 0, and the *SD* is always 1. The shape of the distribution of Z scores is identical to the shape of the original distribution of scores.

For age standardization, the age-specific means and *SD*s would be used rather than the overall sample mean. For example, suppose we have the following information about BPI means and *SD*s for children in a sample who were ages 4, 5, and 6:

Age 5:   Mean: 10.0   *SD:* 2.0
Age 6:   Mean: 12.0   *SD:* 3.0
Age 7:   Mean: 14.0   *SD:* 3.0

Suppose now that we had three children in the three age groups, each of whom had a raw BPI score of 12. Their standard scores would be as follows:

Age 5: $Z = (12 - 10) \div 2 =$ 1.0
Age 6: $Z = (12 - 12) \div 3 =$ 0.0
Age 7: $Z = (12 - 14) \div 3 = -0.67$

Even though all three children have identical raw scores, the standard scores tell us that the 5-year-old has more behavioral problems, relative to other same-aged children, than the 6- or 7-year-old.

Sometimes it is more convenient to work with standard scores that do not have negative numbers or decimals. Standard scores can be further transformed to have any desired mean and standard deviation. As an example, SAT and GRE scores are transformed Z scores that have a mean of 500 and an *SD* of 100. Many widely used cognitive and personality tests (such as the Wechsler IQ test) are standardized to have a mean of 100 and an *SD* of 15. The formula for converting raw scores to such a standard score scale is:

$$\text{Standard Score}_{100,15} = \left(\left(\frac{X - \overline{X}}{SD} \right) \times 15 \right) + 100$$

In other words, the Z score $((X - \overline{X}) \div SD)$ is multiplied by 15, and then 100 is added to that value. If we converted the three BPI Z scores to have a mean of 100 and an *SD* of 15, we would obtain the following:

Age 5: $\text{Standard Score}_{100,15} = (1.0 \times 15) + 100$ = 115.0
Age 6: $\text{Standard Score}_{100,15} = (0.0 \times 15) + 100$ = 100.0
Age 7: $\text{Standard Score}_{100,15} = (-0.67 \times 15) + 100 =$ 90.0

If we wanted to transform Z scores to scores on a scale like the GRE or SAT, we would substitute the *SD* of 100 for 15 as the multiplier in the preceding formula, and the mean of 500 would replace the addend of 100. For example, the standard score for the 5-year-old would be:

$$\text{Age 5: Standard Score}_{500,100} = (1.0 \times 100) + 500 = 600.0$$

Similar transformations could be done using any desired mean and SD.[5]

PARAMETERS AND STATISTICS

As noted in Chapter 2, descriptive indexes based on data from a population are referred to as parameters rather than statistics. Researchers generally compute statistics because they work with samples, but they are typically interested in using the statistics to make inferences about the parameters.

It is conventional in statistics to use Greek letters to symbolize population parameters. While it is rare to see these Greek symbols in research reports, they are nevertheless important to learn as we move into discussions about inferential statistics. Table 3–2 presents the symbols and pronunciations for the mean, standard deviation, and variance, for both statistics and parameters.

The table also summarizes the formulas for computing these indexes. The formula for the mean is the same for population and sample data, but the formulas for the two main indexes of variability are different. Statisticians have demonstrated that if $N - 1$ is used in the denominator with data from a sample, the variability statistics (SD and variance) are better estimators of the parameters than if N were used.

THE COMPUTER AND INDEXES OF CENTRAL TENDENCY/VARIABILITY

Although indexes of central tendency and variability are not difficult to compute, their calculation can be time consuming if the sample size is large. Computers can readily be used to calculate all major descriptive statistics.

When a researcher is using a computer to analyze data, the command to compute an index of central tendency is usually simple. Because of this fact, the researcher typically computes all three indexes rather than making an a priori decision about which is preferable. For the heart rate data presented in Table 2–1, the command to compute all three indexes using SPSS/PC would simply be:

```
FREQUENCIES VARIABLES = HARTRATE
/STATISTICS = MEAN MEDIAN MODE.
```

---

[5]The most commonly used tranformed standard scores are those with means of 500 with SDs of 100, means of 100 with SDs of 15, and means of 50 with SDs of 10. Standard scores with means of 50 and SDs of 10 are sometimes referred to in the research literature as **T-scores.**

TABLE 3–2. NAMES, SYMBOLS, AND FORMULAS FOR DESCRIPTIVE STATISTICS AND PARAMETERS

		STATISTIC			PARAMETER	
Index Name	Symbol	Pronunciation	Formula	Symbol	Pronunciation	Formula
Mean	$\overline{X}$ (M)	X bar	$\dfrac{\Sigma X}{N}$	μ	Mew	$\dfrac{\Sigma X}{N}$
Standard Deviation*	SD (s)		$\sqrt{\dfrac{\Sigma(X-\overline{X})^2}{N-1}}$	σ	Sigma	$\sqrt{\dfrac{\Sigma(X-\overline{X})^2}{N}}$
Variance*	Var (s^2)		$\dfrac{\Sigma(X-\overline{X})^2}{N-1}$	σ^2	Sigma squared	$\dfrac{\Sigma(X-\overline{X})^2}{N}$

*The formulas for the SD and Var statistics have N (rather than $N-1$) in the denominator when these statistics are computed with sample data for descriptive purposes, rather than for making inferences about the population parameters.

In this example, the computer would produce a full frequency distribution for HARTRATE (as in Figure 2–1), followed by the information that the mode is 66.000, the median is 66.000, and the mean is 65.390. In this situation, we would probably report only the mean in a research report because the values of all three indexes are fairly close and the distribution is not skewed.

It should be noted that the computer is totally ignorant about the levels of measurement of variables in a data set. If we instructed the computer to calculate the mean marital status of subjects (for example, using the data in Table 2–3), it would certainly proceed to do so, but the information would not make sense; the mean for the data in Table 2–3 is 1.876, a meaningless number. The ease with which a computer can perform calculations should not lead researchers to forego thoughtful consideration of what is appropriate for the variable's level of measurement.

The commands for instructing a computer to calculate indexes of variability also are simple. For the heart rate data presented in Table 2–1, the SPSS/PC command to compute the range, the *SD,* and the variance[6] would be as follows:

    FREQUENCIES VARIABLES = HARTRATE
    /STATISTICS =RANGE STDDEV VARIANCE.

---

[6]The *SQR* is not a routinely available statistic in most statistical software packages, but nevertheless can be computed easily by instructing the computer to show the values of specified percentiles of a distribution. For example, in SPSS/PC, the following subcommand could be added to the basic FREQUENCIES command:

    /NTILES = 4.

This subcommand would yield the values of the four quartiles for the distribution, from which the *SQR* could be readily calculated.

HARTRATE

Mean	65.390	Std err	.469	Median	66.000
Mode	66.000	Std dev	4.694	Variance	22.038
Kurtosis	-.541	S E Kurt	.478	Skewness	-.109
S E Skew	.241	Range	20.000	Minimum	55.000
Maximum	75.000	Sum	6539.000		

Valid cases   100   Missing cases   0

FIGURE 3–6. COMPUTER PRINTOUT OF BASIC DESCRIPTIVE STATISTICS

Normally, a researcher instructs the computer to calculate indexes of central tendency and variability simultaneously. In fact, researchers are most likely to use a command such as the following:

> FREQUENCIES VARIABLES = HARTRATE
> /STATISTICS = ALL.

The STATISTICS subcommand in this example (again, in SPSS/PC) instructs the computer to calculate and display all the descriptive statistics associated with SPSS's FREQUENCIES program. Figure 3–6 presents the printout that resulted from this command for the heart rate data. This figure shows 14 different statistics, including many that were discussed in this chapter (e.g., the mean, mode, median, range, *SD,* and variance) and some that were discussed in the previous chapter (e.g., indexes of kurtosis and skewness).

Computers can also be used to compute standard scores. In SPSS/PC, the Z-score transformation is achieved with the following command:

> DESCRIPTIVES HARTRATE
> /OPTIONS = 3.

This instruction would create a new standard score variable (which automatically would be named ZHARTRAT) for the heart rate data. ZHARTRAT, which would be computed to have a mean of 0 and an *SD* of 1, would be created for every subject and added to the file for subsequent analysis.

RESEARCH APPLICATIONS OF CENTRAL TENDENCY AND VARIABILITY

Descriptive indexes of central tendency and variability are widely used by researchers. This section examines some of the major applications of such indexes and discusses methods of effectively displaying such information in a research report.

The Uses of Central Tendency and Variability Indexes

For variables that are measured on an interval or ratio scale (and for many ordinal-level variables as well), researchers fairly routinely compute indexes of central tendency and variability, paying particular attention to the mean and *SD*. We have already seen that the mean and *SD* have an important application in the creation of standard scores. A few of the other major reasons for using such indexes are described here.

1. *Answering Research Questions.* When a study is descriptive, researchers are sometimes able to answer their research questions directly through the computation of descriptive statistics such as indexes of central tendency and variability. For example, one of the aims of a study by McDonald (1993) was to describe the types and amounts of narcotic analgesics administered to postoperative appendectomy patients by nurses. She reported the means, standard deviations, and ranges for the amounts of eight specific narcotic analgesics received by the sample of 180 patients.

2. *Understanding the Data.* Even when a study is not primarily descriptive, researchers often develop a better understanding of their data by examining their main study variables descriptively. Means and *SD*s are almost always computed for all major interval- and ratio-level variables prior to pursuing more complex analyses. In research reports, researchers often present indexes of central tendency and variability to help orient the reader before going on to report the results of inferential statistics. For example, Heidrich (1994) used multivariate statistical analyses to examine the relationships among actual and ideal self-conceptions, physical health, and depression in elderly women. Before reporting her main statistical findings, however, she presented a descriptive table with the means and *SD*s for her measures of actual and ideal self-conceptions at two points in time.

3. *Describing the Research Sample.* As noted in Chapter 2, it is important to carefully determine the major background characteristics of the research sample so that the findings can be properly interpreted. Many subject characteristics are more succinctly described through indexes of central tendency than through frequency information. For example, Rudy and her colleagues (1993), in their study of body satisfaction in edentulous clients, presented the means, modes, medians, and ranges for three ratio-level background variables of their subjects: their age, number of years of schooling, and number of years edentulous.

4. *Addressing Missing Data Problems.* When a researcher encounters missing data in a data set, a decision must be made regarding how to handle this problem. One approach is to drop the case and another is to drop the variable. These are extreme solutions that researchers usually prefer to avoid.[7] When missing values are reasonably random and when the extent of the problem is not large, researchers sometimes perform a **mean substitution.** That is, they calculate a mean based on the

---

[7]The handling of missing data is a complex topic. While some strategies are described in this book, missing data techniques are described more fully in Polit and Hungler (1995), Cohen and Cohen (1975), and Little and Rubin (1990).

cases that are not missing, and then replace the missing values with the value of the mean. For example, if a subject's age were missing and the mean age of all other sample members were 39, the value of 39 could be substituted for the missing values code. (If the distribution were highly skewed, it might be preferable to substitute the median.)

The Presentation of Central Tendency and Variability in Research Reports

Measures of central tendency and variability are reported in the vast majority of research reports. They are usually reported either directly in the text or in tables. Occasionally, means are presented in graphic form.

Decisions about presenting information in tables or in the text must be based primarily on efficiency. If only one or two descriptive statistics are being reported (for example, the sample's mean age and mean number of days hospitalized), it is probably better to present this information in the text. However, if there are descriptive statistics for multiple variables that are conceptually related, a table is likely to be the most effective method of presentation. Typically, researchers report, at a minimum, means and *SD*s, and they often present ranges as well. (If the number of cases varies from one variable to the next, the *N*s should also be presented.) As an example, Haq (1993) studied client satisfaction with nurses among older adults at a nursing center. She presented means, *SD*s, modes, and ranges for the four subscales of the Client Satisfaction Survey (CSS) and the total scale. Her table, an adapted version of which is presented in Table 3–3, suggests that all of the subscale scores were moderately, negatively skewed since all of the modes are greater than the means.

Graphs are most likely to be used to display central tendency information when the researcher wants to emphasize contrasts. In particular, graphs are often used for plotting means over time. Almost invariably, the means are plotted on the *Y* (vertical) axis, while the time periods are plotted along the *X* (horizontal) axis. Occasionally, researchers display this information in a histogram type format with bars drawn to a height indicating

TABLE 3–3. EXAMPLE OF A TABLE WITH INDEXES OF CENTRAL TENDENCY AND VARIABILITY

Client Satisfaction Survey Scale	Mean	*SD*	Mode	Range
Technical/Professional	26.1	2.6	28	16–28
Educational Relationship	23.3	3.6	26	10–28
Trusting Relationship	33.7	4.3	37	12–37
Goal Congruency	16.7	2.7	20	7–20
Total Scale	99.9	11.6	108	60–113

*Originally Table 2 in Haq's (1993) report. The table was titled **CSS Total Scores and Subscale Scores (N = 156).***

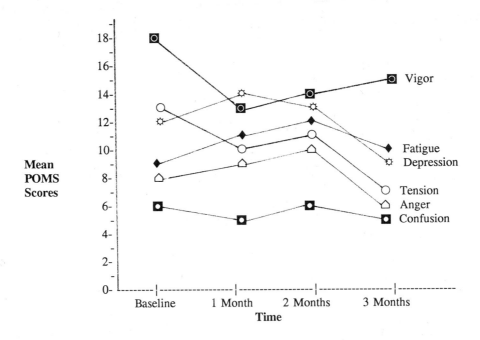

Mood States in Radiation Patients Over Time

FIGURE 3–7. EXAMPLE OF A GRAPH PLOTTING MEANS OVER TIME

a mean value. More often, however, means are plotted using dots that are connected by a straight line, creating what is referred to as a **line graph.** For example, suppose we were interested in studying the mood states of cancer patients who received radiation therapy over a 3-month period. Using the Profile of Mood States (POMS), which consists of six subscales, we could collect data on patients' moods prior to radiation and then at 1, 2, and 3 months after treatment. Mean scores on the POMS could then be displayed in a graph, such as the one shown in Figure 3–7.

Tips on Preparing Tables with Central Tendency and Variability Indexes

As with any table, it is important to present tables of descriptive statistics clearly and succinctly. We offer some suggestions for enhancing the presentation of central tendency and variability indexes in tables.

- It is usually preferable not to combine in one table variables for which different types of descriptive statistics are appropriate. For example, if some variables are better described with percentages (nominal-level variables), while others are better described using means (interval- or ratio-level variables), two separate tables may be necessary. The exception is that a single table is often used for displaying the background characteristics of a sample, regardless of the level of measurement of the variables.

- Readers can usually compare numbers down a column more readily than across a row. For this reason, the names of the variables being described are usually listed along the left in the first column. The descriptive statistics being presented are named across the top row. Table 3–3 exemplifies this format.

- Means and *SD*s are usually reported to one or two decimal places. Greater precision is almost never necessary. Within a column of information, the level of precision should be the same.

- There are no specific rules for ordering the variables that appear in a table of descriptive statistics. If there is a meaningful conceptual ordering (for example, dependent variables might be ordered to correspond to a set of hypotheses), this is a highly effective approach. If the values of the statistics themselves can be meaningfully ordered, this is advantageous to the reader. For example, DiIorio, vanLier, and Manteuffel (1994) studied clinicians' recommendations for how to relieve nausea and vomiting during pregnancy. Sample members rated the frequency with which they recommended 33 specific relief measures on a four-point scale. The researchers presented a table with the mean ratings of each method, ranked from highest to lowest.

- Researchers have adopted several different conventions for displaying means and *SD*s in tables. One option is to list the means and *SD*s in separate columns, as in Table 3–3. Sometimes, to save space, researchers place the *SD* in parentheses directly next to the mean. For example, the first entry in Table 3–3 would then be 26.1 (2.6). A third method is to present the *SD* next to the mean, preceded by "±" (e.g., 26.1 ± 2.6).

- In tables that present information on central tendency and variability, it is often possible and desirable to display other types of information at the same time. For example, in addition to the actual range of score values, researchers sometimes include the theoretical range (i.e., the minimum and maximum scores that are possible for the measure being used). When the variables in the table have been measured by psychosocial scales (e.g., measures of depression, self-esteem, and so on), researchers sometimes present the reliability coefficients[8] of the scale in the same table as the means and *SD*s. For example, Cox (1993) used two scales in her study of family functioning in relation to pet attachment. She presented a table with the means, *SD*s, ranges, theoretical ranges, and reliability coefficients for the scales and all subscales.

RESEARCH EXAMPLE

Indexes of central tendency and variability are reported in the vast majority of research reports. Below we provide a brief summary of the descriptive statistics reported in a recent study.

---

[8]**A reliability coefficient** is a quantitative index of how reliable or consistent a measure is. Formulas for most reliability coefficients are not presented in this textbook, although some are discussed in subsequent chapters. Interested readers should consult a research methods textbook (e.g., Polit and Hungler, 1995) or a book on psychometric methods (e.g., Nunnally, 1978; Guilford, 1964). Statistical software packages such as SPSS have commands for computing reliability coefficients.

TABLE 3–4. EXAMPLE OF A TABLE WITH VARIOUS DESCRIPTIVE STATISTICS

Variable	Mean	SD	Possible Range	Actual Range	Reliability Coefficient
Pain Intensity	58.40	15.04	0–100	7.1–82.6	n/a
Distress (Profile of Mood States scale)	20.67	12.64	0–72	0–53	.93
Disability (Sickness Impact Profile scale)	19.88	9.69	0–100	0–42	.78
Helplessness	2.21	1.02	0–5	0.14–4.67	.70
Resourcefulness	2.92	0.72	0–5	1.50–4.31	.42
Catastrophizing	2.44	1.07	0–5	0.22–4.67	.84
Coping	3.05	0.73	0–5	1.44–4.78	.66

Adapted from Table 1, Wells (1994). The table was titled **Sample Means and Variance Indicators.**

Wells (1994) studied patients' perceived control over pain in relation to levels of distress and disability in a sample of 71 patients with chronic nonmalignant pain. Descriptive statistics were used in the text to characterize the research sample. For example, Wells reported that the mean age of the sample was 45.5 years ($SD = 11.8$) and that the mean duration of the patients' pain was 3.8 years.

Although Wells used primarily inferential statistics to address her research questions, she began the results section of her report by presenting basic descriptive statistics for the key variables in the study. Table 1 of her report, reproduced here as Table 3–4, shows five pieces of information for each major dependent and independent variable: the mean, the standard deviation, the possible range of scores on the measure, the *actual* range of scores on the measure, and (for all but one scale) the reliability coefficient.

SUMMARY

A distribution of data for a quantitative variable can be described in terms of its shape, its central tendency, and its variability. Indexes of **central tendency** yield a number that describes a "typical" or average data value, usually from the center of the distribution. Indexes of **variability** yield a quantitative measure of how dispersed or spread out the data values in a distribution are.

The three most widely used indexes of central tendency are the mode, the median, and the mean. The **mode** is the score value that occurs most frequently in a distribution. The **median** is the point in the distribution above which and below which 50% of the cases fall (i.e., the score at the 50th **percentile**). The **mean** is the arithmetic average, computed by adding together all score values and dividing by the number of cases. Unless data are severely skewed, the mean is generally the preferred index of central tendency because of its stability and its utility in other statistical procedures.

The most widely used indexes of variability or dispersion are the range and the standard deviation. The **range** is simply the highest score minus the lowest score. The **standard deviation** is an index that indicates how much, on average, the scores deviate from the mean. It is calculated by first summing all the squared **deviation scores** (each subject's raw score minus the mean), dividing by the number of subjects minus 1, and then taking the square root. The **variance** is an index of variability equal to the standard deviation, squared.

Indexes of central tendency and variability are widely used by researchers to describe their main research variables and the sample characteristics. They are also used in other applications, such as in the calculation of **standard scores,** which are scores that are expressed as relative distances from the mean, in standard deviation units. Standard scores (sometimes referred to as **Z scores**) are used to enhance comparisons and the interpretability of data values.

EXERCISES

The following exercises cover concepts presented in this chapter. Exercises indicated with a dagger (†) can be checked against answers appearing in Appendix A. Additionally, Chapter 3 of the accompanying *Applications Manual* offers supplementary exercises, including ones that require computer analysis of a data set on diskette.

† 1. The following set of numbers represent the scores of 30 psychiatric inpatients on a widely used measure of depression (the Center for Epidemiologic Studies Depression scale). What are the mean, the median, and the mode for these data?

```
41   27   32   24   21   28   22   25   35   27
31   40   23   27   29   33   42   30   26   30
27   39   26   34   28   38   29   36   24   37
```

If the values of these indexes are not the same, discuss what they suggest about the shape of the distribution.

† 2. Find the medians for the following distributions:
a. 1   5   7   8   9
b. 3   5   6   8   9   10
c. 3   4   4   4   7
d. 3   4   4   4   6   20
e. 2   4   5   5   8   9

† 3. For which distribution in Exercise 2 would the median be preferred to the mean as the index of central tendency? Why?

† 4. The following 10 data values are diastolic blood pressure readings. Compute the mean, the range, the *SD,* and the variance for these data.

130   110   160   120   170
120   150   140   160   140

† 5. For each blood pressure value in Exercise 4, compute a *Z* score. Then, transform these *Z* scores to standard scores with a mean of 500 and an *SD* of 100.

Bivariate Description

Most research questions are about relationships between two or more variables. For example, when scientists study whether smokers are more likely than nonsmokers to develop lung cancer, they are asking if there is a relationship between smoking and lung cancer. When nurse researchers ask whether primiparas are more likely than multiparas to request epidural analgesia, they are studying the relationship between parity and requests for pain relief.

The descriptive statistics we have discussed thus far do not concern relationships; they are used to describe one variable at a time. Most of the remainder of this book describes inferential statistical tests that allow us to make inferences about relationships within the population. This chapter discusses methods of *describing* relationships by means of **bivariate descriptive statistics.** The three most typical situations are when there are two nominal variables, a nominal variable and an interval or ratio variable, or two interval or ratio variables.

CROSSTABULATION: DESCRIPTION OF TWO NOMINAL VARIABLES

Suppose we were interested in comparing men and women patients with regard to their rate of readmission into a psychiatric hospital within 1 year of discharge. In this example, there are two research variables—gender and readmission status—and both are dichotomous, nominal-level variables. Two independent frequency distributions would tell us, first, how many men and women there were in the sample, and second, how many sample members, overall, were readmitted within 1 year of discharge. To describe the relationship between the two variables, we would **crosstabulate** the two variables in a two-dimensional arrangement that is often referred to as a contingency table.

A **contingency table** (or **crosstabulation table**) is essentially a two-dimensional frequency distribution. A hypothetical contingency table for this example is presented in Table 4–1.

To construct a contingency table, we array the categories of one variable across the top horizontally (in this example, gender), and the categories of the second variable along the left vertically (here, readmission status). This creates the **cells** for the contingency table—that is, the unique combinations of the two variables. The number of cells is the number of categories of the first variable multiplied by the number of categories of the second. There are four cells (2 × 2) in the present example.

Next, cases are allocated to the appropriate cell. That is, men who were readmitted are tallied in the upper left cell, women who were readmitted are tallied in the upper right cell, and so on. Once all of the sample members have been categorized in the correct cell, frequencies and percentages can be easily computed for each cell. In this example, we see that men were somewhat more likely than women to be readmitted to a psychiatric hospital within 1 year of discharge (30% versus 20%, respectively).

Contingency tables are easy to construct and they communicate considerable information. The commands for instructing the computer to prepare a contingency table are straightforward as well. However, students sometimes need assistance in reading the printouts for computer-generated contingency tables. Note that in Table 4–1, the percentages were based on gender: 30.0% of the men (15 ÷ 50) and 20.0% of the women (10 ÷ 50) were readmitted. We could also have calculated percentages based on readmission status. For example, we could say that 6 0.0% of all the patients readmitted were men (15 ÷ 25), or that 53.3% of those *not* readmitted were women (40 ÷ 75). The computer can be instructed to compute all possible percentages.

As an example, suppose we were interested in comparing women who had a cesarean delivery and those who had a vaginal delivery with regard to whether they experienced postpartum depression. A fictitious contingency table for this example

TABLE 4–1. CONTINGENCY TABLE FOR GENDER/READMISSION STATUS EXAMPLE

READMISSION STATUS	GENDER		
	Male	Female	**TOTAL**
Readmitted	15 (30.0%)	10 (20.0%)	25 (25.0%)
Not Readmitted	35 (70.0%)	40 (80.0%)	75 (75.0%)
TOTAL	50	50	100

DEPRESS   EXPERIENCED POSTPARTUM DEPRESSION?   by   DELIVERY   TYPE OF DELIVERY

```
                      DELIVERY        Page 1 of 1
              Count
              Row Pct |CESAREAN VAGINAL
              Col Pct |                       Row
              Tot Pct |     1   |      2   | Total
DEPRESS       --------+---------+---------+
                 1    |    11   |    12   |    23
  YES                 |   47.8  |   52.2  |   23.0
                      |   57.9  |   14.8  |
                      |   11.0  |   12.0  |
                      +---------+---------+
                 2    |     8   |    69   |    77
  NO                  |   10.4  |   89.6  |   77.0
                      |   42.1  |   85.2  |
                      |    8.0  |   69.0  |
                      +---------+---------+
              Column       19        81       100
               Total     19.0      81.0     100.0
```

Number of Missing Observations: 0

FIGURE 4–1.   COMPUTER PRINTOUT OF A CONTINGENCY TABLE

(Figure 4–1) has been created to demonstrate how to read a printout from a cross-tabulation.[1] Let us begin by examining the column and row percentages of this printout. In the bottom row we see that there were 19 women (19.0%) with a cesarean delivery and 81 (81.0%) with a vaginal delivery. In the far right column we see that there were 23 women (23.0%) who experienced depression, and 77 women (77.0%) who did not. These are sometimes referred to as the **marginal frequencies.** Both the row totals and the column totals add up to the grand total—i.e., the total sample size of 100 (100% of the cases), shown in the bottom right corner.

As in the previous example, there are four cells (2 × 2) in this contingency table because both variables are dichotomous. In the printout, each cell contains four pieces of information, which we describe here for the first (upper left) cell. According to the printout, 11 of the 100 women in this sample had a cesarean delivery *and* experienced postpartum depression. The next number is the row percentage: 47.8% (11 ÷ 23) of the women who were depressed had a cesarean delivery. The third number in the cell is the column percentage: 57.9% (11 ÷ 19) of the women with a cesarean delivery experienced depression. Finally, the fourth number is the total percentage: of the 100 sample members, 11.0% had a cesarean delivery and were depressed. In the upper left hand

---

[1]The SPSS/PC command that produced Figure 4–1 is as follows:

```
CROSSTABS TABLES=DEPRESS BY DELIVERY
   /CELLS=COUNT ROW COLUMN TOTAL.
```

corner, the printout provides a reminder of how to read these numbers by indicating the order of the information in a cell:

Count
Row Pct
Col Pct
Tot Pct

The most meaningful pieces of information in this table are the column percentages for the cells. They tell us that substantially more of the women with a cesarean delivery (57.8%) than with a vaginal delivery (14.8%) experienced postpartum depression. When the computer is instructed to display the independent variable along the top, as in this example,[2] it is usually the column percentages that are of greatest interest.

Although we have indicated that contingency tables such as these are used when there are two nominal-level variables, they are also appropriate if either or both variables are ordinal-level with a small number of categories. For example, we could crosstabulate smoking status (nonsmoker, smokes $\leq$ 1 pack per day, smokes > 1 pack per day) and age group (<30, 31-50, 51+) to create a nine-cell contingency table that would describe the relationship between smoking behavior and age. Both of these variables, as defined in this example, are ordinal.

COMPARISON OF GROUP MEANS: DESCRIPTION OF A NOMINAL VARIABLE AND AN INTERVAL OR RATIO VARIABLE

Suppose that we wanted to compare women who were put on antepartal hospital bed rest with women who were not with regard to weight gain during pregnancy. The dependent variable in this example (weight gain) is a ratio-level variable and the independent variable (bed rest status) is nominal-level. This is a very common research situation that can be addressed by computing separate means on the dependent variable for the two groups of women. A printout for this fictitious example (Figure 4–2) shows the mean, SD, and number of cases for the sample as a whole (labeled "For Entire Population") and then separately for women on bed rest and those not on bed rest.[3] This table indicates that the 50 women not on bed rest gained, on average, nearly 5 pounds more

---

[2]The researcher controls the order of the variables in a computer-generated contingency table. For example, when the reasearcher instructs the computer to crosstabulate VARY BY VARX (in SPSS), the variable after the "BY" is displayed along the top row, and the other variable is displayed down the left column.

[3]The SPSS/PC command that created the printout in Figure 4–2 is as follows:
    MEANS TABLES=WGTGAIN BY BEDREST.

```
Summaries of    WGTGAIN      POUNDS GAINED WHILE PREGNANT
By levels of    BEDREST

Variable         Value  Label                    Mean      Std Dev    Cases

For Entire Population                          13.1950     4.4062      100

BEDREST            1   BED REST                10.9660     2.6785       50
BEDREST            2   NO BED REST             15.4240     4.6810       50

   Total Cases =      100
```

FIGURE 4–2.   COMPUTER PRINTOUT OF GROUP MEAN COMPARISON FOR TWO GROUPS

than the 50 women who were put on antepartal hospital bed rest. There was also considerably more variability in weight gain among those not on bed rest.

This approach would also be appropriate if the dependent variable was measured on an ordinal scale that approached interval-level properties. For example, we might want to compare the two groups of women with respect to scores on a psychological scale (e.g., coping, body image, and so on). Such scales yield measures that are ordinal but that are often treated as interval variables.

CORRELATION: DESCRIPTION OF THE RELATIONSHIP BETWEEN TWO INTERVAL- OR RATIO-LEVEL VARIABLES

Correlation procedures are an extremely useful way of describing the direction and magnitude of a relationship between two variables. For example, correlation procedures can be used to address the question, To what extent are respiratory function and anxiety levels among patients with chronic obstructive pulmonary disease related? Or, What is the magnitude of the relationship between cardiac output measurements obtained via the thermodilution cardiac output technique and the direct Fick method?

Variables are said to be correlated with one another when there is a relationship between them. Correlations between two variables can be plotted graphically. More often, researchers describe correlations through the calculation of an index that summarizes the extent and direction of a relationship. We describe graphic procedures first because they help us to explore why correlation coefficients are useful in describing **linear** (straight line) **relationships.**

Scatterplots

The relationship between two variables that have been measured on an interval or ratio scale can be displayed graphically on a **scatterplot** (sometimes referred to as a **scatter diagram**). This type of graph plots the values of one variable *(X)* on the abscissa or X axis, and simultaneously plots the values of a second variable *(Y)* on the ordinate or *Y* axis. As an example, suppose that for every hour that students volunteered to work at a school-based clinic, a sponsor donated $1 toward the school's athletic fund. Figure 4–3 presents data for the hours worked *(X)* and the dollar amounts donated *(Y)* for 10 students. The first student volunteered 1 hour, and the amount of the donation was therefore $1. The tenth student volunteered 10 hours, resulting in a $10 donation. These data are also shown graphically in the scatterplot in Figure 4–3. Each dot on the scatterplot represents a data point for the two variables (e.g., the dot at the intersection of 1 hour on the *X* axis and $1 on the *Y* axis is the data point for student 1). As indicated in this graph, there is a straight line relationship between *X* and *Y*. Algebraically, we can say that $X = Y$. That is, the value of *X* is always equal to the value of *Y*. If a student worked 20 hours, the donation would be $20. The relationship between *X* and *Y* is described as a **perfect relationship,** because we need only know the value of *X* to know or predict the value of *Y*, and vice versa.

Researchers virtually never study variables that are perfectly related to one another, and so scatterplots of actual research data are rarely so orderly and comprehensible as the one in Figure 4–3. Figure 4–4 presents a scatterplot with some fictitious data for two variables for which the relationship is strong, but not perfect. Let us say that *X* represents nursing students' test scores on a 10-question midterm statistics test and *Y* represents their scores on a 10-question final exam. (The letters on the graph correspond to subjects a through j, and are shown here to help identify each data point.) Although we cannot perfectly predict values of *Y* based on values of *X*, it is neverthe-

Student	Data Hours (X)	Donation (Y)
1	1	$1
2	2	$2
3	3	$3
4	4	$4
5	5	$5
6	6	$6
7	7	$7
8	8	$8
9	9	$9
10	10	$10

FIGURE 4–3.   SCATTERPLOT FOR VOLUNTEER/DONATION EXAMPLE

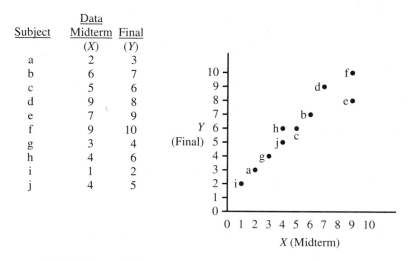

Subject	Data Midterm (X)	Final (Y)
a	2	3
b	6	7
c	5	6
d	9	8
e	7	9
f	9	10
g	3	4
h	4	6
i	1	2
j	4	5

FIGURE 4–4.   SCATTERPLOT OF STUDENTS' TEST SCORES

less true that students who performed well on the midterm also tended to do well on the final exam.

Scatterplots are useful in showing both the magnitude and direction of relationships. The scatterplot in Figure 4–4 illustrates a strong **positive relationship.** The relationship is strong because the data points fall fairly closely together along a straight diagonal line; the relationship is positive because high values on X are associated with high values on Y. Scatterplots of positive relationships show points that extend from the lower left corner of the graph to the upper right one. Figure 4–5 (A) shows another example of a positive relationship, but one that is quite weak; the points are scattered in a fairly loose fashion, though the general trend is in a distinctly positive direction. Figure 4–5 (B) shows a scatterplot of a positive correlation that is moderately strong.

Researchers sometimes observe a **negative relationship** (also referred to as an **inverse relationship**) between variables. This occurs when high values on one variable are associated with low values on another. For example, researchers have generally found that depression and self-esteem are negatively related—people who have high levels of self-esteem tend to have low levels of depression, and vice versa. Scatterplots of negative relationships have points that slope from the upper left corner to the lower right one. Figure 4–5 (D) shows a scatterplot of a perfect negative relationship between two variables, and Figure 4–5 (E) illustrates a negative relationship that is strong, but not perfect.

When variables are totally uncorrelated, the points on the graph are scattered all over in a random fashion, such as in the scatterplot in Figure 4–5 (C). In this situation, a person with a high score on X is about equally likely to have a low or a high score on Y.

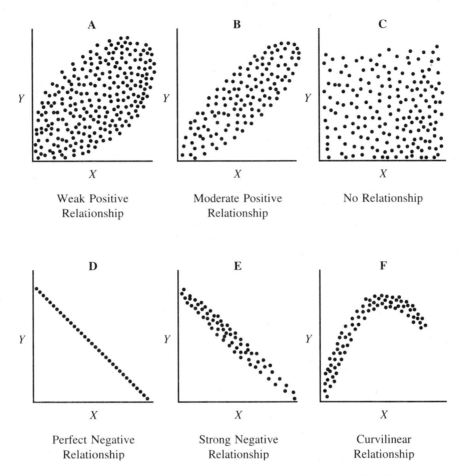

FIGURE 4–5.   SCATTERPLOTS SHOWING VARIOUS RELATIONSHIPS

For example, if we were to construct a scatterplot showing the relationship between nurses' height and their salaries, we might expect a graph such as this one; there is no reason to expect tall nurses to earn more (or less) than short nurses.

One other type of relationship is shown in Figure 4–5 (F). This scatterplot illustrates what is known as a **curvilinear relationship.** In this situation, a straight line does not adequately characterize the relationship between the variables. Scores on *Y* increase as the scores on *X* increase, but only to a certain point, and after that point the scores on *Y* decline. As an example, there may be a curvilinear relationship between the number of hours slept and perceptions of energy levels; perceived energy would likely increase with increasing amounts of sleep, but at some point a large number of hours of sleep might reflect a physiological condition associated with low energy.

Correlation Coefficients: General Principles

Although correlations between two variables can readily be graphed, researchers are much more likely to describe correlations by means of a statistic known as a **correlation coefficient.** Correlation coefficients, like scatterplots, indicate both the magnitude and direction of a linear relationship between two variables. Because they are expressed numerically, correlation coefficients are more precise about magnitude than scatterplots, to which we usually attach broad verbal labels such as "weak" or "moderate" or "strong."

Correlation coefficients are indexes whose values range from 1.00 through .00 to +1.00. All negative values (from −1.00 to −.01) indicate a negative relationship, while all positive values (from +.01 to +1.00) indicate a positive relationship. A correlation coefficient of .00 indicates no relationship between the variables.

The **absolute value** (the numerical value without any sign) of the correlation coefficient indicates the strength of the relationship. The smaller the absolute value, the weaker is the relationship. For example, −.90 indicates a very strong relationship, while +.45 indicates a moderate one. When two variables are perfectly and positively correlated (as in the case of the data shown in Figure 4–3), the correlation coefficient is +1.00. Perfect negative correlations are expressed as −1.00.

Pearson's r

The most widely used correlation index is the **Pearson product-moment correlation coefficient** (also known as **Pearson's r**), a statistic that is appropriate when two variables are measured on an interval or ratio scale, or on a level that approximates interval characteristics. Other correlation indexes are described later in this book.

Correlation coefficients are usually calculated by computer rather than manually. However, manual computation, though laborious, is not difficult. There are several alternative formulas for computing Pearson's r. We offer the following equation:

$$r_{xy} = \frac{\Sigma(X - \overline{X})(Y - \overline{Y})}{\sqrt{[\Sigma(X - \overline{X})^2]\,[\Sigma(Y - \overline{Y})^2]}}$$

where r_{xy} = the correlation coefficient for variables X and Y
Σ = the sum of
X = an individual value for variable X
$\overline{X}$ = the mean for variable X
Y = an individual value for variable Y
$\overline{Y}$ = the mean for variable Y

TABLE 4-2. CALCULATION OF PEARSON'S r

Subject	1 X	2 $(X - \bar{X})$	3 $(X - \bar{X})^2$	4 Y	5 $(Y - \bar{Y})$	6 $(Y - \bar{Y})^2$	7 $(X - \bar{X})(Y - \bar{Y})$
a	2	−3	9	3	−3	9	9
b	6	1	1	7	1	1	1
c	5	0	0	6	0	0	0
d	9	4	16	8	2	4	8
e	7	2	4	9	3	9	6
f	9	4	16	10	4	16	16
g	3	−2	4	4	−2	4	4
h	4	−1	1	6	0	0	0
i	1	−4	16	2	−4	16	16
j	4	−1	1	5	−1	1	1
	$\Sigma X = 50$		$\Sigma = 68$	$\Sigma Y = 60$		$\Sigma = 60$	$\Sigma = 61$
	$\bar{X} = 5.0$			$\bar{Y} = 6.0$			

$$r_{xy} = \frac{\Sigma(X - \bar{X})(Y - \bar{Y})}{\sqrt{[\Sigma(X - \bar{X})^2][\Sigma(Y - \bar{Y})^2]}}$$

$\Sigma(X - \bar{X})(Y - \bar{Y}) = 61$
$\Sigma(X - \bar{X})^2 \quad = 68$
$\Sigma(Y - \bar{Y})^2 \quad = 60$

$$r_{xy} = \frac{61}{\sqrt{68 \times 60}} = \frac{61}{\sqrt{4080}} = \frac{61}{63.8745} = .955$$

Although this formula looks complex, it basically involves manipulating deviation scores for the two variables.[4] An example is completely worked out in Table 4–2, using the data on nursing students' scores on the statistics midterm and final exam, plotted in Figure 4–4.

The first step in computing r with this formula is to compute the means for X and Y, which are shown as 5.0 and 6.0, respectively (columns 1 and 4 in Table 4–2). Deviation scores are then obtained for each subject (columns 2 and 5), and then each deviation score is squared (columns 3 and 6). The **crossproducts** of the two deviation scores are calculated in column 7. That is, the deviation score for variable X is multiplied by the deviation score for variable Y for each subject. The individual values in columns 3, 6, and 7 are then summed, and these sums constitute the elements required in the correlation formula. As shown at the bottom of Table 4–2, the value of r in this example is .955, which is a very strong, positive correlation.

---

[4]In fact, we can simplify the appearance of the formula by using the symbols for deviation scores:

$$r_{xy} = \frac{\Sigma xy}{\sqrt{(\Sigma x^2)(\Sigma y^2)}}$$

When a computer is used to calculate the Pearson r statistic, the command is usually quite simple. For example, in SPSS/PC, the command for correlating two variables named VARX and VARY would be:

CORRELATION VARIABLES=VARX VARY.

Interpretation of Correlation Coefficients

Although the numerical value of a correlation coefficient is a direct reflection of magnitude, there are no straightforward guidelines for interpreting the strength of a correlation coefficient. For example, researchers who have examined the relationship between cardiac output measurements obtained via the thermodilution cardiac output technique and the direct Fick method have generally found correlations in the vicinity of .95. In this context, if a correlation of .80 between the two methods of measuring cardiac output were observed in a new study, the correlation would be considered low. On the other hand, the correlation between self-esteem and depression is probably in the vicinity of $-.40$, and in this situation, a correlation of $-.80$ would be considered extremely high. Correlations between variables of a psychosocial nature rarely exceed .50.

Scatterplots are sometimes useful in interpreting a correlation coefficient when the magnitude is modest. A low correlation coefficient could reflect a weak relationship between two variables, *or* a relationship that is not linear. For example, two computer-generated scatterplots[5] are presented in Figure 4–6. These scatterplots use standard scores as the data values rather than actual raw scores, so the means of all variables are 0. The top graph, which plots VARX against VARY, suggests a relationship that is quite weak. There is only the barest suggestion that the variables are positively correlated and, in fact, the correlation coefficient for these two variables is $+.19$. The correlation coefficient for the two variables in the bottom graph of Figure 4–6 (VARY and VARZ) is quite similar ($r = +.20$), but the nature of the relationship is clearly different. VARY and VARZ have a fairly strong positive relationship at all points below the mean. Above the mean of 0, however, the two variables appear to be related in a loosely negative direction. Because the relationship is not linear, the correlation coefficient does not adequately summarize the pattern.

An interesting feature of a correlation coefficient is that its square is a direct indication of the proportion of the variability in one variable that can be accounted for or explained by variability in a second variable. For example, if the correlation coefficient

---

[5]The SPSS/PC command that created the scatterplots in Figure 4–6 is as follows:

```
REGRESSION VARIABLES=VARX VARY VARZ
  /DEPENDENT=VARY
  /METHOD=ENTER
  /SCATTERPLOT=(VARY, VARX) (VARY, VARZ).
```

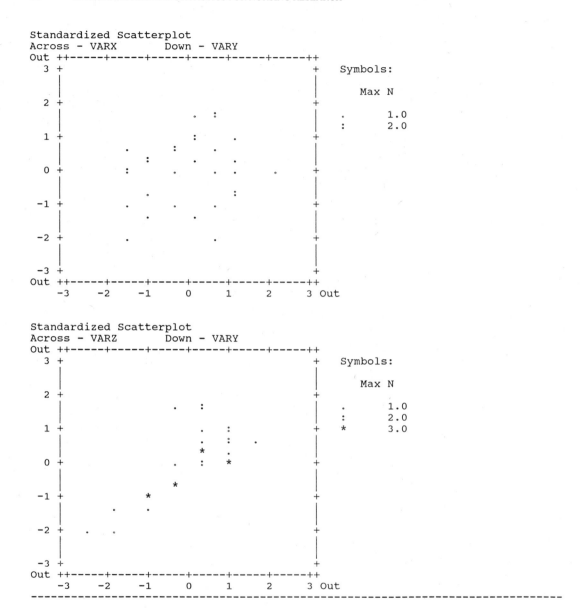

FIGURE 4–6.   COMPUTER PRINTOUT OF TWO SCATTERPLOTS

describing the relationship between SAT scores *(X)* and nursing students' grades *(Y)* is .50, we can then say that 25% $(.50^2)$ of the variability in the students' grades is explained by variability in SAT scores. This relationship is depicted graphically in Figure 4–7. In this figure the two circles represent the total amount of variation in the two variables, and the hatched area indicates how much of the variation in grades is accounted

SAT Scores (*X*)   Nursing Students' Grades (*Y*)

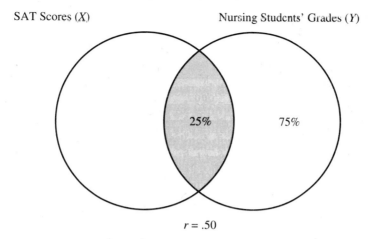

$r = .50$

FIGURE 4–7.   ILLUSTRATION OF PERCENTAGE OF EXPLAINED VARIABILITY IN TWO CORRE-LATED VARIABLES

for by variation in the abilities measured by the SAT (i.e., 25%). The remaining 75% of the variability in grades is accounted for by other factors (e.g., motivation, prior experience, idiosyncracies of faculty grading, and so on). If the correlation between the two variables were perfect (if the student with the highest SAT scores obtained the highest grades, the second highest scorer got the second highest grades, and so on), the two circles would overlap completely. This concept is examined in much greater depth in subsequent chapters.

It must be emphasized that when a researcher determines that two variables are correlated, this does not imply that one variable *caused* the other. For example, if we determine that there is a negative correlation between self-esteem and depression, we cannot conclude that having low self-esteem causes people to become depressed. Nor can we conclude that being depressed reduces people's self-esteem. Either of these might be true, but it might also be that both are caused by some other factor (e.g., receiving a failing grade on an important test). Researchers must always be cautious when drawing inferences from correlations. Even a very strong correlation between two variables provides no evidence that one variable caused the other.

RESEARCH APPLICATIONS OF BIVARIATE DESCRIPTIVE STATISTICS

Bivariate descriptive statistics are a useful means of summarizing the relationship between two variables. This section examines some of the major applications of bivariate descriptive statistics and discusses methods of effectively displaying such information in a research report.

The Uses of Bivariate Descriptive Statistics

The majority of research investigations concern the relationship between two or more variables. In most cases, these studies rely on inferential statistics that are discussed in subsequent chapters of this book. Nevertheless, bivariate descriptive statistics are also used widely by researchers. A few of the major uses for these statistics are described here.

1. *Answering Research Questions.* Descriptive research (or studies that incorporate descriptive questions) often use the methods described in this chapter to answer their research questions. For example, Prattke and Gass-Sternas (1993) described differences between wives and husbands undergoing artificial insemination by donor (AID). They presented a table in which gender of spouse was crosstabulated with three categories of appraising AID (as a harm/loss or threat, as a challenge, or as a benefit). The table revealed that husbands were substantially more likely than wives to view AID as beneficial.

2. *Understanding the Data.* As with other descriptive statistics, bivariate descriptive statistics are often used in preliminary analyses to help the researcher better understand the data when more complex analyses are planned. Many sophisticated multivariate techniques build on correlational techniques and it is almost always useful to first look at correlations descriptively. In research reports, correlations among all major study variables are sometimes displayed prior to presenting the results of inferential statistics. For example, Duckett, Henly, and Garvis (1993) used multivariate procedures to predict how long a mother breastfed her infant, but they first presented a descriptive correlation matrix that showed all the intercorrelations among variables hypothesized to be predictors of breastfeeding duration.

3. *Describing the Research Sample.* As indicated in the previous two chapters, researchers almost always describe the major background characteristics of their subjects. Often, the researcher describes background traits for subgroups within the sample rather than for the sample as a whole. In other words, the researcher crosstabulates background characteristics with a variable that is relevant to the study, such as treatment group (experimental versus control). For example, Allan, Mayo, and Michel (1993) undertook a qualitative study that compared the body size values of white women and African American women. Their table describing sample characteristics crosstabulated race with five background variables: education, socioeconomic status, marital status, age group, and weight group (normal, overweight, and obese).

4. *Developing and Refining an Instrument.* When researchers decide to develop and refine a new instrument to measure a construct of interest, correlation procedures are often used during the process. For example, suppose a researcher was interested in measuring loneliness among nursing home residents and found no suitable self-report scale. The researcher might begin by developing an **item pool** of 30 to 40 items and then administering them on a trial basis to a sample of 100 subjects in a nursing home. A score on the scale would be computed for each subject by adding together responses to all items. The researcher might then want to evaluate whether each item was contributing properly to the scale. This is usually done by computing

correlation coefficients between responses to individual items and the total scale score, and between all possible pairs of items. Items are often discarded (or revised) if the item-total correlation coefficient is less than .50 or if an interitem correlation is less than .30. As a research example, Kidd and Huddleston (1994) developed a scale to measure risky driving practices. They developed a pool of items based on in-depth, qualitative interviews with patients who sustained injuries during a motor vehicle crash. In a pilot test of their instrument, 9 of their original 19 items were deleted based on low interitem and item-total correlations.

The Presentation of Bivariate Descriptive Statistics in Research Reports

Bivariate descriptive statistics are often reported directly in the text of a research report. For example, a researcher might report that 50% of the experimental group and 52% of the control group were women. Or, a researcher might report that the correlation between subjects' preoperative heart rate and scores on an anxiety scale was +.43. However, whenever bivariate statistics are being described for multiple variables simultaneously, the information is usually more conveniently presented in tables than in the text.

When a contingency table results in only four cells, as in Table 4–1, the information can be efficiently summarized in a sentence (e.g., "Twenty percent of the women, compared with 30% of the men, were readmitted to the psychiatric hospital within 1 year of discharge"). However, when there are six or more cells, tables may be less confusing and more informative than a textual presentation. For example, Metheny and her colleagues (1993) studied the effectiveness of pH measurements in predicting feeding tube placement. They presented a contingency table (reproduced here as Table 4–3) that crosstabulated tube site (nasogastric or nasointestinal) with three categories of pH values. The table shows that there was a substantially greater likelihood of low pH values with nasogastric tube placements than with nasointestinal tube placements.

Tables are especially effective for summarizing crosstabulations for multiple variables. For example, Nyamathi and her colleagues (1993) compared their two research groups (impoverished minority women in a specialized AIDS education program and

TABLE 4–3. EXAMPLE OF A 2 $\times$ 3 CONTINGENCY TABLE

pH Meter Reading	Tube Site	
	Nasogastric ($n = 405$)	Nasointestinal ($n = 389$)
pH 0 to 4.0	63.5%	4.9%
pH > 4.0, ≤ 6.0	21.7%	8.0%
pH > 6.0	14.8%	87.1%

*Originally Table 2 in Metheny et al.'s (1993) report. The table was titled **Overall Percentage Distribution of pH-Meter Readings by Tube Site, Nasogastric or Nasointestinal.***

TABLE 4–4. EXAMPLE OF A TABLE WITH MULTIPLE CROSSTABULATIONS

	Research Group			
	Specialized ($n = 448$)		Traditional ($n = 410$)	
Demographic Variable	n	Percent	n	Percent
Site				
Homeless shelter	292	65.2	249	60.7
Drug recovery program	155	34.6	162	39.5
Race				
Black	364	81.3	333	81.2
Hispanic	84	18.7	77	18.8
Serostatus				
HIV positive	7	1.6	6	1.5
HIV negative	441	98.4	404	98.5

*Originally Table 1 in Nyamathi et al.'s (1993) report. The table was titled **Demographic Characteristics of Women, by Group (N = 858)**.*

those in a more traditional AIDS education program) in terms of several variables, including race, site from which they were recruited into the study, and serostatus. A portion of their table is shown here in Table 4–4. This format is also equally useful for presenting means and *SD*s of multiple variables for two or more comparison groups.

Occasionally, researchers present three-dimensional contingency tables. A three-dimensional crosstabulation involves crossing two nominal (or ordinal) variables separately for subgroups of the sample. An example from the study by Metheny et al. (1993) is shown in Table 4–5. In this table, the researchers crosstabulated tube site and cate-

TABLE 4–5. EXAMPLE OF A 2 × 3 × 2 CONTINGENCY TABLE

	Tube Site	
pH Meter Reading	Nasogastric	Nasointestinal
Acid Inhibitors Absent	($n = 185$)	($n = 197$)
pH 0 to 4.0	73.5%	5.6%
pH > 4.0, ≤ 6.0	15.7%	8.1%
pH > 6.0	10.8%	86.3%
Acid Inhibitors Present	($n = 219$)	($n = 189$)
pH 0 to 4.0	55.3%	4.2%
pH > 4.0, ≤ 6.0	26.9%	7.9%
pH > 6.0	17.8%	87.8%

*Originally Table 3 in Metheny et al.'s (1993) report. The table was titled **Percentage Distribution of pH-Meter Readings by Tube Site, Controlling for Acid Inhibitors**.*

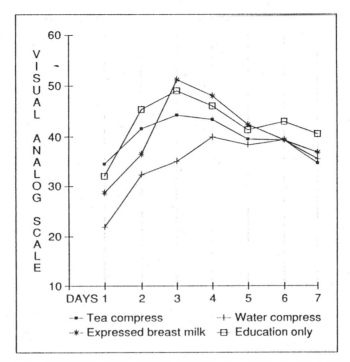

FIGURE 4–8.   EXAMPLE OF PLOTTED MEANS FOR FOUR GROUPS OVER TIME

Originally Figure 2 in Buchko et al.'s (1994) report. The figure was titled Group Comparison of Means for Pain Intensity Measured on a Visual Analog Scale for the First 7 Days Postpartum.

gories of pH values (as in Table 4–3), but in this case they did so separately for patients receiving or not receiving acid-inhibiting agents. The top panel of the table shows crosstabulations for patients who did not receive acid inhibitors, while the bottom panel crosses tube site and pH values for patients who did receive them. In this example, the three-way crosstabulation is useful in illuminating an interesting pattern: a higher percentage of patients without acid inhibitors (73.5%) than with them (55.3%) had low pH values (≤ 4.0) with the nasogastric tube site.

Descriptive crosstabulations of two variables are not usually presented in graphic form, unless there is also a time dimension. In particular, when an interval-level or ratio-level variable has been measured at multiple points in time for two or more groups, researchers sometimes display the means graphically. As an example, Buchko and a team of coresearchers (1994) compared pain intensity among four groups of breastfeeding primiparous women who had been given different comfort measures to alleviate nipple

TABLE 4–6. EXAMPLE OF A CORRELATION MATRIX

Pain Dimension	Correlations					
	1	2	3	4	5	6
1. Sensory						
2. Affective	.71					
3. Evaluative	.32	.33				
4. Miscellaneous	.61	.67	.45			
5. Total pain	.93	.85	.49	.82		
6. Pain intensity	.33	.42	.56	.34	.44	
7. Visual analog rating	.49	.51	.51	.48	.58	.68

Originally Table 4 in Neill's (1993) report. The table was titled **Correlation Between Pain Dimensions for All Subjects (N = 89).**

soreness. As shown in Figure 4–8, mean pain ratings were graphed over a 7-day period for the four groups. A table with this same information would be much less effective in communicating both group differences and the overall pattern over time.

As we have seen, correlations between two variables can be displayed graphically in a scatterplot. However, scatterplots are rarely included in research reports because correlation coefficients summarize linear relationships more succinctly and also more precisely.

Correlation coefficients are often displayed in a two-dimensional matrix format, with a list of variables along both the top row and in the left-hand column of the table. The correlation coefficients between the two sets of variables are then placed at the intersections of each column and row. Usually, the same variables are listed in both the columns and rows of the **correlation matrix,** thereby showing the correlations between all combinations of variables in a highly efficient manner. For example, Neill (1993) studied various aspects of pain within several different ethnic groups. Her report included a correlation matrix (Table 4–6) that presented the intercorrelations among seven different dimensions of pain for the entire research sample. This table lists the seven variables in the first column, and the top row designates the numbers corresponding to the variables. (Variable 7, the visual analog pain rating, does not appear twice because it would be redundant to do so.) The first (upper left) entry in the table indicates the correlation between the sensory (variable 1) and affective (variable 2) dimensions of pain ($r_{12} = .71$), and so on. This table shows that all pain measures were positively correlated. Total pain was substantially correlated with sensory pain ($r_{15} = .93$); however, the correlation between the sensory and evaluative dimensions of pain was rather modest ($r_{13} = .32$).

Tips on Preparing Tables with Bivariate Descriptive Statistics

As with any tabular presentation, it is important to construct tables of bivariate descriptive statistics so that they are clear, informative, and concise. We offer some suggestions to improve the presentation of tables displaying bivariate statistics.

- In Chapter 3 it was noted that readers can normally make comparisons more easily reading down a column than reading across a row. However, when bivariate descriptive statistics are being displayed, it may be necessary to have a format that requires crossrow comparisons. When two or more groups are being compared, the main interest is a cross-group comparison, and the groups are usually displayed along the top row. In part, this is done to economize on space; the number of groups is usually fewer than the number of categories of the second variable (for a contingency table) or the number of variables (for a table displaying group means on multiple variables). Moreover, in a contingency table, it is psychologically easier to read a table with percentages that add to 100% down a column rather than across a row, as in Table 4–3.
- Researchers vary in the level of precision shown in tables with bivariate descriptive statistics. It is usually adequate to present means and percentages to one decimal place (e.g., $M = 32.1$; 45.8%).
- Traditionally, correlation coefficients are shown in tables to two decimal places, without a zero before the decimal point (e.g., $r = .61$, $r = -.06$). Greater precision is almost always unnecessary. When the correlation coefficient is positive, the plus sign is usually omitted.
- When correlations are presented in a correlation matrix, the diagonal (i.e., the intersection of variable 1 with variable 1, variable 2 with variable 2, etc.) can be left blank, as in Table 4–6. Alternatively, the diagonal can contain dashes (—) or the values 1.00, which indicate that all variables are all perfectly correlated with themselves. The other correlations can appear either above or below the diagonal.

RESEARCH EXAMPLE

Bivariate descriptive statistics appear in many research reports. Here we briefly describe a report for a recent methodologic study.

Hagerty and Patusky (1995) conducted a study to develop and rigorously test a self-report instrument designed to measure sense of belonging in adults, the Sense of Belonging Instrument (SOBI). The SOBI is a 27-item instrument with two separate scales, SOBI-P (psychological state of sense of belonging) and SOBI-A (antecedents or precursors of sense of belonging). The reliability and validity of the instrument were tested through a series of studies with three subject groups: community college students, patients in treatment for major depression, and Roman Catholic nuns.

The researchers believed that if the SOBI were a good measure of the sense-of-belonging construct, the scores of the three groups would not be similar. They displayed the means, *SD*s, and *n*s on the SOBI-P and SOBI-A separately for the three subject groups. Group differences were especially marked on the SOBI-P; for example, the mean score for depressed patients was 43.5, compared to 63.8 for the nuns.

The researchers also examined the correlations between the SOBI scales and other measures of similar constructs—social support, loneliness, and reciprocity. Their table displaying the correlations for the three groups is reproduced here as Table 4–7. This table indicates that the SOBI-P had moderately high correlations with measures of the three other constructs in all but one case

TABLE 4–7. CORRELATIONS BETWEEN SOBI-P, SOBI-A, AND OTHER MEASURES

	SOBI-P			SOBI-A		
Measure	Students	Depressed Patients	Nuns	Students	Depressed Patients	Nuns
Social Support	.56	.42	.58	.32	.44	.26
Reciprocity	.57	.22	.59	.36	.56	.37
Loneliness	−.72	−.76	−.62	−.41	−.33	−.13

Originally Table 3 in Hagerty and Patusky's (1995) report.

(the correlation with reciprocity among depressed patients). All correlations were in the expected direction—i.e., positive correlations with social support and reciprocity and negative correlations with loneliness. Correlations for the SOBI-A tended to be much more modest in magnitude, with absolute values ranging from a low of .13 to a high of .56. The researchers concluded that the SOBI-P is a good measure of sense of belonging but that the SOBI-A requires additional development and investigation.

SUMMARY

Bivariate descriptive statistics are used to describe relationships between two variables. A **contingency table** is a two-dimensional frequency distribution that **crosstabulates** the frequencies of two nominal-level (or ordinal-level) variables. The number of **cells** in a contingency table is equal to the number of categories of the first variable multiplied by the number of categories of the second (e.g., $2 \times 3 = 6$ cells). Each cell contains information about the counts and percentages for the specified crosstabulated categories.

When one variable is nominal-level and the second variable is interval-level or higher, the relationship can be described by computing means and *SD*s for each category of the nominal-level variable (e.g., mean blood pressure for men versus women).

Correlation procedures are used to describe the magnitude and direction of **linear relationships** between two variables measured on an interval or ratio scale. Such relationships can be shown graphically on a **scatterplot,** which plots values of one variable along the X axis and simultaneously plots values of the second variable on the Y axis. If the correlation between the two variables is strong, the points on the graph will tend to cluster closely along a straight diagonal line. Lines sloping from the lower left corner to the upper right corner reflect **positive relationships**—high values on the first variable are associated with high values on the second. Lines sloping from the upper left to the lower right reflect **negative relationships**—high values on one variable are associated with low values on the other.

Researchers usually compute a **correlation coefficient** to efficiently summarize the magnitude and direction of linear relationships. Correlation coefficients range from

−1.00 for a perfect negative relationship through 0.00 for no relationship to +1.00 for a perfect positive relationship. A **perfect relationship** occurs when the values of one variable can be used to perfectly predict the values of the second. The greater the absolute value of the coefficient, the stronger is the relationship. The most widely used correlation coefficient is the **Pearson product-moment correlation,** also referred to as **Pearson's *r.***

EXERCISES

The following exercises cover concepts presented in this chapter. Exercises indicated with a dagger (†) can be checked against answers appearing in Appendix A. Additionally, Chapter 4 of the accompanying *Applications Manual* offers supplementary exercises, including ones that require computer analysis of a data set on diskette.

† 1. The following data designate whether patients in two groups (experimental and control) have complied with a medication regimen (1 = yes, 2 = no) after the experimental group participated in a special intervention designed to promote perceived mastery over health events:

Experimental:	1	2	2	1	1	1	2	1	2	1	2	1	1	1	2
Control:		2	2	1	2	2	2	1	2	1	2	2	1	1	2	2

Construct a contingency table for these data, computing both row and column percentages for each of the four cells.

† 2. The following data represent the birth weights (in ounces) of infants born to teenaged mothers versus older mothers:

Teenaged Mothers:	107	110	89	97	120
	79	119	101	109	94
Older Mothers:	121	98	118	103	109
	108	117	82	111	100

Compute the mean birth weights for the two groups, and the overall birth weight for the sample.

3. Below are values for diastolic and systolic blood pressure for 10 people:

Diastolic:	90	80	90	78	76	78	80	70	76	74
Systolic:	130	126	140	118	114	112	120	110	114	116

Construct a scatterplot that shows the relationship between the variables. Verbally describe the direction and magnitude of the relationship.

† 4. Compute the correlation coefficient (Pearson's *r*) to summarize the relationship for the blood pressure data presented in Exercise 3. How accurate was your verbal description of the scatterplot, as compared to the value of the coefficient?

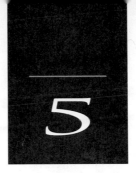

Statistical Inference

Descriptive statistics allow researchers to learn about the characteristics, behaviors, and experiences of their samples. However, most research questions are not about the attributes of the particular individuals who comprise a sample, but rather about some larger group of people.

Suppose, for example, that a researcher were testing the hypothesis that transcutaneous nerve stimulation is an effective means of reducing pain from a surgical incision during wound dressing. Fifty patients in an experimental group are given electrical stimulation before and during wound dressing, while another group of 50 patients in a control group get no special treatment. Subjects in both groups rate their pain on a visual analogue scale, where the values can range from 0 (no pain) to 100 (maximum pain). Using descriptive statistics, the researcher determines that the mean pain rating in the experimental group is 72.0, while the mean rating in the control group is 77.0. At this point, the researcher can *only* conclude that the particular 50 people in the experimental group perceived less pain than the particular 50 people in the control group. The researcher does *not* know whether the 5-point average difference in pain ratings would be observed in a new sample of subjects, and therefore cannot conclude that the transcutaneous nerve stimulation is an effective treatment for alleviating pain. Because researchers almost always want to be able to generalize beyond their sample to some broader population, they apply inferential statistics. **Inferential statistics** allow researchers to draw conclusions about population parameters, based on statistics from a sample.

We all make inferences regularly—and every inference contains some degree of uncertainty. For example, when we eat at a new restaurant and are served a dish that we do not enjoy, we may make the inference that the restaurant is mediocre. Our conclusion may be erroneous—perhaps we ordered the one dish on the menu that is below the restaurant's normal standards. We would only know for certain about the overall quality of the restaurant by tasting every dish on the menu.

Similarly, when a researcher makes inferences using inferential statistics, there is always a risk of error. Only by obtaining information from populations can researchers be sure that their conclusions are perfectly accurate. Because researchers can seldom collect data from the entire population in which they are interested, they use a statistical framework that allows them to determine how likely it is that the conclusions based on sample data are valid. This framework uses the **laws of probability.**

FUNDAMENTALS OF PROBABILITY

In the hypothetical study to test the effectiveness of the transcutaneous nerve treatment for alleviating pain, there are two mutually exclusive possibilities:

H_0: The experimental treatment is *not* effective in reducing pain.
H_1: The experimental treatment *is* effective in reducing pain.

The first possibility is what is referred to as the **null hypothesis.** The null hypothesis (often symbolized in statistics books as H_0) states that there is no relationship between the independent variable (the transcutaneous nerve treatment) and the dependent variable (pain). The **alternative hypothesis** (H_1) is the actual **research hypothesis,** which states the expectation that there *is* a relationship between the independent and dependent variables. In the population (all surgical patients), only one of these possibilities is correct.

The researcher in this example observed a 5-point average difference in pain ratings between the experimental and control groups. Does this difference allow the researcher to reject the null hypothesis? By using inferential statistics, the researcher would be able to determine *how probable it is that the null hypothesis is false.*

Probability is a very complex topic, with many different rules for different situations. In this section we present only an overview of probability theory, to establish a basis for understanding the fundamental principles of statistical inference.[1]

Probability of an Event

When we flip a normal, two-sided coin, one of two possible outcomes can occur: we can obtain a head, or we can obtain a tail. The probability (p) of some event, such as obtaining a head on a coin toss, can be defined as the following ratio:

---

[1]A fuller explication of probability is presented in several statistical textbooks, such as those by Jaccard and Becker (1990), Hays (1988), and McCall (1990).

$$p(\text{event}) = \frac{\text{number of ways the specified event can occur}}{\text{total number of possible events}}$$

Thus, in the coin toss example, we can use this ratio to determine the probability that heads will come up:

$$p(\text{heads}) = \frac{1 \text{ head}}{2 \text{ possible events (heads or tails)}} = \frac{1}{2}$$

Proportions are often used to express probabilities, so we can say that the probability of heads (or tails) is .50. (In everyday parlance, we often say that there is a 50-50 chance of having the coin come up heads.) On a six-sided die, the probability of rolling, say, a 3 is 1/6, or .17. In a normal, shuffled deck of 52 cards, the probability of randomly drawing the queen of spades is 1/52, or .02. A probability always ranges from 0 (completely impossible) to 1.00 (completely certain).

The probability of an event can also be interpreted with a "long-run" perspective. For example, in 100,000 coin tosses, we would expect 50,000 heads. Over the long run, with a large enough number of trials, the proportion of heads should be .50.

Some readers may have noticed that probability is similar in form to relative frequencies, as discussed in Chapter 2. For example, in the frequency distribution of patients' marital status shown in Table 2–3, the relative frequency of single patients was:

$$\frac{\text{number of times the event "single" occurred}}{\text{number of possible occurrences of marital status}} = \frac{55}{250}$$

In other words, the relative frequency of single patients is .22. Thus, the probability of randomly selecting a given value from a known distribution equals the relative frequency of that value. In this example, the probability of randomly selecting a single person from the sample of 250 patients is .22.

Probability of Consecutive Events

Another situation in which probability can be used is for predicting the probability of consecutive events. For example, we might be interested in determining the probability of obtaining heads twice in a row on two consecutive, independent coin tosses. The **multiplicative law** in probability provides a formula for this situation:

$$p(\text{A and then B}) = p(\text{A}) \times p(\text{B})$$

where A is the first independent event
      B is the second independent event

TABLE 5–1. PROBABILITIES IN COIN TOSS EXAMPLE

Toss No.	Possible Outcomes and Probabilities				Total Probability
1	H = .500	T = .500			1.000
2	HH = .250	HT = .250	TH = .250	TT = .250	1.000
3	HHH = .125				
4	HHHH = .063				
5	HHHHH = .031				
6	HHHHHH = .016				
7	HHHHHHH = .008				
8	HHHHHHHH = .004				
9	HHHHHHHHH = .002				
10	HHHHHHHHHH = .001				

H = heads
T = tails

In the coin toss example, the probability of two consecutive heads is:

p(heads and then heads) = p(heads) $\times$ p(heads)
p(heads and then heads) = .50 $\times$ .50 = .25

In the same fashion, the probability of three consecutive heads is:

p(three consecutive heads) = p(heads) $\times$ p(heads) $\times$ p(heads)
p(three consecutive heads) = .50 $\times$ .50 $\times$ .50 = .125

Knowing this formula, we could construct a table that shows the probability for all possible outcomes in consecutive coin tosses. Table 5–1 presents a partial listing of outcomes, focusing primarily on the probability of obtaining consecutive heads. In the first toss, the probability of heads (H) and tails (T) is, in each case, .50. The last column shows that the probability of obtaining *either* heads or tails is 1.00—that is, it is completely certain that one of these outcomes will occur. In the second toss, the probability of two consecutive heads (HH) is .250, as is the probability of heads then tails (HT), tails then heads (TH), or two tails (TT). From the third toss on, the table shows only the probabilities for consecutive heads. The probability of five consecutive heads, for example, is .031. Fewer than five times out of 100 would we expect to obtain five heads in a row.

We can use this table to test the hypothesis that a coin is biased (for example, that it has two heads, or is weighted to turn up heads more often than tails). Our hypotheses may be stated formally as follows:

H_0: The coin is fair.
H_1: The coin is biased.

To test the hypothesis that the coin is biased, we obtain some data by tossing the coin 10 times. Let us assume that we obtained 10 heads. We can now consult Table 5–1 to learn how probable this outcome is. The table indicates that the probability of getting 10 consecutive heads is .001. That is, by chance alone we would obtain 10 heads on 10 consecutive tosses only once in 1000 times. We might then decide to reject the null hypothesis, concluding that there is a high probability that the coin is biased.

This example is very similar to the procedures used in statistical inference. The researcher uses probability tables to assess whether an observed outcome (e.g., a 5-point difference in average pain ratings) is likely to have occurred by chance alone, or whether the outcome probably reflects a true outcome that would be observed with other samples from the same population. Based on the information in the probability tables, the researcher makes a decision to accept or reject the null hypothesis.

Probability as an Area

As indicated in a previous section, probability is similar in form to relative frequencies. And, just as relative frequencies can be graphed in histograms or frequency polygons, so too can probabilities be graphed in **probability distributions.** For example, suppose we graphed the probability of obtaining 1, 2, 3, 4, 5, and 6 dots on the roll of a single die. For each number, the probability would be 1/6, or .167. Figure 5–1 presents a histogram of the probability of obtaining 1 to 6 dots on a single roll of one die.

The area within the histogram is exactly 1.0 (i.e., 6 $\times$ .167), the total of all the probabilities that a die will yield a number between 1 and 6. From this distribution, then, we can readily determine various probabilities by considering the area under the his-

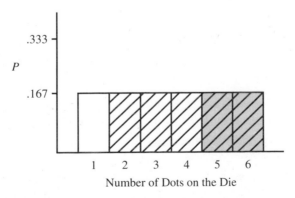

FIGURE 5–1.   PROBABILITY DISTRIBUTION OF DOTS IN THE ROLL OF ONE DIE

togram. For example, the probability of rolling a 5 *or* a 6 (shown as the shaded area on Figure 5–1) is .333 (2/6). The probability of obtaining a number greater than 1 on a single roll (the hatched area) is .833 (5/6).

Probability distributions can also be constructed for continuous variables, and are sometimes referred to as **probability density functions.** Suppose, for example, that we collected data on the heights of a population of 1000 sixth grade children and constructed a frequency polygon, such as the one in Figure 5–2. The mean of this distribution of heights is 60.0 inches, and the *SD* is 5.0 inches. What is the probability that a randomly selected student from this population would be, say, 65 inches tall or taller? The shaded area in the right tail of this figure, corresponding to heights equal to or greater than 65 inches, is approximately 16% of the total area under the curve in this distribution. The proportion of sixth grade students who are 65 inches or taller can be regarded as the probability that one student selected at random from this population of 1000 children will be at least 65 inches tall. In other words, $p = .16$ in this example.

How did we determine that heights of 65 inches or greater account for 16% of the distribution? When data values are normally distributed (or approximately so), the area under a curve can be determined by converting raw scores to standard scores and consulting an appropriate table. Using the formulas presented in Chapter 3, we can calculate the standard scores (which are referred to as *z* scores when the data are normally distributed) as:

$$z = \frac{X - \overline{X}}{SD} = \frac{65.0 - 60.0}{5.0} = \frac{5.0}{5.0} = 1.0$$

Table B–1 in Appendix B presents information on the area in a normal distribution for various *z* scores.[2] In this example, we would first find the *z* score of 1.00 in column 1 of this table. Then, moving across that row, column 2 tells us that the proportion of values equal to or greater than a *z* of 1.00 is .159 (i.e., roughly 16% of the area). Column 3 tells us that the proportion of values between a *z* of 0.0 and 1.0 (here, between 60 and 65 inches tall) is .341. We could use Table B–1 to determine the probability of randomly selecting a student between any two height intervals in the distribution.

SAMPLING DISTRIBUTIONS

Suppose that we were unable to measure the height of all 1000 sixth grade students in our hypothetical population, but that instead we had to rely on data from a sample. If we randomly selected 25 children and measured their height, would the obtained sample

---

[2]Table B–1 is an abbreviated table that shows only a selected number of *z* score values. For *z* scores falling between values shown in this table (e.g., a *z* of .13), interpolation can be used as a rough estimate, or a fuller table in other statistics textbooks can be consulted, such as the one presented in Jaccard and Becker (1990).

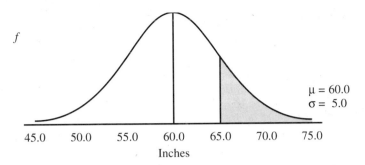

f

μ = 60.0
σ = 5.0

45.0   50.0   55.0   60.0   65.0   70.0   75.0

Inches

FIGURE 5–2. HYPOTHETICAL DISTRIBUTION OF HEIGHTS FOR A POPULATION OF SIXTH GRADERS

mean be exactly 60.0 inches? We *might* by chance obtain a mean of 60.0, but it would also be possible to obtain such means as 60.6, or 59.8, or 61.2. A sample statistic is often unequal to the value of the corresponding population parameter because of **sampling error.**

Sampling error reflects the tendency for statistics to fluctuate from one sample to another. The amount of sampling error is the difference between the obtained sample value and the population parameter. A researcher does not, of course, know the amount of sampling error; if the population parameter were known, there would be no need to draw a sample. However, inferential statistics allow researchers to estimate how close to the population value the calculated statistic is likely to be. The concept of **sampling distributions,** which are actually probability distributions, is central to estimates of sampling error.

Characteristics of Sampling Distributions

For the sake of understanding sampling distributions, we must imagine an activity that would never actually occur in practice. Suppose that we randomly selected 25 sixth graders from the population of 1000 students, and calculated the mean height. Now consider replacing the 25 students, drawing another sample of 25 children, and calculating another mean. Table 5–2 shows the means and the amount of sampling error (that is, the sample mean minus the population mean of 60.0) for 20 such samples. We can see that the sampling error ranges from very small amounts (0.1 inch) to much larger amounts (2.1 inches). Now suppose we repeated the process of selecting new samples of 25 students and calculating their mean height over and over again for an infinite number of times. If we did this and treated each sample mean as a new "data point," we could plot these sample means in a frequency polygon. The hypothetical distribution, shown in Figure 5–3, is referred to as a sampling distribution of the mean. A **sampling distribution of the mean** is a theoretical probability distribution of the means of an infinite

TABLE 5–2. HYPOTHETICAL SAMPLE MEANS OF CHILDREN'S HEIGHTS IN 20 RANDOM SAMPLES OF 25 STUDENTS

Sample Mean	Sampling Error	Sample Mean	Sampling Error
$\overline{X}$	$\overline{X} - \mu$	$\overline{X}$	$\overline{X} - \mu$
61.0	1.0	59.9	−0.1
59.4	−0.6	60.4	0.4
58.9	−1.1	61.1	1.1
62.1	2.1	59.7	−0.3
60.3	0.3	60.2	0.2
59.8	−0.2	58.0	−2.0
60.1	0.1	61.7	1.7
59.6	−0.4	59.6	−0.4
58.8	−1.2	59.1	−0.9
60.9	0.9	59.4	−0.6

number of samples of a given size from a population. There is a different sampling distribution for every sample size. For example, the sampling distribution of the mean for samples of 25 students is different from the sampling distribution of the mean for samples of 50 students from the same population.

Sampling distributions are theoretical because, in practice, no one draws an infinite number of samples from a population. Their characteristics can be modeled mathematically, however, and have been defined by a formulation known as the **central limit theorem.** This theorem stipulates that the mean of the sampling distribution is identical to the population mean of raw scores. In other words, if we calculated the mean heights for an infinite number of samples of 25 students drawn from the population of 1000 sixth graders, the average of all the sample means would be exactly 60.0, as shown in

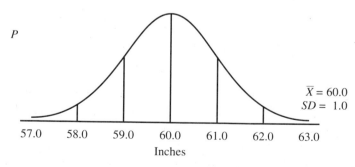

FIGURE 5–3.   SAMPLING DISTRIBUTION OF HEIGHTS FOR SAMPLES OF 25 SIXTH GRADERS

Figure 5–3. Moreover, the average sampling error—the mean of the $(\overline{X} - \mu)$s—would always equal 0. We can see that in Table 5–2, some of the sample means overestimated the population mean, and others underestimated it. With an infinite number of samples, the overestimates and underestimates would cancel each other out.

Another feature of sampling distributions is that if the raw scores in the population are normally distributed, the sampling distribution of the mean will also be normal. Moreover, even if the population distribution of raw scores is *not* normal, the sampling distribution will increasingly approach a normal distribution as the size of the sample on which it is based gets larger. Because sampling distributions usually approximate a normal distribution, we can make probability statements about the likelihood of obtaining various sample means based on information about the area under the curve. However, before we can do so, we need to determine the standard deviation of the sampling distribution.

By comparing the distribution of population values of actual heights in Figure 5–2 with the sampling distribution in Figure 5–3, we can readily see the similarities: both are normal distributions and both have a mean of 60.0. However, the distribution of sample means is much less widely spread out than the distribution of original heights. Logically, this makes sense. It would be fairly unlikely, for example, to select at random a single sixth grader who is 70.0 inches tall or taller. (In fact, Table B–1 informs us that for a z of 2.0—i.e., a score that is 2 *SD* above the mean—p would equal .023). But drawing a random sample of 25 students whose *average* height was 70.0 inches or greater would be *much* less likely, because that would require selecting a large number of "improbable" (exceptionally tall) cases. Thus, it is clear that the sample *SD* cannot be used as an estimator of the *SD* of the sampling distribution.

Standard Error of the Mean

The standard deviation of a sampling distribution of the mean has a special name: the **standard error of the mean** *(SEM)*. The term contains the word "error" because the various sample means that compose the distribution contain some error as estimates of the population mean—i.e., sampling error. The term also contains the word "standard," which signifies that the standard error of the mean is an index of the average amount of error for all possible sample means. The smaller the *SEM,* the more accurate are the sample means as estimates of the population value. The larger the *SEM,* the higher is the probability that the sample mean will yield a poor estimate of the population mean.

Since sampling distributions are usually approximately normal, we can use the *SEM* to estimate the probability of obtaining a sample mean within a specified range. Figure 5–3 shows that the *SEM* for the sampling distribution of sample means for the heights of 25 sixth graders is 1.0. As indicated in Chapter 3, 95% of the values in a normal distribution lie within about ± 2 *SD*s of the mean. Thus, we can estimate that the probability is .95 that the mean height of a sample of 25 students will lie between 58.0

and 62.0 inches. In other words, about 95% of all the sample means randomly selected from the population would be within 2 inches of the true parameter, given a sample of 25 students.[3] Only 2½% of the sample means would be less than 58.0 and only 2½% would be greater than 62.0 inches—a total of 5% of the area of the sampling distribution, located in the two tails.

With information about the *SEM,* then, researchers can interpret a sample mean relative to the population mean. However, since researchers do not actually construct sampling distributions, how can the *SEM* be calculated? How, for example, did we determine that the *SEM* for the distribution in Figure 5–3 is 1.0? Fortunately, statisticians have developed a formula that allows researchers to estimate the *actual SEM* (symbolized as $\sigma_{\bar{x}}$) based on data from a single sample:

$$s_{\bar{x}} = \frac{SD}{\sqrt{N}}$$

where $s_{\bar{x}}$ = estimated standard error of the mean
SD = standard deviation of the sample
N = number of cases in the sample

In our current example, suppose that the *SD* for our sample of 25 students is 5.0. We can use this formula to calculate the following estimate of the *SEM:*

$$s_{\bar{x}} = \frac{5.0}{\sqrt{25}} = 1.0$$

Thus, the estimated standard deviation of the sampling distribution is 1.0.

The smaller the *SEM,* the greater the confidence that researchers have in their estimates of the population value. From the formula for the *SEM,* it can be seen that there is a way for researchers to decrease the value of the *SEM* and thus improve the accuracy of their estimates of the population mean: they need only increase the size of their sample. In our present example, suppose that we drew a sample of 100 sixth graders rather than 25. With a sample of 100 students and the same *SD* of 5.0, the estimated *SEM* would be:

$$s_{\bar{x}} = \frac{5.0}{\sqrt{100}} = 0.50$$

---

[3]We can use Table B–1 to estimate the probability for any range of sample means. For example, suppose we wanted to determine the probability of selecting a sample with a mean within one-half a standard deviation of the population mean. Remember that the z scores correspond to *SD* units, so that one-half a standard deviation unit from the mean is equivalent to a z of .50. With a z of .50, column 3 of Table B–1 tells us that the area between the mean and this z value is .192. Multiplying by 2 to get the area below and above the mean, the estimated *P* of selecting a sample of 25 students whose mean height is within ±.5 *SD* of the population mean—i.e., between 59.5 and 60.5 inches—is (.192 × 2) or .384.

As the sample increases, there is a higher probability that the sample mean will be close to the value of the population mean. This is because having a large number of cases promotes the likelihood that extreme cases (very short children and very tall ones) will cancel each other out.

The formula for the *SEM* also indicates that the greater the homogeneity of the population (i.e., the smaller the *SD*), the smaller is the standard error of the mean. If the *SD* of the sample had been 2.5 inches rather than 5.0 inches, the estimated *SEM* would be:

$$s_{\bar{x}} = \frac{2.5}{\sqrt{100}} = 0.25$$

Thus, small sample sizes and a heterogeneous population lead to large *SEM*s, and conversely large sample sizes and a homogeneous population increase the likelihood that sampling errors will be small. Researchers cannot control population heterogeneity, but they can increase the accuracy of their inferences by using large samples.

ESTIMATION OF PARAMETERS

Researchers use inferential statistics to address two broad goals. One goal is to estimate the value of population parameters. In the example we have been discussing, we were trying to estimate the mean height of the population of 1000 sixth graders by measuring a sample of 25 students. A second goal is to test hypotheses. Hypothesis testing is far more common than parameter estimation and will be elaborated upon in a subsequent section. In both cases, the overall purpose is the same: to use data from a sample to draw inferences about populations, and in both cases the concepts of sampling distributions and standard errors are central features.

Estimation procedures are used when the researcher has no a priori hypothesis about the value of a parameter and wishes to estimate that value through sample statistics. In most cases, estimation involves estimating the population mean, but the procedures can be adapted to apply to other parameters.

Point Estimation

Estimates can be either point estimates or interval estimates. **Point estimation** involves the calculation of a single value to estimate the parameter. For example, if we drew a sample of 25 students and calculated the mean height to be 61.0 inches (the first sample mean in Table 5–2), this would represent our point estimate of the population mean.

The problem with point estimates is that they offer no context for interpreting their accuracy. How much confidence can the researcher place in the value of 61.0 as an estimate of the parameter? A point estimate gives no information regarding the probability that it is correct or close to the population value.

Interval Estimation

An alternative to point estimation is to estimate a range of values that has a high probability of containing the population value. For example, it is clearly more likely that the
population mean lies between 59.0 and 63.0 than that it is *exactly* the calculated sample
mean of 61.0. This is referred to as **interval estimation** because the estimate is an interval of values, not a single value.

When researchers use interval estimation, they construct a **confidence interval**
(sometimes abbreviated *CI*), and the values at the boundaries of the interval are the **confidence limits.** The degree of confidence that the researcher expresses in the interval is
based on a probability that the interval contains the population parameter. For example,
the researcher might say that the probability is .95 that the population mean lies between
59.0 and 63.0.

Probability distributions such as those we discussed earlier are used to construct
confidence intervals, using the *SEM* as the basis for establishing the confidence limits.
Let us assume for the moment that we know that the true value of the standard error of the
mean ($\sigma_{\bar{x}}$) in this example is 1.0, and that we also know that the heights in the population
of 1000 students are normally distributed. We can then use the normal distribution to construct a confidence interval. By convention, researchers most often calculate a 95% confidence interval. As noted earlier, 95% of the scores in a normal distribution lie within
about ± 2 *SD*s from the mean. More precisely, 95% of the scores lie within 1.960 *SD*s
above and below the mean. We can now build a 95% *CI* by using the following formula:

$$95\% \; CI = \bar{X} \pm (1.96 \times \sigma_{\bar{x}})$$

where $\bar{X}$ = value of the sample mean
$\quad \sigma_{\bar{x}}$ = actual *SEM* of the sampling distribution

This statement indicates that the researcher is 95% confident that the population
mean lies between the confidence limits, and that these limits are equal to 1.960 times
the true standard error, above and below the sample mean. In the present example, the
confidence limits would be:

$$95\% \; CI = 61.0 \pm (1.96 \times 1.0)$$
$$95\% \; CI = 61.0 \pm 1.96$$
$$95\% \; CI = 59.04 \leq \mu \leq 62.96$$

The last statement stipulates that the confidence is 95% (i.e., the probability is .95)
that the population mean (μ) is greater than 59.04 but less than 62.96. We can also interpret this in terms of long-range performance: out of 100 sample means based on a sample
of 25 students, 95% of such confidence intervals would contain the population mean.

The researcher can control the risk of being wrong by establishing different **confidence levels.** Although the 95% confidence level is most widely used, the researcher

sometimes wants to take less of a risk of making an error. With a 95% confidence level, there is a 5% risk of an error. With a 99% confidence level, there is only 1 chance in 100 of making an error. However, there is a trade-off: the price for lower risk is a loss of precision—that is, the confidence interval is wider. In a normal distribution, 99% of the scores lie within 2.575 *SD*s of the mean. Thus, the formula for a 99% *CI* is:

$$99\% \ CI = \overline{X} \pm (2.58 \times \sigma_{\bar{x}})$$

In the present example, the 99% confidence interval would be:

$$99\% \ CI = 61.0 \pm (2.58 \times 1.0)$$
$$99\% \ CI = 61.0 \pm 2.58$$
$$99\% \ CI = 58.42 \le \mu \le 63.58$$

In using a 99% confidence interval, the researcher reduces the risk that the interval will fail to contain the population mean, but the interval is larger. With the 95% interval, the range between the confidence limits was just under 4 inches. With a 99% confidence interval, the range of possible values for the population mean is more than 5 inches, which is about a 30% decrease in precision. In most research situations, a 95% confidence interval is adequate, but when important decisions about individual human beings are being made, a 99% confidence interval—and perhaps an even more stringent criterion, such as a 99.9% confidence interval—may be advisable.

Interval Estimation and the *t* Distribution

In the preceding example, we stipulated an assumption that generally does not hold true in real-world situations: we assumed we knew that the true *SEM* ($\sigma_{\bar{x}}$) for the sampling distribution was 1.0. This assumption made it possible for us to use the values from the normal distribution (1.96 for the 95% confidence interval) in calculating the confidence limits. This is because when $\sigma_{\bar{x}}$ is known and we calculate a *z* score for the sample mean, we are calculating the *exact* number of *SEM*s that the sample mean is from the mean of the sampling distribution (which is always equal to μ, the population mean). When we use an estimated *SEM* ($s_{\bar{x}}$), we need a different distribution.

In most cases, especially if the sample size is large, the normal curve will provide a reasonably good approximation. In the present example, however, the sample size of 25 is not particularly large. And, in any event, scientists usually strive for precision rather than approximation. Thus, when the true *SEM* is not known but rather is estimated from sample data—as will almost always be the case—a different theoretical distribution, known as the *t* **distribution,**[4] should be used to compute confidence intervals.

---

[4]The *t* distribution is a theoretical distribution that was developed by W. S. Gossett, who wrote under the name of Student. For this reason, the distribution is sometimes referred to as **Student's *t* distribution.**

In standard form, the *t* distribution is very similar to a normal distribution; it is bell-shaped and symmetrical, and has a mean of 0.0. However, the exact shape of the *t* distribution is influenced by the number of cases in the sample. There is a different *t* distribution for every sample size. Figure 5–4 shows that when $N = 5$, the shapes of the *t* and the normal distributions differ: the tails of the *t* distribution are fatter, for example, which means that you have to go out farther into the tails to capture 95% of the area. This, in turn, implies that the confidence interval developed on the basis of the *t* distribution will be wider. Figure 5–4 also shows that when the sample size is 30 (or larger), the normal and *t* distributions are quite similar.

Statisticians have developed tables that tell us the area under the *t* distribution for different sample sizes and probability levels. Such a table is presented in Table B–2 of Appendix B. To use this table, you must first select a confidence (probability) level. In this table, the probabilities are specified as *the probability of making an error.* Thus, values for the 95% confidence level are shown in the third column, under the heading .05. Values for the 99% confidence level are presented in the fifth column, under the heading .01. To use the table for the *t* distribution, we must enter at the appropriate row. Each row designates a number of **degrees of freedom** (labeled with the abbreviation *df* in the first column of the table). We will explain the concept of degrees of freedom later in this chapter. Here, it is important only to know that the number of degrees of freedom is equal to the sample size, minus 1.

Now we are in a position to construct the appropriate confidence interval for the example of 25 sixth grade students whose mean height is 61.0 inches. The formula for the confidence intervals when the true *SEM* is estimated from sample data is:

$$95\% \ CI = \overline{X} \pm (t \times s_{\bar{x}})$$

where $\overline{X}$ = value of the sample mean
   t = tabled *t* value at .05 level for $df = N - 1$
   $s_{\bar{x}}$ = calculated *SEM* for the sample data

In our example, the calculated value of $s_{\bar{x}}$ is 1.0, and Table B–2 tells us that the value of *t* for the 95% confidence interval with 24 degrees of freedom $(25 - 1)$ is 2.06. Thus,

$$95\% \ CI = 61.0 \pm (2.06 \times 1.0)$$
$$95\% \ CI = 61.0 \pm 2.06$$
$$95\% \ CI = 58.94 \leq \mu \leq 63.06$$

We can be 95% confident that the mean height of our population of sixth grade students is between about 58.9 and 63.1. If we return to the sample means presented in Table 5–2, we see that, in fact, only 1 of the 20 sample means would *not* have a 95% confidence interval that captures the population mean of 60.0. The confidence limits for the

$N = 5$ $N = 30$

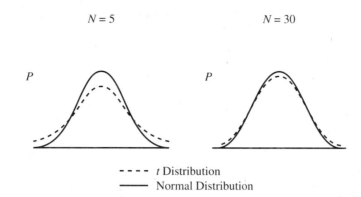

- - - - *t* Distribution
———— Normal Distribution

FIGURE 5–4. COMPARISON OF THE NORMAL AND *t* DISTRIBUTIONS WITH *N* = 5 AND *N* = 30

sample mean of 62.1 (the fourth mean in the first column) would be 60.04 and 64.16. Researchers generally accept the risk that their confidence intervals do not include the population mean 5% of the time.

HYPOTHESIS TESTING

Hypothesis testing is a more common application of inferential statistics than estimation. Hypothesis testing involves using sampling distributions and the laws of probability to make an objective decision. The decision concerns whether to accept or reject the null hypothesis. Although we have already seen a few examples of null hypotheses in this chapter, we need to elaborate on this concept because of its importance in hypothesis testing.

The Null Hypothesis

Researchers usually have one or more research hypotheses that indicate an expected relationship between variables. The predicted relationship can be expressed verbally in a number of ways. The following are all examples of research hypotheses that predict a relationship between an independent and a dependent variable:

1. Patients cared for by primary nurses will be *more* satisfied with their nursing care *than* patients cared for by team nurses.
2. Length of time in labor will be *different* for women in an upright position *from* that for women in a recumbent position.
3. Catecholamine production (measured by vanillymandelic acid excretion) is *related to* a patient's level of stress.

The italicized phrases in these hypotheses (more than, different from, related to) embody the nature of the predicted relationship. These are the types of hypothesis that researchers typically seek to support with their data. However, a research hypothesis cannot be tested directly. It is the null hypothesis, which states the *absence* of a relationship, that is subjected to statistical testing. For instance, in the third example the researcher would test the null hypothesis that catecholamine production is *un*related to patients' stress levels.

The procedures used to test hypotheses are based on rules of negative inference. *Hypothesis testing begins with the assumption that the null hypothesis is true.* For example, in the coin toss example discussed earlier in this chapter, we assumed that the coin was fair. We then collected data through coin tosses and used the results to inform our decision about the likelihood that this assumption was valid. We concluded, after obtaining 10 heads in a row, that the coin was probably biased and therefore rejected the null hypothesis.

The null hypothesis is analogous to the basic assumption of innocence in the American system of criminal justice; just as an accused criminal is assumed to be innocent until proven guilty, so too in research situations variables are assumed to be "innocent" of any relationship until there is sufficient evidence to the contrary. In the justice system, the null and alternative hypotheses may be formally stated as follows:

H_0: The accused is innocent of committing the crime.
H_1: The accused is guilty of committing the crime.

In criminal proceedings, the concept of *reasonable doubt* is an important one, and again there is a parallel in statistical inference. When a judge instructs a jury to find a defendant innocent if there is a reasonable doubt that he or she did not commit the crime, the judge is, in effect, asking the jurors to decide if $p = 1.0$ that the accused is guilty. In our justice system, however, there is no objective cutoff point for determining reasonable doubt. In hypothesis testing, researchers establish a fixed probability as their criterion for "guilt" and "innocence."

Another important difference between hypothesis testing and the justice system concerns the language associated with the decisions. Lawyers and judges often talk about requiring *proof* that the accused is guilty. Researchers, however, never use the term proof, unless they are in a position to obtain data from a population—in which case, inferential statistics would not be needed. The rejection of a null hypothesis does not constitute proof that the research hypothesis is valid; it constitutes evidence that the null hypothesis is *probably* incorrect. There remains a possibility that the null is true even though it is rejected.

Type I and Type II Errors

Because statistical inference is based on data that are incomplete, there is always a risk of error. Figure 5–5 summarizes the four possible outcomes of statistical decision-making. When the null hypothesis is true (i.e., there is no relationship between the inde-

The real situation is that H_0 is:

		True	False
	True (Accepts H_0)	Correct decision Probability = $1 - \alpha$	Type II error Probability = β
The researcher decides that H_0 is:	False (Rejects H_0)	Type I error Probability = α	Correct decision Probability = $1 - \beta$

FIGURE 5–5.   THE FOUR OUTCOMES OF STATISTICAL DECISION MAKING

pendent and dependent variables in the population) and the researcher concludes that the null is true, the correct decision has been made, as depicted in the upper left box of the figure. Similarly, when the null hypothesis is really false and the researcher decides to reject the null (lower right box), the correct decision again is made.

The figure shows that there are two types of errors that the researcher can commit. The first is the incorrect rejection of a true null hypothesis. For example, the null may state the absence of a relationship between patient satisfaction and type of nursing care (primary versus team). If the researcher incorrectly rejects this null hypothesis, erroneously concluding on the basis of sample data that patient satisfaction is higher with, say, primary nursing, then a **Type I error** would have been committed.

The researcher can also commit an error by incorrectly accepting a false null hypothesis. For example, if the researcher concludes that patients are equally satisfied with both types of nursing care, when in fact patient satisfaction in the population is really higher with one type, then a **Type II error** would have been committed.

Controlling the Risk of Errors

Obviously, the researcher does not realize when a Type I or Type II error has been committed. Only by knowing the population values would the researcher be able to definitively conclude that the null hypothesis is true or false.

However, the researcher can control the probability of committing an error. Type I errors can be controlled through the **level of significance,** which is the probability level established by the researcher as the accepted risk of making a Type I error. Inferential statistics always involve a comparison of a computed statistic against the probability in a theoretical distribution. The level of significance, symbolized as **α (alpha),** indicates the size of the area in the theoretical probability distribution that corresponds to the rejection of the null hypothesis.

The most widely accepted standard for the level of significance is the .05 level. This corresponds to the 95% confidence level we discussed in the previous section. With a .05 significance level, we are accepting the risk that out of 100 samples, we would reject a true null five times. Conversely, with $\alpha = .05$, the probability is .95 $(1 - \alpha)$ that a true null hypothesis will be accepted. These probabilities, shown in the two left-hand boxes in Figure 5–5, always total 1.0.

Researchers sometimes establish a stricter level of significance. With an α of .01, the risk is that in only 1 out of 100 samples would we erroneously reject a true null hypothesis. And with the stringent significance level of .001, the risk is even lower: in only 1 out of 1000 samples would we be in error by rejecting the null hypothesis. In our example of tossing the coin to test for bias, we could have used this very conservative .001 criterion and still rejected the null hypothesis that the coin was fair.

Researchers can also exert some control over Type II errors, but the situation with Type II errors is much more complex. The probability of committing a Type II error is symbolized as β **(beta);** the probability of correctly rejecting the null hypothesis when it is false $(1 - \beta)$ is referred to as the **power** of the statistical test. The risk of a Type II error is affected by many factors, such as sample size, the research design, the strength of the underlying relationship between variables, and the type of statistical test being used. Moreover, the probability of committing a Type II error increases as the risk of making a Type I error decreases. In other words, when researchers establish a very strict criterion for α, they increase the probability of committing a Type II error.

Although we will say more about power and the control of Type II errors in subsequent chapters, we note here that many researchers accept a very high risk of erroneously accepting a false null hypothesis. Polit and Sherman (1990) found, for example, that the majority of the nursing studies they examined had a β much greater than .20. With β equal to .20, there is a 1 in 5 probability that a researcher will fail to reject a null hypothesis that is false. The most straightforward method of reducing the risk of a Type II error is to increase the size of the sample: the larger the sample, the more powerful the statistical test will be.

Establishing Probable and Improbable Results

By establishing the significance level, the researcher is formulating a decision rule. The decision is to reject the null hypothesis if the statistic being tested falls at or beyond a **critical region** on the theoretical distribution, and to accept the null hypothesis otherwise. The decision rule should be established before the data are analyzed, so that the decision to reject or accept the null hypothesis is not influenced by subjective biases.

The critical region, established by the significance level, indicates what is improbable for a null hypothesis. An example should help to clarify this process. Suppose that we were interested in determining whether people with a fertility problem had positive or negative attitudes toward in vitro fertilization (IVF). We might ask a sample of 100 infertility patients to express their attitude toward IVF on a rating scale that ranged from 0 (extremely negative) to 10 (extremely positive). Our goal in this example is to determine whether the mean attitude for the population of infertility patients is different from 5.0, the score on the rating scale that represents a neutral feeling. The null and alternative hypotheses are:

$H_0: \mu = 5.0$
$H_1: \mu \neq 5.0$

Suppose the data from the sample of 100 patients result in a mean rating of 5.50 with an *SD* of 2.0. This mean is consistent with the alternative hypothesis (H_1), but can we automatically reject the null hypothesis? Because of sampling error, we need to test for the possibility that the mean of 5.5 occurred simply by chance, and not because the population generally has a positive attitude toward IVF.

Since hypothesis testing involves an assumption that the null hypothesis is true, we can construct a sampling distribution that assumes that the population mean is 5.0. Next, we need to estimate the standard deviation of the sampling distribution—the *SEM*—using the sample *SD:*

$$s_{\bar{x}} = \frac{2.0}{\sqrt{100}} = \frac{2.0}{10} = 0.2$$

The resulting sampling distribution is presented in Figure 5–6. Because we are using the estimated *SEM* rather than the actual *SEM,* the *t* distribution rather than the nor-

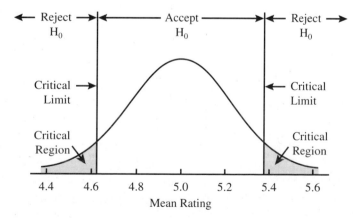

FIGURE 5–6.   CRITICAL REGIONS IN THE SAMPLING DISTRIBUTION FOR ATTITUDES TOWARD IVF EXAMPLE

mal distribution is appropriate for establishing the critical regions. In Table B–2, we find that for a significance level of .05 and $df = 99$ $(100 - 1)$, the t value is approximately 1.99. The limit of what is "probable" if the null hypothesis were correct is, thus, just under 2 standard deviations (1.99 SDs) on the sampling distribution. The boundaries of the critical region for rejecting the null hypothesis are established by multiplying the estimated SEM by the t value—i.e., $1.99 \times .2 = .398$. As shown in Figure 5–6, the limits of what is probable if the null hypothesis were true are the points corresponding to .398 above and below the hypothesized population mean of 5.0. If our sample mean falls inside the critical limits (i.e., between 4.602 and 5.398), we would conclude that the null hypothesis has a 95% probability of being true. However, our sample mean of 5.5 is beyond the critical limit—it lies in the shaded region on the distribution that indicates what is "improbable" if the null hypothesis were true. We can now accept the alternative hypothesis that patients are not, on average, neutral in their attitudes toward IVF.

Test Statistics

In practice, researchers do not actually construct a sampling distribution and draw the critical region on the distribution. Rather, they compute a **test statistic,** using an appropriate formula, and then compare the value of the test statistic to a value in the relevant table. The selection of an appropriate test statistic is made on the basis of such factors as the nature of the hypothesis and the level of measurement of the variables.

In subsequent chapters, we describe numerous test statistics that can be used to test various types of hypotheses. Here, we illustrate the procedure of using test statistics by pursuing the example of patients' attitudes toward IVF. We can test the hypotheses using the **one-sample t-test.** For this test statistic, the formula is as follows:

$$t = \frac{\overline{X} - \mu}{s_{\overline{x}}}$$

where $\overline{X}$ = value of sample mean
μ = hypothesized value of population mean
$s_{\overline{x}}$ = estimated SEM

The obtained value of t resulting from this formula is then compared to the values in Table B–2 for the designated significance level and degrees of freedom. If the absolute value[5] of the computed t statistic is greater than the tabled value, then the null hypothesis is rejected. In the example at hand, the computed value of t is:

---

[5]The absolute value of a number is the number without any sign. Thus, the absolute value of both $+2.50$ and -2.50 is 2.50. We would designate the absolute value of -2.50 symbolically as $|-2.50|$.

$$t = \frac{5.5 \quad 5.0}{0.2} = 2.50$$

As indicated earlier, the tabled value of t for $df = 99$ and $\alpha = .05$ is 1.99. Therefore, since 2.50 is greater than 1.99, we reject the null hypothesis that the population mean is 5.0.

Statistical Significance. When researchers calculate a test statistic that is beyond the tabled value, they say that their results are **statistically significant.** It is important to understand the precise meaning of this term. The word *significant* in this context should not be interpreted to mean *important* or *useful* or *meaningful* or *clinically relevant.* In statistics, significant means that the obtained results are probably not attributable to chance (i.e., attributable to random fluctuations and sampling error), at the specified level of probability.

A result that is **statistically nonsignificant** is one that could have been obtained simply by chance. In other words, a nonsignificant result is one that, on the relevant theoretical distribution, does not lie in the critical region for rejecting the null hypothesis.

There is a definite prejudice in research circles for results that are statistically significant. Researchers are often disappointed if their substantive predictions—their research hypotheses—are not supported by the data. Moreover, reviewers and editors for research journals are less likely to accept manuscripts of research reports where statistically significant results are not reported. This prejudice is not arbitrary; it reflects the fact that nonsignificant results are ambiguous. Inferential statistics are designed to disconfirm the null hypothesis, and consequently there is never any justification for interpreting an accepted null hypothesis as evidence of a *lack* of relationship among variables. Because of the basic framework for hypothesis testing, researchers whose substantive hypotheses are the null case (i.e., they hypothesize no relationship among variables) will not be able to make the required inferences with traditional inferential statistics.

While there is a strong preference for statistical significance, we must caution that significance does not necessarily mean that the results are of importance to the health care community and their clients. We noted earlier that researchers can reduce the standard error by increasing the size of their sample. With a large enough sample, almost all findings are statistically significant, but that does not mean that they have practical value.

One-Tailed versus Two-Tailed Tests. In most situations, researchers use what are called two-tailed tests. A **two-tailed test** is one that uses both tails of a sampling distribution to determine the critical region for rejecting the null hypothesis. For example, the critical region in Figure 5–6 is found in both tails of the sampling distribution—values above 5.398 and below 4.602. The area corresponding to 5% of the probability distribution (for an α of .05) is comprised of 2½% at the lower end and 2½% at the upper end.

There are situations, however, when a two-tailed test is unnecessarily conservative. When the researcher has a strong basis for predicting a specific *direction* for the alternative hypothesis, a one-tailed test may be appropriate. A **one-tailed test** is one in which the critical region is in only one end of the distribution.

For the sake of illustration, suppose that we had a firm basis for hypothesizing not only that infertility patients' attitudes toward IVF are not neutral, but also that they are positive. This is referred to as a **directional hypothesis.** Our hypotheses in this example might be formally stated as follows:

H_0: $\mu = 5.0$
H_1: $\mu > 5.0$

Originally, we predicted simply that the population mean would not be neutral—not equal to 5.0. This implies that we were prepared to find mean ratings that reflected either negative attitudes or positive ones, and therefore it was necessary to look at both tails of the sampling distribution. In a one-tailed test, the critical region defining improbable values is entirely in one tail of the distribution—the tail corresponding to the direction of the alternative hypothesis. Because the entire 5% of "improbable" values is at one end with a one-tailed test, it is easier to reject the null hypothesis.

Figure 5–7 illustrates this concept with the example at hand. With a two-tailed test, the mean sample rating had to exceed 5.398 in order to be considered statistically significant at the .05 level. With a one-tailed test, the mean sample rating has to exceed only 5.332 to reject the null hypothesis. This value represents the hypothesized mean (5.0), plus the standard error (0.2) times the tabled value for a one-tailed test with $\alpha = .05$ and *df* = 99. Column 2 of Table B–2 (i.e., the column headed by .10, which is equivalent to .05

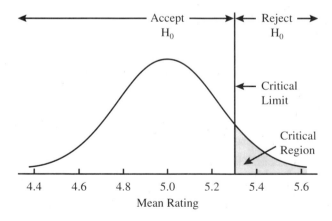

FIGURE 5–7.   CRITICAL REGION FOR A ONE-TAILED TEST: ATTITUDES TOWARD IVF EXAMPLE

for a one-tailed test, as shown in the bottom row of the table) indicates that the tabled t value is approximately 1.66. The critical limit is thus $5.0 + (0.2 \times 1.66) = 5.332$.

Most researchers use two-tailed tests even when their substantive hypotheses are directional. In research reports, if the researcher does not stipulate that the statistical tests were one-tailed, then it should be assumed that two-tailed tests were used. This is a conservative approach that reduces the risk of committing a Type I error. However, the result is also that the risk of a Type II error then increases. Thus, when theory or prior research evidence strongly suggests that findings opposite to those in the directional hypothesis are virtually impossible, a one-tailed test—which will yield greater statistical power—may be justified. For example, suppose we were to test the following null hypothesis:

H_0: Hand-washing has no effect on bacteria counts.

In this situation, the appropriate alternative hypothesis is clearly directional—i.e., that hand-washing reduces bacteria. It would make little sense to test the null hypothesis against the tail of the distribution implying the possibility that hand-washing *increases* bacteria.

The decision to use a one-tailed test must always be based on a solid foundation of theory or prior empirical evidence. It is also essential to establish the decision to use a one-tailed or two-tailed test *before* the analyses are performed. It is inappropriate to compute a test statistic and then decide, based on the result, that a one-tailed test should be used.

Assumptions. The use of statistical tests always requires that certain statistical assumptions be made. An **assumption** is a statement about conditions in the population that are accepted as true but that are not proved.

Assumptions vary according to the test statistic being used, and we will note the assumptions associated with specific tests in subsequent chapters. However, one assumption that is common to virtually all statistical tests is the assumption that the subjects in the sample have been independently and randomly sampled from the population of interest. A **random sample** is a sample drawn in such a way that every element in the population has an equal chance of being selected. Random samples have a greater likelihood than samples drawn by other means of being representative of the population. Sampling errors can and do occur in random samples, but such sampling errors are simply the result of chance factors rather than the result of **systematic bias.** Samples that are not selected by random procedures are likely to harbor systematic bias. When samples are biased, it is inappropriate to generalize the findings from the sample to the population.

In most nursing research—or, for that matter, in most research with human subjects, regardless of the discipline—the research samples are *not* randomly selected. In our hypothetical example of 100 infertility patients, it is unlikely that we could have obtained our sample by selecting 100 patients at random from *all* infertility patients in the United States. More likely, we would have obtained our sample from clients at a local infertility clinic. Even if we defined our population very narrowly as all the patients at that one clinic (which would probably not satisfy our underlying goals for conducting the study), the chances are pretty high that the sample would not be random. Some people, for example, would refuse to participate in the study, and non-participation is rarely random.

Since it is essential for the assumption of independent and random observations to be met for the statistical test to be valid, what should researchers do? First, random sampling procedures should be adopted whenever feasible. Second, if random sampling is not possible, the researcher should consider what is reasonable to assume as the population. In essence, the researcher needs to ask, From what population can this group be assumed to be a reasonably random (representative) sample? Third, the interpretation of the findings from nonrandom samples should be conservative and cautious. In deciding whether the results of the statistical inference can be generalized to the population, the researcher should look for evidence of similarities between sample characteristics and population characteristics. A final piece of advise is to **replicate** studies—that is, to repeat the study with a new sample of subjects.

For the one-sample *t*-test, there is an additional assumption beyond the assumption of independent, random sampling. It is assumed that the values on the target variable are normally distributed in the population. Fortunately, statisticians have been able to demonstrate that in most situations the *t*-test is **robust** to violations of the normality assumption. By robust, we mean that the accuracy of our decisions (the frequency of making Type I and Type II errors) is not strongly diminished when the underlying distribution of the variable is not normal. Generally, small deviations from normality can be tolerated regardless of the size of the sample. Larger deviations can be tolerated as the sample size increases. Thus, if a sample is small (under 30 cases) and there is evidence that the distribution is bimodal or severely skewed, a one-sample *t*-test should not be used.

Parametric and Nonparametric Tests. There are numerous statistical tests, and these tests can be classified in two broad groups. Most tests described in this book belong to the class known as parametric tests. **Parametric tests** are ones that involve the estimation of at least one parameter. The one-sample *t*-test is parametric because it involves the estimation of the population mean. Parametric tests, in general, assume that the variables are normally distributed in the population, and most parametric tests have other assumptions as well. Parametric statistics are usually applied only when the dependent variable is measured on an interval level or higher.

A second class of tests is called **nonparametric tests,** which do not test hypotheses about specific population parameters. These tests are sometimes referred to as **distribution-free tests** because they require no assumption about the shape of the distribution of the variables in the population. There are nonparametric tests that are appropriate for all four levels of measurement, although nonparametric tests are most frequently applied when the variables are measured on a nominal or ordinal scale. Nonparametric tests are generally much easier computationally than parametric tests.

The use of parametric and nonparametric tests is controversial. Some people argue that if the assumptions for a parametric test are not met, then a nonparametric test should be selected instead. Since parametric tests are generally robust to violations of the assumptions underlying them, however, others argue that parametric tests are usually appropriate when the violations are modest.

Since nonparametric tests are easier to compute and have less restrictive assumptions, why would a researcher ever chose a parametric test? First, the ease of computation is not much of an issue in this era when most statistical analyses are performed by computer. Second, parametric tests are much more powerful. By powerful, we refer to the concept of power discussed earlier: the likelihood of correctly rejecting a false null hypothesis. With a given set of data, a parametric procedure has a higher probability of correctly rejecting the null hypothesis than when a nonparametric procedure is applied to the same set of data.

It seems sensible to adopt a moderate position in this controversy. When deviations from normality appear to be modest, and when the measures of the variables are *approximately* interval-level, it is probably safe to use a parametric test. However, when the sample distribution of a variable is markedly skewed or multimodal—especially if the sample size is small—or if the variables cannot possibly be construed as interval-level, a nonparametric test may be preferable.

Between-Subjects Tests and Within-Subjects Tests. Another distinction in statistical tests concerns the nature of the comparisons being made. Hypothesis testing involves making some type of comparison.[6] When using a one-sample *t*-test, for example, the research is comparing a sample mean against a hypothesized value. If the hypothesis concerned the relationship between gender and coping skills, the researcher would compare men to women with regard to coping.

When the comparison involves separate groups of people, the research design is referred to as a **between-subjects design,** and the statistical test must be a between-subjects test (sometimes referred to as a **test for independent groups**). For example, when men are compared to women, a test for independent groups is required because the people in the male group cannot be the same people as those in the female group. As another example, if a researcher were interested in comparing the effects of two therapies (relaxation therapy versus music therapy) on perceptions of pain, and randomly as-

---

[6]The term *comparison* suggests an examination of group differences. But, in fact, whenever a researcher tests a hypothesis about a relationship between variables, the analysis essentially involves making comparisons. For example, when a researcher asks if there is a relationship between cholesterol levels and heart rate, this can be conceptualized as asking whether people with high cholesterol levels have different heart rates than people with low cholesterol levels. Correlational questions essentially involve comparisons of relative value on a continuum.

signed subjects to either the relaxation group or the music group, again a test for independent subjects would be required because people in the relaxation group did not receive the music therapy and vice versa.

There are other research designs, however, that involve using a single group of subjects. For example, the researcher in the example of the two pain therapies might expose half the subjects to the relaxation therapy first, followed by music therapy, while the other half would get the therapies in the reverse order. In this situation, the comparison of the two therapies is not independent, because the same subjects are in both groups. Another example involves a design wherein subjects are compared before and then after some intervention to determine if there were any changes. Such designs are often referred to as **repeated measures designs** or **crossover designs.** The appropriate statistical tests for such designs are **within-subjects tests** (sometimes referred to as **tests for dependent groups**).

The majority of research situations call for between-subjects tests. However, both types of statistical tests are described in subsequent chapters.

Steps in Hypothesis Testing

The remainder of this book describes various statistical tests, each of which is appropriate for a given research situation. Each test has its own computational formula, and a table corresponding to a relevant theoretical distribution. The overall process of testing hypotheses, however, is basically the same regardless of which test is used.

When the test statistic is being calculated manually, the steps in hypothesis testing are as follows:

1. *Determine the appropriate test statistic.* The selection of the correct test depends on several factors, including the nature of the comparison to be made, the number of groups being compared, the level of measurement of the independent and dependent variables, and the extent to which assumptions for parametric tests have been met. The tables that appear in the inside covers of this book provides some guidance for selecting an appropriate statistical test. The entries in these tables will be more understandable as you progress through the book and become familiar with alternative statistical procedures.
2. *Establish the level of significance.* It is important to set the criterion for the decision rule (rejection of the null hypothesis) before the analyses are undertaken. In most cases, the level of significance will be .05.
3. *Determine whether to use a one-tailed or two-tailed test.* In most cases, a two-tailed test will probably be appropriate. However, if there is a firm basis for hypothesizing not only the existence of a relationship but also the direction of that relationship, a one-tailed test may be warranted.
4. *Calculate the test statistic.* Using the data collected for the research, the test statistic is then computed, using the formula associated with the selected statistical test.

5. *Determine the degrees of freedom.* Degrees of freedom *(df)* is a concept used in statistical testing to indicate the number of components that are free to vary about a parameter. This is a difficult concept to grasp, but fortunately the formulas for determining degrees of freedom are very easy. It is not essential to understand the underlying principles of the *df* concept, but a simple illustration may clarify what is meant by "free to vary about a parameter." Suppose we knew that the mean value of five numbers was 10.0. How many raw data values (*X*s) would we need to know to have complete information on the set of data? The answer is four (*N* − 1); once we know the first four values, the fifth value is fixed, given that the mean is 10.0. For example, if the first four *X*s were 8, 10, 12, and 14, the fifth number would not be free to vary; it would have to be 6.

6. *Compare the computed test statistic against a tabled value.* Each statistical test has an associated theoretical distribution. Tables have been developed to indicate probability levels associated with different values in the distribution for different degrees of freedom. Most tables are set up to show the critical limit of the test statistic only for significance levels that are most commonly used—usually .05, .01, and .001. Thus, to use the tables you must first locate the appropriate α and degrees of freedom, and then retrieve the value of the critical limit. Then this tabled value is compared to the absolute value of the computed statistic. If the absolute value of the computed statistic is greater than the tabled value, the result is statistically significant, at the specified probability level. If the computed statistic is smaller, then the results are nonsignificant.

When a computer is used to perform the statistical analyses, the researcher still needs to make the up-front decisions (steps 1 through 3). First, the appropriate statistical test must be selected so that the correct instructions can be given to the computer. Next, the researcher should decide in advance what the significance criterion will be and whether a one-tailed or two-tailed test is appropriate. The next three steps are then carried out by the computer. The computer will calculate the test statistic, determine the degrees of freedom, and specify the actual probability that the null hypothesis is true. For example, the computer might indicate that the probability is .018 that the music therapy group and the relaxation therapy group had comparable pain ratings. This means that fewer than 2 times out of 100 (18 times out of 1000) would a group difference as large as that observed be found simply as a result of chance. The computed probability must then be compared to the established significance criterion. If α was set at .05, this result would be statistically significant because .018 reflects an outcome that is less probable than the criterion. If α was set at .01, however, the result would be nonsignificant at the specified level of significance. Note, though, that the computer-generated probability levels are usually specified for a two-tailed test. If a one-tailed test is used, the researcher must divide the probability value in half. In the present example, the *p* value would be .009 for a one-tailed test (.018 ÷ 2). Thus, the one-tailed test would pass the significance criterion of .01, while a two-tailed test would not.

THE COMPUTER AND ONE-SAMPLE *t*-TESTS AND CONFIDENCE INTERVALS

Confidence intervals can be built easily around sample means by instructing the computer to compute the *SEM*. The standard error usually is computed routinely by the computer when descriptive statistics are requested. For example, Figure 3—6 presented a computer printout of descriptive statistics for the heart rate data used for examples in Chapters 2 and 3. This figure shows that the *SEM* (Std err) is .469. Consulting Table B–2 for the appropriate value in the *t* distribution for *df* = 99 and α = .05, we find the value is about 1.98. Thus, the confidence intervals are .93 (.469 $\times$ 1.98 = .93) above and below the mean of 65.39, or the 95% confidence limits are 63.46 and 66.32.[7]

Most software packages also allow researchers to perform one-sample *t*-tests. This usually involves creating a variable to represent the hypothesized population mean, and then comparing that value to the sample mean. Figure 5–8 presents a printout for a one-sample *t*-test in which the hypothesis being tested is that the mean population heart rate is 60.0.[8] The mean sample heart rate (HARTRATE) of 65.39 is tested against the hypothesized heart rate (HYP@HR) of 60.00. Panel A of this figure shows basic descriptive information for both "variables," i.e., the mean, the *SD,* and the standard error of the mean. Panel B shows the mean difference, the *SD* of the difference, the *SEM* of the difference, and the 95% confidence interval around the mean difference. Then, the *t*-value of 11.48 is presented. With 99 *df,* this *t* is highly significant: $p < .000$. We do not know *exactly* what the probability is in this case because the computer prints only to three decimal places. We *do* know, however, that $p < .0005$. We can reject the null hypothesis that the mean population heart rate is 60.0. In fewer than 5 out of 10,000 samples would we have obtained a mean of 65.39 if the population mean really were 60.0.

RESEARCH APPLICATIONS

Although hypothesis testing is far more frequent than estimation procedures, it must be admitted that one-sample *t*-tests are not frequently used.[9] This is because researchers rarely have a fixed value against which a computed sample mean is to be tested.[10] Our

---

[7]In SPSS it is possible to use the ONEWAY procedure for computing confidence intervals, but the ONEWAY procedure requires dividing the sample into at least two groups. Then confidence intervals are computed for each group and the entire sample.

[8]The SPSS/PC commands that produced the printout in Figure 5–8 are as follows:

    COMPUTE HYP@HR = 60.
    T-TEST PAIRS = HARTRATE HYPHR.

[9]In fact, no example of a one-sample *t*-test could be readily located in the recent nursing research literature.

[10]An exception is when there are **norms** for a variable. A norm is a standard based on either population values or information from a large, representative sample. For example, there are norms for many psychological tests (e.g., most IQ tests have a mean of 100). There are also norms for many physiological variables, such as heart rate, blood pressure, birth weight, and so on.

```
- - - t-tests for paired samples - - -
```

	Variable	Number of pairs	Corr	2-tail Sig	Mean	SD	SE of Mean
A	HARTRATE				65.3900	4.694	.469
		100	.	.			
	HYP@HR				60.0000	.000	.000

	Paired Differences Mean	SD	SE of Mean	t-value	df	2-tail Sig
B	5.3900	4.694	.469	11.48	99	.000
	95% CI (4.458, 6.322)					

FIGURE 5–8. COMPUTER PRINTOUT OF A ONE-SAMPLE *t*-TEST

example of comparing the mean sample rating of IVF attitudes against the theoretical neutral rating of 5.0 was contrived so that we could use the simplest possible case for illustrating hypothesis testing procedures. More commonly used statistical tests for two or more variables are described in subsequent chapters. When a researcher is using inferential statistics in a one-sample situation, it is much more likely that estimation procedures will be used.

The Uses of Estimation of the Mean

All of the uses to which a mean can be put, as described in Chapter 4, also apply to point estimates and confidence intervals around a mean. In practice, however, the use of confidence intervals about a mean is not widespread. For example, researchers often show background characteristics of their sample by presenting mean values (e.g., mean age, mean educational level) without building a confidence interval around the means.

Some journals, however, use confidence intervals extensively. The *American Journal of Public Health,* for example, encourages the construction of tables that present means with their corresponding confidence intervals. When preparing a research report for publication, researchers should examine the journals that are of interest to determine the usual modes of presentation.

Presentation of Parameter Estimates of Means in Research Reports

Point estimates and interval estimates of means often can be reported in the text of a report. The following is an example of a statement that could be made to report a confidence interval: "The mean birth weight for the infants whose mothers were addicted to heroin was 2025 grams (95% *CI* = 2010, 2040)." This indicates that there is a 95%

probability that the mean population birth weight for infants of heroin-addicted mothers lies between 2010 and 2040 grams.

Tables are convenient for displaying confidence intervals for multiple means simultaneously. Such a tabular presentation is illustrated later in this chapter in the section on research examples.

Confidence intervals—or, alternatively, information about *SEM*s—can also be presented in graphic form. When means are plotted in a graph, which occurs most typically when there is a time dimension, there are several conventions for displaying information about the accuracy of those means. One commonly used convention is illustrated by a graph presented in a study by Miaskowski, Franck, Putris, and Levine (1993). These researchers studied the antinociceptive and motor side effects associated with intrathecal administration of the selective μ-opioid agonist DAMGO in rats. They plotted means for nociceptive activity and motor coordination over a 4-hour period following intrathecal (IT) administration of DAMGO. The graph, reproduced here as Figure 5–9, uses circles to indicate the mean values, and **error bars** or brackets around the means to designate the standard error of the mean. A similar convention can be used to display confidence intervals graphically.

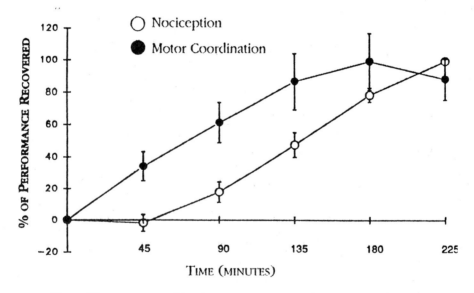

NOTE. The recovery of nociceptive activity and motor coordination as a percentage of peak analgesic and motor coordination effect was calculated. Each point in the figures represents the mean ± SEM. Some error bars are contained within the symbols. $N = 13$

FIGURE 5–9.   EXAMPLE OF A GRAPH WITH MEANS AND *SEM*S

Originally Figure 3 in Miaskowski et al.'s (1993) report. The graph was titled Time Course of Nociceptive Activity and Motor Coordination Following IT Administration of DAMGO (μg) Measured as Percentage Recovery from Peak Effect.

Tips on Preparing Tables with Information on Statistical Significance

In this section we offer general guidance on presenting information about statistical tests in tables.

- Tables that present information on tests of statistical significance vary in content, and we will be presenting many examples for specific tests in the chapters that follow. In most cases, however, there is a column headed by the name of the test statistic. The entries in the column are the values of the computed statistic. Table 5–3 illustrates this procedure with a hypothetical example of a series of one-sample t-tests that tested null hypotheses about the neutrality of attitudes toward alternative solutions to a fertility problem.
- When the number of cases on which the test statistic is based varies from one variable to another, there is usually a column designating the degrees of freedom. In this example, the df is shown in a footnote to the table because df was 99 for all four tests.
- When statistical tests have been performed, the table almost invariably presents information about probability values. Often, as in Table 5–3, there is a separate column for the p values. By convention, significant p values usually are displayed as being below the commonly used cutoff values of .05, .01, and .001, as appropriate, or as *NS* (nonsignificant). Even when the researcher sets α at .05, lower probability values are displayed when they are observed. For example, the entries for both the third and fourth variable in the table could have been $p < .05$, but this would have provided less information about how unlikely it was that the null hypothesis was true than by showing the more stringent probability levels. (Of course, if we had set $\alpha = .01$ in this example, we would have had to put *NS* in the p column for both the first and second variables.) Now that computers are widely used and provide information on the *actual* probability, it is also possible to put this information in tables.
- A widely used alternative to having a separate column for p values is to place asterisks next to the value of the test statistic to designate the probability levels. In most cases, one asterisk is used to represent $p < .05$, two asterisks designate $p < .01$, and three asterisks designate $p < .001$. (There should always be a key at the bottom of the table explaining what the asterisks represent.) In Table 5–3, for example, the entries under the t column could have been 2.50* for the first variable, 2.78** for the third variable, and 9.41*** for

TABLE 5–3. FICTITIOUS EXAMPLE OF A TABLE WITH ONE-SAMPLE t-TESTS

Variable	Mean	SD	t	p
Attitude Toward In Vitro Fertilization	5.50	2.00	2.50	<.05
Attitude Toward Artificial Insemination by Donor	5.25	2.25	1.11	NS
Attitude Toward Adoption	4.50	1.80	2.78	<.01
Attitude Toward Remaining Childless	3.40	1.70	9.41	<.001

$df = 99$

One-Sample t-Tests Testing Neutrality of Attitudes Toward Infertility Alternatives

the fourth variable. When this system is used, statistics with no associated asterisks are understood to be nonsignificant.

RESEARCH EXAMPLE

Confidence intervals are most likely to be used when there is a strong descriptive interest in the mean value of an attribute that has substantive importance—that is, when there is knowledge to be gained by estimating the population parameter. A research example that presented confidence intervals is summarized below.

> As we saw in Chapter 4, Metheny and her colleagues (1993) studied the extent to which pH values of aspirates from feeding tubes could be used to differentiate between gastric and intestinal tube placement. The researchers based their analyses on a total of 794 pH meter measurements, of which 405 were from nasogastric tubes and 389 were from nasointestinal tubes. Acid inhibitors were present for about half the readings.
> The mean pH meter readings in this study were of substantive interest, and so the researchers presented a table with mean pH values for gastrointestinal aspirates under different conditions. The table, which is reproduced here as Table 5–4, included the 99% confidence limits around the mean. As this table shows, the 99% *CI* is fairly small, indicating a small *SEM* (e.g., the 99% *CI* for all nasogastric aspirates ranges from 3.26 to 3.78). This table demonstrates that it is straightforward for researchers to add *CI* information in tables that present means and standard deviations.

SUMMARY

Researchers use **inferential statistics** in their studies to generalize from sample data to a broader population. Researchers are not able to make inferences about population values directly from sample data due to **sampling error,** which results from the tendency of sample statistics to fluctuate from one sample to another, simply as a function of chance.

TABLE 5–4. EXAMPLE OF A TABLE WITH CONFIDENCE INTERVALS

Readings	*M*	*SD*	99% *CI*	Number
All nasogastric (NG)	3.52	2.02	3.26 to 3.78	405
All nasointestinal (NI)	7.05	1.26	6.88 to 7.22	389
NG, acid inhibitors absent	3.12	1.90	2.76 to 3.48	185
NG, acid inhibitors present	3.84	2.06	3.48 to 4.20	219
NI, acid inhibitors absent	6.94	1.31	6.70 to 7.18	197
NI, acid inhibitors present	7.15	1.21	6.92 to 7.38	189

*Originally Table 1 in Metheny et al.'s (1993) report. The table was titled **Means, Standard Deviations, and 99% Confidence Intervals for pH-Meter Readings on Gastrointestinal Aspirates.***

Inferential statistics use theoretical **sampling distributions** and the **laws of probability** as a basis for establishing "probable" and "improbable" research outcomes. The **sampling distribution of the mean** is a hypothetical distribution of the means of an infinite number of samples of a given size from a population. The standard deviation of this distribution is known as the **standard error of the mean** *(SEM);* it is an index of the average amount of error in a sample mean as an estimate of the population mean. The smaller the *SEM,* the more accurate are the estimates of the population value.

Statistical inference encompasses two broad approaches: estimation procedures and hypothesis testing. **Estimation** is used when the researcher has no a priori hypothesis about the value of a parameter. **Point estimation** involves the calculation of a single value, while **interval estimation** yields a range of values (a **confidence interval**) within which the population value is expected to lie, at a given level of probability.

Hypothesis testing, which is used when the researcher has an a priori research hypothesis, begins with an assumption that the null hypothesis is true. The **null hypothesis** (H_0) is typically a statement about the absence of a relationship between variables, while the **research hypothesis** (or **alternative hypothesis, H_1**) is the hypothesis the researcher is seeking to support. Based on a calculated **test statistic,** the researcher makes a decision to accept or reject the null hypothesis. Because decision making is based on sample data, there is always a possibility that the decision is incorrect. When the researcher incorrectly rejects a null hypothesis that is true, a **Type I error** is committed; when the researcher incorrectly accepts a false null hypothesis, a **Type II error** is committed. The researcher establishes the **level of significance,** which is the probability of making a Type I error. The two most commonly used levels of significance (often symbolized as α) are .05 and .01. With α equal to .05, the researcher accepts the risk that in 5 samples out of 100 the null hypothesis will be rejected when it is true. The probability of committing a Type II error (symbolized as β) is more difficult to control, but large samples reduce the risk of a Type II error—that is, they increase the **power** of the statistical test.

Hypothesis testing involves several steps. First, the researcher selects an appropriate statistical test. The selection is based on several factors, such as the level of measurement of the variables and the degree to which the data are likely to support the assumptions for a parametric test. A **parametric test** involves the estimation of a parameter, the use of data measured on an interval scale or higher, and assumptions about the distribution of the variables. A **nonparametric test** has less restrictive assumptions, and is more likely to be used when the key variables are nominal- or ordinal-level. Researchers also decide whether a **one-tailed test** (suitable for a **directional hypothesis**) is defensible, or whether a **two-tailed test**—which uses both ends of the theoretical distribution to define the **critical region** of "improbable" values—is more appropriate.

Once the researcher makes the preliminary decisions, a test statistic is calculated using the sample data. After determining the correct **degrees of freedom** *(df),* the researcher then consults the appropriate table. If the absolute value of the test statistic is greater than the tabled value, the result is said to be **statistically significant,** at the specified level of probability. This means that the obtained result is not likely to be the result of chance factors. A **nonsignificant** result is one in which deviations from the null hypothesis are likely to have occurred simply by chance.

One statistical test was described in this chapter. The **one-sample *t*-test** is used when the researcher tests the null hypothesis that the sample mean is equal to some specified value, and when the *SEM* must be estimated from sample data. A *t* **distribution** is one that is similar to a normal distribution, but that has fatter tails when the sample size is small. When there is information about the *actual* (not estimated) *SEM, z* scores and the normal distribution can be used to test hypotheses about a single mean.

EXERCISES

The following exercises cover concepts presented in this chapter. Exercises indicated with a dagger (†) can be checked against answers appearing in Appendix A. Additionally, Chapter 5 of the accompanying *Applications Manual* offers supplementary exercises, including ones that require computer analysis of a data set on diskette.

† 1. What is the probability of drawing a spade from a normal, shuffled deck of 52 cards? What is the probability of drawing five spades in a row (i.e., the probability of getting a flush in five-card poker)?

2. Draw a histogram that graphs the probability of drawing a spade, a club, a heart, or a diamond from a normal deck of 52 cards. Shade in the area showing the probability of drawing a red card.

† 3. Given a normal distribution of scores with a mean of 100 and an *SD* of 10, compute *z* scores for the following raw values: 95, 115, 80, 130.

† 4. Based on Figure 5–2, which shows a normal distribution of students' heights with a mean of 60.0 and an *SD* of 5.0, approximately what is the probability of randomly selecting a student whose height is less than 50 inches? (Use the tabled values for the normal distribution in Table B–1.)

† 5. If a sampling distribution of the mean had an *SEM* equal to 0.0, what would this suggest about the sample means drawn from the population—and about the scores in the population?

† 6. Compute the mean, the standard deviation, and the estimated standard error of the mean for the following sample data: 3, 3, 4, 4, 4, 5, 5, 5, 5, 5, 5, 6, 6, 6, 7, 7.

† 7. Population A and Population B both have a mean height of 70.0 inches with an *SD* of 6.0. A random sample of 30 people is selected from Population A, and a random sample of 50 people is selected from Population B. Which sample mean will probably yield a more accurate estimate of its population mean? Why?

† 8. Suppose we obtained data on vein size after application of a nitroglycerin ointment in a sample of 60 patients. The mean vein size is found to be 7.8 mm with an *SD* of 2.5. Using the *t* distribution in Table B–2 (because information on the true *SEM* is

not available), what are the confidence limits for a 95% confidence interval? For a 99% confidence interval?

† 9. Suppose you wanted to test the hypothesis that the average speed on a highway— where the maximum legal speed is 55 mph—is not equal to 55 mph (i.e., H_0: $\mu =$ 55; H_1: $\mu \neq$ 55). Speed guns are used to measure the speed of 50 drivers, and the mean is found to be 57.0, $SD = 8.0$. What is the calculated value of t for a one-sample t-test? With $\alpha = .05$, is the sample mean significantly different from the hypothesized mean of 55.0, using a two-tailed test, i.e., can the null hypothesis be rejected?

† 10. For the problem in Exercise 9, would the obtained result be statistically significant with $\alpha = .05$ for a one-tailed test (i.e., for H_1: $\mu > 55$)?

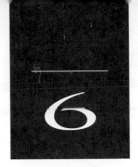

Testing the Difference between Two Means: The Two-Sample *t*-Test

In the preceding chapter, we looked at a statistical test for drawing inferences about the mean of a population. A much more common situation involves inferences about the *difference* between two populations means. For example, a researcher might be interested in knowing if the mean body temperature of a population receiving a specialized treatment is different from the mean temperature of a control population not receiving the treatment. Or, a researcher might want to determine the difference between the mean stress levels of preoperative male patients and those of preoperative female patients. Another researcher might want to compare the mean weight of a population of patients before versus after an innovative weight-loss intervention. In all of these situations, if the researchers are making comparisons based on sample data with the intent of generalizing to broader populations—i.e., drawing inferences about group differences in the populations—then the **two-sample *t*-test** is the appropriate statistical test.

BASIC CONCEPTS FOR THE TWO-SAMPLE *t*-TEST

Let us suppose that we wished to determine whether the ingestion of caffeinated coffee affects intraocular pressure (IOP) in nonglaucomatous people. Fifty subjects are randomly assigned to an experimental group that ingests 40 ounces of hot black coffee, while 50 subjects are randomly assigned to a control group that receives 40 ounces of hot water. Thirty minutes later, the IOP of all 100 subjects is measured. The mean IOP of those in the experimental group is found to be 15.5 mm Hg, while the mean IOP of those in the control group is 13.5 mm Hg. Can we now conclude that the ingestion of caffeinated coffee versus hot water (the independent variable) is related to IOP levels (the dependent variable)?

As we saw in the previous chapter, a mean from a sample is almost never exactly the same as the population mean because of sampling error. Thus, the two populations in question (a hypothetically infinite number of ingestors of caffeinated coffee and a hypothetically infinite number of ingestors of hot water) *could* have the same mean IOPs even though the sample means are different by 2.0 mm Hg. A mere inspection of the two sample means is inadequate for reaching conclusions about the populations.

The Null and Alternative Hypotheses

In the present example, there are two competing possibilities: either the ingestion of caffeinated coffee is related to the IOP of nonglaucomatous people, or it is not. The null hypothesis posits that there is no relationship between the two variables. We can state the null hypothesis formally as:

$$H_0: \mu_1 = \mu_2$$

where μ_1 = population mean for the first group (those receiving caffeinated coffee)
μ_2 = population mean for the second group (those receiving hot water)

The alternative hypothesis is that there *is* a relationship between the independent and dependent variables—that is, that the two population means are not equal:

$$H_1: \mu_1 \neq \mu_2$$

Two things about these hypotheses should be noted. First, the hypotheses are about the population parameters (μ), not about the statistics $(\overline{X})$. The researcher uses sample data to draw conclusions about what is true in the population. Second, the alternative hypothesis in this case is stated as a nondirectional hypothesis. That is, it does not specify whether μ_1 is expected to be greater than μ_2 or vice versa. Thus, in this example, a two-tailed test would be applied.

The next task before us is to determine whether the null hypothesis has a high probability of being incorrect, using statistical inference. By showing that the null hypothesis is improbable, we can accept the alternative hypothesis that the population means are unequal.

Sampling Distribution of a Mean Difference

A two-sample t-test follows the same hypothesis-testing logic that we discussed in Chapter 5. The test statistic is based on a theoretical sampling distribution that allows the researcher to conclude whether an observed difference between two sample means is "probable" or "improbable," given the null hypothesis. The relevant sampling distribution is the **sampling distribution of the difference between two means.**

A sampling distribution, as we have already seen, is a theoretical distribution of an infinite number of sample values drawn from a population. In the present situation, the distribution is based not on individual sample means, but rather on differences between the means of samples drawn from two different populations. That is, the sampling distribution plots the distribution of an infinite number of mean differences (M_{Diff}) for samples of a specified size, where M_{Diff} is defined as follows:

$$M_{\text{Diff}} = \overline{X}_1 - \overline{X}_2$$

In the example of the IOP, our sample difference score would be:

$$M_{\text{Diff}} = 15.5 - 13.5$$
$$M_{\text{Diff}} = 2.0$$

If we measured the IOPs of a new sample of 50 people drinking caffeinated coffee and 50 drinking hot water, new means—and a new difference score—would be obtained. If all possible difference scores were computed and graphed in a frequency distribution, the result would be a sampling distribution of the difference between the two means. Just as the mean of a sampling distribution of the mean is always equal to the population mean, so too *the mean of a sampling distribution of the difference between two means is always equal to the difference between two population means.* Thus, by knowing the standard deviation of such a distribution, we can determine differences that are in the tail and that are, therefore, improbable when the null hypothesis is true.

The standard deviation of such a sampling distribution is referred to as the standard error of the difference between two means or, more commonly, the **standard error of the difference**. The standard error of the difference summarizes how much sampling error will occur, on average, when two group means and M_{Diff} are computed.

A relatively large standard error of the difference makes it difficult for researchers to reject the null hypothesis, even when it is false. When the standard error is small, by contrast, it is easier to have confidence in any one sample difference as an estimate of the population difference. Similar to the standard error of the mean, the standard error of the difference is influenced by two factors: the size of the samples (n_1 and n_2) and the variability of scores in the populations. The standard error becomes smaller as the sample size increases and the variability of scores in the populations decreases.

The *t* statistic for testing the difference between two group means uses an estimate of the standard error of the difference in its formula, as we discuss in a subsequent section. Let us first consider the underlying requirements for the *t*-test.

Assumptions and Requirements for the *t*-Test

The *t*-test for comparing group means is appropriate when the independent variable consists of two levels of a nominal-level variable (i.e., when there are two and only two groups) and when the dependent variable approximates interval-scale characteristics or higher. In our example about intraocular pressure, there were two levels of the independent variable—caffeinated coffee versus hot water—and a ratio-level dependent variable, IOP measures.

Strictly speaking, the use of a t-test for testing differences between two group means is justified only if several assumptions are met. First, the subjects are presumed to be randomly sampled. This assumption is true of virtually all statistical tests, as previously discussed. Second, the variable is presumed to be normally distributed within each of the two populations. The t-test is robust with regard to the assumption of normality. That is, the results are reasonably accurate even if the assumption is not satisfied, especially if the sample sizes are reasonably large.

A third assumption stipulates that the variances of the two populations are equal. That is, it is assumed that:

$$\sigma^2_1 = \sigma^2_2$$

This is known as the **assumption of the homogeneity of variance.** It is usually safe to ignore this assumption when the sample sizes are approximately equal. If the sample sizes are markedly dissimilar (for example, one group is more than 1.5 times greater than the second group) and if there is reason to suspect that the population variances are unequal, the standard formula for the t-test may well produce erroneous results.[1] More specifically, there is a greater risk of committing a Type II error (incorrectly accepting the null hypothesis) when the variation in one population is substantially greater than that in the second. As we will see later in this chapter, there is an alternative formula that can be applied when it is suspected that the assumption of homogeneous variances has been violated.

t-TESTS FOR INDEPENDENT AND DEPENDENT GROUPS

There are two types of situations in which a t-test for comparing two group means is appropriate. The first situation calls for the **independent groups t-test,** which is used when the subjects in the two groups are not the same people nor connected to one another in any systematic way. For example, the independent groups t-test would be used in our example of the subjects randomly assigned to either the caffeinated coffee group *or* the hot water group. No one in the coffee group received the hot water condition, and vice versa. Moreover, the composition of one group was in no way paired or matched to the composition of the other group.

---

[1]Clearly, when there is reason in advance to suspect that the population variances are unequal, it is advisable to design the study in such a way that the samples are of approximately equal size.

A different formula must be used when the people in the two groups are not independent. For example, when the weight of people going through a weight reduction program is measured before and after the intervention, the subjects in the two groups are the *same* individuals, and therefore the two samples are not independent. In such a situation, the **dependent groups *t*-test** is required. In this section we present computational formulas for both types of test.

Independent Groups *t*-Tests

Suppose that we developed a special intervention to alleviate the distress of preschool children who are about to undergo the fingerstick procedure for a hematocrit determination. Twenty children will be used to evaluate the effectiveness of the special treatment, with 10 randomly assigned to an experimental (treatment) group and 10 assigned to a control group that receives no special preparation. The main dependent variable is the child's pulse rate just prior to the fingerstick. The hypotheses being tested are:

$$H_0: \mu_1 = \mu_2 \qquad H_1: \mu_1 \neq \mu_2$$

where μ_1 = population mean for the experimental group
μ_2 = population mean for the control group

To test these hypotheses, we must compute the t statistic. In this example, we need to use the formula for the independent groups *t*-test, since membership in the experimental group is completely independent of membership in the control group. A simplified formula for t is:

$$t = \frac{\overline{X}_1 - \overline{X}_2}{s_{\bar{x}_1 - \bar{x}_2}}$$

The numerator is the difference in means between the two sample groups, and the denominator is the estimated standard error of the difference. This formula is similar to the formula for the one-sample *t*-test presented in Chapter 5, where we saw that the numerator was the mean (minus the hypothesized population mean),[2] and the denominator was the standard error of the mean (*SEM*).

---

[2] A more complete formula for the t statistic—and one that more closely resembles the formula for the one-sample t statistic presented in Chapter 5—is as follows:

$$t = \frac{(\overline{X}_1 - \overline{X}_2) - (\mu_1 - \mu_2)}{s_{\bar{x}_1 - \bar{x}_2}}$$

The added expression in the numerator $(\mu_1 - \mu_1)$ represents the population difference between the two means. However, since the null hypothesis stipulates that the two population means are equal, this expression can be assumed to be zero and dropped from the equation.

Pooled Variance t-Test. The standard error of the difference between means, which is needed to compute the t statistic, is estimated on the basis of the variances of the two samples. If we assume that the variances of the two populations of children (those receiving and those not receiving the special preparation) are equal, we can compute the t statistic using the pooled variance estimate of the standard error of the difference in the denominator. (In our present example, we can use the pooled variance estimate even if the variances are dissimilar because the two sample sizes are equal.) The basic (pooled variance) formula for the independent groups t-test is:

$$t = \frac{\overline{X}_1 - \overline{X}_2}{\sqrt{\left[\frac{(n_1 - 1) s^2_1 + (n_2 - 1) s^2_2}{n_1 + n_2 - 2}\right]\left[\frac{1}{n_1} + \frac{1}{n_2}\right]}}$$

where $\overline{X}_1$ = sample mean of Group 1
$\overline{X}_2$ = sample mean of Group 2
s^2_1 = variance of Group 1
s^2_2 = variance of Group 2
n_1 = number of cases in Group 1
n_2 = number of cases in Group 2

Although this formula looks complex and may seem intimidating, it simply boils down to the computation of the means and the variances of the two groups, and then plugging these values into the equation along with information on the size of the groups.[3]

Some data for our fictitious example about the experimental preparation for the fingerstick are presented in Table 6–1. According to this table, the mean pulse rate of the children in the experimental group was 10.0 bpm lower than that of the children in the control group (95.0 versus 105.0). But does this difference reflect real differences in the populations or is it merely the result of random fluctuation? The t-test will enable us to draw a conclusion, at a specified probability level.

All of the components of the t-test have been computed and are shown at the bottom of Table 6–1. (The actual calculation of the variances—the squared standard deviations—is not shown in the table; the *SD* and variance formulas were presented in Chapter 3.) According to the calculation, the value of the t statistic is 1.85. In order to evaluate whether this is statistically significant (i.e., improbable if the null hypothesis is true), we must first compute the degrees of freedom for the t-test. The *df* formula for the independent groups t-test is:

$$df = n_1 + n_2 - 2$$

---

[3]By convention, N is used to designate the total sample size, while n is used to represent the size of a group within the sample.

TABLE 6–1. EXAMPLE OF THE CALCULATION OF POOLED VARIANCE INDEPENDENT GROUPS t-TEST

Pulse of: Experimental Group (Group 1) X_1 (bpm)	Control Group (Group 2) X_2 (bpm)
100	105
86	95
112	120
80	85
115	110
83	100
90	115
94	93
85	107
105	120
$\Sigma X_1 = 950$	$\Sigma X_2 = 1050$
$\overline{X}_1 = 950 \div 10$	$\overline{X}_2 = 1050 \div 10$
$\overline{X}_1 = 95.0$	$\overline{X}_2 = 105.0$
$s^2_1 = 154.46$	$s^2_2 = 138.67$
$n_1 = 10$	$n_2 = 10$

$$t = \frac{\overline{X}_1 - \overline{X}_2}{\sqrt{\left[\dfrac{(n_1 - 1)s^2_1 + (n_2 - 1)s^2_2}{n_1 + n_2 - 2}\right]\left[\dfrac{1}{n_1} + \dfrac{1}{n_2}\right]}}$$

$$t = \frac{95.0 - 105.0}{\sqrt{\left[\dfrac{(9)\,154.46 + (9)\,138.67}{18}\right]\left[\dfrac{1}{10} + \dfrac{1}{10}\right]}} = \frac{-10.0}{5.41}$$

$$t = -1.85 \quad df = 18$$

Thus, in this example, df is 18 $(10 + 10 - 2)$. Suppose that we have set α equal to .05 for a two-tailed test. Table B–2 in the Appendix indicates that the tabled value of t with $df = 18$ is 2.10. Since this tabled value is greater than the absolute value of the calculated t statistic (-1.85), we must retain the null hypothesis that stipulates that the population means are equal. We cannot conclude that the group difference of 10.0 bpm in the children's pulse rates is attributable to the special preparation, given our hypothesis and decision rule.

Of course, we might well have tested different hypotheses, such as the following, instead:

$$H_0: \mu_1 = \mu_2 \qquad H_1: \mu_1 \leq \mu_2$$

The alternative hypothesis is now directional; it predicts not only that the two groups will have unequal mean pulses, but that the mean pulse rate for the experimental group will be lower than that for the control group. Because we have no expectation that the special preparation would *increase* the preprocedure pulse rate of the children in the experimental group, we can use a one-tailed test. Returning to Table B–2, we find that with $\alpha = .05$ and $df = 18$, the tabled t value for a one-tailed test is 1.73. The absolute value of the calculated t statistic, 1.85, is now greater than the tabled value. Therefore, the null hypothesis can be rejected. The mean pulse rate of the experimental group is significantly lower than that of the control group. This example provides an opportunity to reemphasize the caveat that the decision to use a one-tailed or a two-tailed test should be made *before* the t statistic is computed, not after its value is known.

Separate Variance t-Test. We were able to use the basic pooled variance formula for the t-test in this example because the sample sizes of the two groups were identical. Moreover, we can see in Table 6–1 that the variances of the two groups were reasonably similar (154.5 for the experimental group and 138.7 for the control group). When the assumption of equal population variances is untenable and when the sample sizes are unequal, a different formula for the t statistic must be used. The **separate variance** formula is:

$$t = \frac{\overline{X}_1 - \overline{X}_2}{\sqrt{\dfrac{s^2_1}{n_1} + \dfrac{s^2_2}{n_2}}}$$

There are statistical tests for determining whether the pooled variance or separate variance test should be used, but it is beyond the scope of this book to present these formulas.[4] Suffice it to say that the pooled variance estimate is widely used and is appropriate whenever sample sizes are approximately equal and there are at least five cases in each group.

Dependent Groups *t*-Test

There are several research situations in which an independent groups t-test is inappropriate. One such situation occurs when means are computed for the same group of people at two different points in time (for example, before and after an intervention). In this within-subjects design, the "groups" clearly are not independent; they comprise the same people. Sampling fluctuation is almost always lower in such a dependent group situation. This is because the various attributes of individuals that contribute to sampling fluctuation (e.g., their health, personalities, income, motivation, and so on) have a comparable effect on both means. The t-test for independent groups is, therefore,

---

[4]When the analyses are done on the computer, a test for homogeneity of variance is usually performed as part of the t-test procedure, and the t statistic using both the pooled and separate variance estimates is calculated. A subsequent section presents output from such a computer analysis.

overly conservative or insensitive for testing dependent group differences, since a major source of intersubject variation is controlled.

There are other situations in which a dependent groups t-test is used. Whenever subjects in one group are paired to subjects in the second group on the basis of some attribute, the dependent groups t-test is appropriate. Here are some examples:

- Group 1 = husbands; Group 2 = their wives
- Group 1 = first-born children; Group 2 = their younger siblings
- Group 1 = AIDS patients; Group 2 = their primary caretakers

In another relevant situation, researchers sometimes deliberately pair-match subjects in one group with unrelated subjects in another group to enhance the comparability of the two groups. For instance, people with lung cancer might be pair-matched to people without lung cancer on the basis of age, education, and gender, and then the smoking behavior of the two groups might be compared. In all of these instances, the selection of subjects in the second group is constrained by which subjects are in the first group—their selection is not totally independent. Furthermore, the factors that affect the variability in the dependent variable are also constrained. These situations all call for a dependent groups t-test, which is referred to in some statistics books as a **paired t-test** or a **correlated groups t-test.**

To illustrate the dependent groups t-test, suppose that we wanted to compare direct and indirect methods of blood pressure measurement in a sample of trauma patients. Blood pressure values are obtained from 10 patients via both radial arterial catheter (direct) and the bell component of the stethoscope (indirect). In this example, the hypotheses being tested are as follows:

$$H_0: \mu_1 = \mu_2 \qquad H_1: \mu_1 \neq \mu_2$$

where μ_1 = population mean for the direct method
μ_2 = population mean for the indirect method

To test these hypotheses, we need to perform a dependent groups t-test, because the same people are in both groups. The formula for the t statistic for dependent groups is:

$$t = \frac{\overline{D}}{}$$

where $\overline{D}$ = mean difference between pairs of values
s^2_D = variance of the difference
n = total number of pairs

In this formula, the $\overline{D}$ in the numerator is the difference between all pairs of individual scores, averaged—i.e., the mean of all the $(\overline{X}_1 - \overline{X}_2)$s. The expression in the denominator is the estimate of the standard error of difference. The following equivalent formula can be more readily used for actual calculations:

$$t = \frac{\Sigma D}{\sqrt{\dfrac{n\Sigma D^2 - (\Sigma D)^2}{n-1}}}$$

where D = difference scores between the pairs
n = total number of pairs

Again, although the formula looks complex, the components are not difficult to compute. The main calculation involves computing difference scores between all pairs, and then either squaring each difference score and summing (ΣD^2), or summing the difference scores and then squaring (($\Sigma D)^2$).

Some systolic blood pressure data for our fictitious example are presented in Table 6–2. As the calculations at the bottom of this table show, the mean systolic blood pressure of the 10 patients is 129.3 mm Hg by the direct method and 128.0 mm Hg by the indirect method. We can apply the t-test for dependent groups to determine if the difference of 1.3 mm Hg is statistically significant, or likely to be the result of sampling error.

Table 6–2 shows that the calculated value of t is 1.90. We can consult Table B–2 for the tabled t value once we have calculated the applicable degrees of freedom. For the dependent groups t-test, the formula is:

$$df = n - 1$$

where n = total number of pairs

Thus, in our present example, $df = 9$. With 9 degrees of freedom and $\alpha = .05$ for a two-tailed test, the tabled value of t is 2.26. Since the tabled value is larger than the computed value of t, our decision is to accept the null hypothesis. We cannot conclude that the population mean for the direct blood pressure measurement is different from the population mean for the indirect method, given our decision rule.

OTHER STATISTICAL ISSUES FOR A TWO-SAMPLE MEAN SITUATION

When a researcher analyzes means for two groups, the main research question typically concerns the *existence* of a relationship. That is, the researcher applies the t-test to determine if the independent variable (group status) is significantly related to the dependent variable (the variable for which the means are computed). This section examines other related statistical issues.

TABLE 6–2. EXAMPLE OF THE CALCULATION OF DEPENDENT GROUPS t-TEST

Direct X_1 (mm Hg)	Indirect X_2 (mm Hg)	Difference $(X_1 - X_2)$ D	D^2
130	128	2	4
102	100	2	4
154	155	−1	1
113	110	3	9
139	140	−1	1
125	120	5	25
156	155	1	1
108	105	3	9
161	160	1	1
105	107	−2	4
$\Sigma X_1 = 1293$	$\Sigma X_2 = 1280$	$\Sigma D = 13$	$\Sigma D^2 = 59$
$\bar{X}_1 = 1293/10$	$\bar{X}_2 = 1280/10$	$(\Sigma D)^2 = 169$	
$\bar{X}_1 = 129.3$	$\bar{X}_2 = 128.0$		

$$t = \frac{\Sigma D}{\sqrt{\dfrac{n\Sigma D^2 - (\Sigma D)^2}{n - 1}}}$$

$$t = \frac{13}{\sqrt{\dfrac{(10)59 - 169}{9}}} = \frac{13}{6.84}$$

$$t = 1.90$$

The Nature and Magnitude of the Relationship

As we pointed out in Chapter 1, researchers often want information on two other aspects of a relationship between variables: the *nature* of the relationship and its *magnitude*. In a two-sample mean-difference situation, it is easy to determine the nature of the relationship by simply inspecting the means; the "nature" question simply concerns which group has the higher mean. However, the strength of the relationship cannot be determined by inspecting the group means, nor by examining the value of the t statistic. A significant t value provides no information on whether the relationship is weak, moderate, or strong. Statistical significance simply indicates that the effect in the population is unlikely to be zero. By knowing the magnitude of a relationship, we can avoid the temptation of exaggerating the importance of a statistically significant result for the "existence" question.

There are several statistics that can be used to summarize the strength of the relationship between a dichotomous independent variable and a dependent variable measured on an interval or ratio scale. One that is easy to compute directly from the t statistic is the **point biserial correlation coefficient,** which is usually symbolized as r_{pb}. The point biserial correlation coefficient is much like the Pearson r discussed in Chapter 4. It can range from -1.00 for a perfect negative relationship, through 0.00 for no relationship, to $+1.00$ for a perfect positive relationship. Also, r_{pb} can be directly interpreted as indicating the magnitude of the relationship; the higher the absolute value, the stronger is the relationship.

The point biserial correlation coefficient can be computed using the formula for the Pearson r. However, in the present context it is much easier to use the following formula, which can be applied with both the independent groups and dependent groups t-tests:

$$r_{pb} = \sqrt{\frac{t^2}{t^2 + df}}$$

where t^2 = computed value of t, squared
df = degrees of freedom for the t-test

Let us return to the example we presented earlier in the chapter concerning the pulse rates of children in an experimental program designed to reduce distress before the fingerstick procedure. We can use the information in Table 6–1, where $t = -1.85$ and $df = 18$, to compute the point biserial correlation coefficient:

$$r_{pb} = \sqrt{\frac{(-1.85)^2}{(-1.85)^2 + 18}} = \sqrt{\frac{3.42}{3.42 + 18}} = \sqrt{.16} = .40$$

Thus, the relationship between group status and pulse rate in this example is a moderate one. Like the square of Pearson's r, the square of r_{pb} provides information about the proportion of explained variation in the dependent variable. Thus, we can say in this example that membership in the experimental versus control group accounts for 16% ($.40^2$) of the variation in the children's preprocedure pulse rates.[5] When information on r_{pb} and t are presented together, the reader has fairly comprehensive information regarding the relationship under investigation. In our present example, we can conclude that the experimental population has a lower pulse rate than the control population, assuming a one-tailed test (nature and existence), and that the relationship is moderately strong (magnitude).

Confidence Intervals

In Chapter 5 we discussed the use of confidence intervals to determine the probable range of values within which the mean of a single population is expected to lie. In a sim-

---

[5]The square of r_{pb} is equivalent to another statistic known as **eta squared** (η^2). We discuss eta squared in Chapter 7.

ilar fashion, confidence intervals can be developed for the difference between two population means. The formula is:

$$[\overline{X}_1 - \overline{X}_2) - t(s_{\bar{x}_1 - \bar{x}_2})] \leq \mu_1 - \mu_2 \leq [(\overline{X}_1 - \overline{X}_2) + ts_{\bar{x}_1 - \bar{x}_2}]$$

where $\overline{X}_1$ = sample mean of Group 1
  $\overline{X}_2$ = sample mean of Group 2
  t = tabled t value at a specified probability
  $s_{\bar{x}_1 - \bar{x}_2}$ = estimated standard error of the difference
  μ_1 = population mean of Group 1
  μ_2 = population mean of Group 2

Note that the t in the formula for the confidence limits is the tabled value, not the computed value, of t. For the example of the children's pulse rates in the experimental versus control group, we can use the information in Table 6–1 to determine the lower and upper confidence limits for the 95% confidence interval, assuming a two-tailed test:

$$[(95.0 - 105.0) - (2.10)(5.41)] = -21.36 \text{ (lower limit)}$$
$$[(95.0 - 105.0) + (2.10)(5.41)] = 1.36 \text{ (upper limit)}$$

We can state with 95% confidence that the mean pulse of the experimental population is between 21.36 bpm *less* and 1.36 bpm *more* than that of the control population. It should be noted that zero is within this interval, indicating the possibility that, for a two-tailed test, $\mu_1 = \mu_2$. This is consistent with the fact that the null hypothesis was not rejected when the two-tailed test was used.

Power

In our examples in this chapter, we used very small samples so that the computations would not be laborious. In actual studies, however, the use of small samples is risky. The likelihood of a Type II error (incorrectly accepting a false null hypothesis) is large when the number of cases is small, because a major determinant of a standard error is sample size.

The probability of committing a Type II error (β) is the complement of power ($1 - \beta$). **Power analysis** is a procedure used to estimate the power of a statistical test—that is, the probability of rejecting the null hypothesis. Power analysis typically is used in two situations. One important application is to use power analysis during the design phase of a study to estimate the size of the sample needed to obtain a significant result. Power analysis can also be used to help interpret statistical results, and is especially useful if the results are not significant. As pointed out in Chapter 5, there is considerable ambiguity when the null hypothesis is retained. The researcher *cannot* conclude that the null hypothesis is true, since inferential statistics are designed to disconfirm the null hypothesis. However, when a power analysis is performed, some of the ambiguity can be resolved because inferences about the likelihood of a Type II error can be drawn.

In performing a power analysis to estimate power, three pieces of information must be known or estimated:

1. The significance criterion, α
2. The sample or subsample size, N or n
3. The population effect size, gamma (γ)

The first two components are straightforward, but the third requires some discussion. The **effect size** is, essentially, a measure of the strength of the relationship between two variables in the population.[6] It is an index of how wrong the null hypothesis is. Thus, the higher the value of γ, the greater is power of the test. This simply means that when the relationship between two variables is strong, it is likely that a sample will reflect it. When the relationship is weak, it is possible, as a result of sampling error, that the relationship will fail to be manifested in a sample.

Since researchers typically do not know the value of the population effect size, it must be estimated from sample data. In a two-group situation with mean differences, the formula for the population effect size is:

$$\gamma = \frac{\mu_1 - \mu_2}{\sigma}$$

The population effect size is, in turn, estimated (γ')with the following sample statistics:

$$\gamma' = \frac{\overline{X}_1 - \overline{X}_2}{SD}$$

where $\overline{X}_1$ = sample mean of Group 1
$\overline{X}_2$ = sample mean of Group 2
SD = pooled standard deviation for both groups

The effect size expresses how far apart the two means are, in standard deviation units. In the example concerning the pulse rate of children in an experimental and a control group, we would compute the following estimated effect size[7]:

$$\gamma' = \frac{95.0 - 105.0}{12.85} = -.78$$

---

[6]Effect size is an important concept in studies that quantitatively integrate the results of several research investigations, a procedure that is referred to as **meta-analysis.** Readers interested in meta-analysis should consult such books as those by Glass, McGaw, and Smith (1981) or Hedges and Olkin (1985).

[7]The computation of the pooled *SD* for this example (12.85) is not shown.

Cohen (1977) has designated some benchmarks for qualitative descriptions of the absolute value of effect sizes. According to Cohen's criteria, an effect size of .20 in a two-group mean-difference situation is considered small, .50 is medium, and .80 is large. Thus, the estimated effect size in our present example, which is nearly .8 SD units, is quite substantial.

Now we have all three components for performing a power analysis: $\alpha = .05$, $n = 10$, and the absolute value of $\gamma' = .78$. We can now estimate the power of the *t*-test by consulting a table in Appendix C, but to use the appendix table we must combine the effect size and sample size to create a new index, delta (δ), which in the present situation is:

$$\delta = \gamma' \sqrt{\frac{n}{2}}$$

In our example, then, delta would be:

$$\delta = .78 \sqrt{\frac{10}{2}} = 1.74$$

Table C–1 presents information on the power of a statistical test as a function of δ and α. To use this table, we find the appropriate value of δ in column 1 and the desired value of α along the top row (for a two-tailed test); the power estimate is at the intersection of the appropriate row and column. For a two-tailed *t*-test with $\alpha = .05$ (column 3) and $\delta = 1.74$, we must look at values of δ for 1.7 and 1.8; we find that power is between .40 and .44, or roughly .42.[8] Since power is $(1 - \beta)$, this means that in our fictitious example the estimated probability of a Type II error (β) is about .58. Nearly six times out of ten with $n = 10$, a false null hypothesis would be retained erroneously, despite the fact that the effect size is quite large. And, in our example, that is exactly what did happen for the two-tailed test.

Since power is influenced by the effect size, sample size, and alpha, it should be clear that a larger sample (or a less stringent α) increases power. Let us suppose, for example, that our results were based on a total sample of 100, with 50 subjects per group rather than 10. In this situation, delta would be

$$\delta = .78 \sqrt{\frac{50}{2}} = 3.90$$

With five times as many subjects, the power for a two-tailed test with $\alpha = .05$ is increased from about .42 to .97. In only 3% of the samples with 50 subjects per group

---

[8] For a one-tailed test, the power is higher. In Table C–1, we find the desired level of α for a one-tailed test in the *bottom row* and then read up. For $\delta = 1.74$, the power for a one-tailed test with $\alpha = .05$ (column 2) is between .52 and .56, or approximately .54.

would a false null hypothesis be erroneously accepted, given the effect size of .78. Just as .05 is considered an acceptable criterion for a Type I error, scientists have generally considered .20 as the standard for a Type II error (i.e., a minimum power of .80).

By performing a power analysis, we are in a better position to evaluate and interpret the nonsignificant result obtained with the two-tailed test. Knowing that the effect size is large and that the power is well below the accepted criterion of .80, it would not be prudent to conclude that the experimental intervention has no merit. The safest conclusion is that the experimental intervention should be tested again with a larger sample of subjects.

As noted earlier, power analysis can also be used during the design phase of a study to estimate sample size requirements to minimize the risk of a Type II error. Although Table C–1 can be used to determine sample size needs, we have prepared a simpler table (Table 6–3) that assumes that the desired power is .80 and that $\alpha = .05$.[9] Suppose, for example, that we wanted to replicate the experimental study of the intervention to reduce children's stress (as measured by pulse rate) prior to the finger-stick. We could use the results obtained in the original study to estimate the sample size requirements in the new study to achieve a power of .80. In Table 6–3, we would first look for the estimated effect size ($\gamma' = .78$) in column 1. Here, our effect size is between the two tabled values of .70 and .80. Thus, for a two-tailed test (column 3), we would need between 25 and 32 subjects *per group* (approximately 26) to achieve the desired power. For a one-tailed test (column 2), we would need between 20 and 26 (about 21) subjects per group.

THE COMPUTER AND TWO-SAMPLE *t*-TEXTS

When there are more than 10 subjects per group—as there usually should be to avoid a Type II error—the manual calculation of the t statistic and other related statistics is tedious, time-consuming, and error-prone. Researchers usually use computers to calculate inferential statistics.

Figure 6–1 shows what a computer printout looks like for an independent groups *t*-test, using the data from our fictitious experimental study of children's pulse rates (Table 6–1).[10] Panel A of this printout shows basic descriptive information—the number of subjects, the mean, the standard deviation, and the standard error of the mean for the dependent variable (KIDPULSE)—for each group of subjects (EXPERIMENTAL

---

[9]Table C–1 should be used for values of α other than .05 and power values other than .80.

[10]The SPSS/PC command that produced the printout in Figure 6–1 is as follows:

```
T-TEST GROUPS = GROUP (1, 2)
    /VARIABLES = KIDPULSE.
```

GROUP is the name of the independent variable, and the parenthetical designation (1,2) tells the computer the codes for the two groups being compared (1 = experimental; 2 = control).

TABLE 6–3. ESTIMATED SAMPLE SIZE REQUIREMENTS AS A FUNCTION OF EFFECT SIZE (Γ') FOR $\alpha = .05$ AND POWER $= .80$

(1) γ'	(2) One-Tailed	(3) Two-Tailed	(1) γ'	(2) One-Tailed	(3) Two-Tailed
.05	5000	6272	.50	50	63
.10	1250	1568	.55	41	52
.15	556	697	.60	35	44
.20	313	392	.70	26	32
.25	200	251	.80	20	25
.30	139	174	.90	15	19
.35	102	128	1.00	13	16
.40	78	98	1.10	10	13
.45	62	77	1.25	8	10

NOTE: The sample sizes shown are the number of subjects per group for a two-sample independent groups t-test.

versus CONTROL). The mean group difference (-10.0000) is shown in Panel B, followed by Levene's test for the homogeneity of variance. This statistic tests the hypothesis that $\sigma_1 = \sigma_2$. Since this statistic is not significant ($p = .719$), we can conclude that the variances of the two groups *are* equal. In other words, the variance of the experimental group (12.428^2) is not significantly different from the variance of the control

```
t-tests for independent samples of   GROUP
```

A
```
                              Number
            Variable          of Cases    Mean        SD       SE of Mean
            -------------------------------------------------------------
            KIDPULSE   CHILDS PULSE RATE

            EXPERIMENTAL      10       95.0000     12.428      3.930
            CONTROL           10      105.0000     11.776      3.724
            -------------------------------------------------------------
```

B
```
       Mean Difference = -10.0000

       Levene's Test for Equality of Variances: F= .134   P= .719
```

C
```
      t-test for Equality of Means                        95%
   Variances  t-value   df    2-Tail Sig   SE of Diff   CI for Diff
   ----------------------------------------------------------------------
    Equal     -1.85     18       .081        5.414       (-21.377, 1.377)
    Unequal   -1.85     17.95    .081        5.414       (-21.377, 1.377)
   ----------------------------------------------------------------------
```

FIGURE 6–1 COMPUTER PRINTOUT FOR INDEPENDENT GROUPS t-TEST

group (11.776^2). Panel C shows the results of the t-test, with the first row presenting information on the pooled variance estimate (i.e., for the equal variance assumption) and the second row showing information for the separate variance estimate (for the unequal variance assumption). If the test for homogeneity of variance *had* been statistically significant, the separate variance estimate would have been the appropriate test. In the present case, the value of t is -1.85 and the two-tailed significance is .081 for both estimates. With $\alpha = .05$ for a two-tailed test, this p value is not statistically significant. (For the one-tailed test, the printed value of p would be halved; i.e., the one-tailed significance would be .0405, which is statistically significant when α is .05.) The next column shows that the estimated standard error of the difference is 5.414. The final column shows the 95% confidence interval (*CI*) for the population mean difference, with the limits of -21.377 and $+1.377$. All of this information corresponds to the manual calculations previously shown in Table 6–1 and in the text. Clearly, using the computer removed much of the drudgery of performing the calculations.

Figure 6–2 presents a computer printout for a dependent groups t-test, using the fictitious data for the direct and indirect blood pressure measurements for 10 subjects (Table 6–2).[11] Once again, the top panel provides basic descriptive information for the dependent variable (blood pressure readings), for the two levels of the independent variable (the two methods of obtaining the measurements, labeled DIRECT and INDIRECT). Panel B shows that the mean paired group difference is 1.3000; the calculated value of t is 1.90, and the exact probability value is .090 for a two-tailed test with 9 *df*—the same results that we obtained through manual computation. Thus, as we concluded earlier, the difference in the two blood pressure measurements is not statistically significant at the .05 level. The bottom entry in Figure 6–2 indicates that the 95% confidence interval for the population difference in blood pressure measurements extends from $-.248$ to $+2.848$.

RESEARCH APPLICATIONS OF THE TWO-SAMPLE *t-TEST*

Researchers use two-sample t-tests extensively. This section examines some of the major applications of t-tests and related statistics, and discusses methods of effectively presenting the information in a research report.

The Uses of *t*-Tests

Many of the dependent variables of interest to nurse researchers are measured on a ratio scale or on a scale that approximates interval characteristics. For example, the majority of biophysiologic measures are ratio-level variables (e.g., blood pressure, heart rate, vi-

---

[11]The SPSS/PC command that produced the printout in Figure 6–2 is as follows:

    T-TEST PAIRS = DIRECT INDIRECT.

```
- - - t-tests for paired samples - - -
```

A

Variable	Number of pairs	Corr	2-tail Sig	Mean	SD	SE of Mean
DIRECT DIRECT BLOOD PRESSURE				129.3000	22.351	7.068
	10	.996	.000			
INDIRECT INDIRECT BLOOD PRESSURE				128.0000	23.017	7.279

B

Mean	Paired Differences SD	SE of Mean	t-value	df	2-tail Sig
1.3000	2.163	.684	1.90	9	.090
95% CI (-.248, 2.848)					

FIGURE 6–2. SPSS COMPUTER PRINTOUT FOR DEPENDENT GROUPS *t*-TEST

tal capacity, bacterial counts), and most measures of psychosocial phenomena are treated as interval-level variables (e.g., scales of depression, stress, and social support). Thus, because the comparison of two group means is common, there are many research situations in which the *t*-test is an analytic option. A few of the major reasons for using the *t*-test are described here.

1. *Answering Research Questions.* The central hypotheses of a research investigation can often be tested by means of a *t*-test. Examples of two-group comparisons include comparing experimental versus control groups, vaginal versus cesarean deliveries, normotensive versus hypertensive patients, men versus women, teenage mothers versus older mothers, and smokers versus nonsmokers. As an actual research example, McCorkle and her colleagues (1994) used *t*-tests to compare two groups of cancer patients (those receiving posthospital home care services versus those not receiving the services) in terms of such outcomes as symptom distress, mental health status, and health perceptions.

2. *Testing for Selection Bias.* It is often important to investigate the extent to which groups being compared are similar with regard to attributes that are extraneous to the research situation. For example, if we were comparing postpartum depression among women who had a vaginal versus a cesarean delivery, it would be important to know whether the two groups were similar with regard to other factors that might affect postpartum depression (e.g., family income, marital satisfaction, predelivery depression, and so on). When the groups being compared are dissimilar on characteristics that are related to the dependent variable, the bias known as **selection bias** can confound the results. Researchers often test for such biases to enhance the interpretability of the findings. When the interval-level or ratio-level background characteristics of two comparison groups are being analyzed for selection bias, the independent groups *t*-test is usually appropriate. As an actual research example, Wineman, Durand, and Steiner (1994) conducted a study in which the substantive

research question concerned the coping behaviors of persons with multiple sclerosis versus those with a spinal cord injury. To test for possible selection biases, the researchers used *t*-tests to compare the two groups with regard to such background characteristics as age, number of years since diagnosis, and functional ability.

3. *Testing for Other Biases.* Selection bias is one of the most pervasive problems in scientific research, but other biases are also important and can often be analyzed using *t*-tests. For example, in studies that involve the collection of data at several points in time, the researcher often tests for **attrition bias**—that is, the nonrandom loss of subjects from the study over time. A test for attrition bias often involves a comparison of the characteristics of subjects who remained in the study with those of subjects who did not remain, using a *t*-test. Another example is a test for **nonresponse bias.** Let us suppose that 100 patients were asked to participate in a study but only 70 agreed to do so. To examine whether nonresponse was systematically related to the patients' characteristics (i.e., whether those who volunteered to participate were a biased subset of all those who were invited), a *t*-test could be used to compare the background characteristics of the two groups. The same procedure can be used to test for nonresponse bias with regard to specific research questions among subjects in a study. That is, the people responding to a question can be compared to those with missing data for that question. Procedures for handling missing data problems vary depending on whether the missing data are random or are systematically related to characteristics of the nonresponders, and so it is often wise to test for nonresponse bias. Another bias that sometimes arises when data for a study are collected over an extended time period is **cohort bias**—that is, systematic differences between those who entered a study early and those who entered later. To test for such a bias, the researcher can divide the sample in half based on time of enrollment, and then perform a *t*-test that compares the characteristics of the two cohorts.

4. *Validity Assessments.* When a new instrument is being developed to measure an abstract construct, the researcher usually wants to determine whether the instrument is really measuring what it is supposed to be measuring—that is, whether the instrument has **construct validity.** One approach to construct validation is to use the **known groups technique,** which is a method of examining whether the new measure discriminates between groups that are expected to be different with regard to the underlying construct. For example, an instrument to assess functional ability would be considered suspect if it failed to discriminate between people with and without emphysema. In this example, a *t*-test would be used to compare the mean functional ability scores of the two groups; statistically significant differences would provide one piece of evidence regarding the instrument's validity.

Table 6–4 presents actual research examples in which two-sample *t*-tests were used for various purposes in recent studies.

The Presentation of *t*-Tests in Research Reports

When there are only two or three *t*-tests to report, it is more efficient to present the results in the text of the report rather than in a table. However, tables are extremely effi-

TABLE 6–4. RESEARCH EXAMPLES OF TWO-SAMPLE *t*-TESTS

Question	Purpose of *t*-Test	Results
Is there a difference in the number of bacterial colonies present on skin cultures following air drying versus blot drying povidone-iodine—prepared skin sites? (Workman, 1995)	To address a substantive question	No differences in number of bacterial colonies ($t(18) < 1.0$, $p = .23$)
Are the characteristics of those in the experimental group (caregivers and care receivers in a special intervention) comparable to those in the control group? (Archbold et al., 1995)	To test for selection bias	Caregivers in experimental group were older than those in control group ($t(20) = 2.6$, $p < .05$)
Are the characteristics of infants who remain in a longitudinal study for a 24-month follow-up comparable to those of infants who dropped out of the study? (Koniak-Griffin, Ludington-Hoe, & Verzemnieks, 1995)	To test for attrition bias	No significant differences for most traits, but infants who remained had higher 4-month development scores than dropouts ($t(48) = -2.62$, $p = .01$)
Are the characteristics of patients who agreed to participate in a study of the use of Emergency Medical Services comparable to those who declined? (Meischke et al., 1995)	To test for nonresponse bias	Patients who agreed to participate were younger than those who did not ($t(3615) = 8.2$, $p < .05$)
Is the Braden Scale effective in discriminating those who do and do not develop pressure sores? (Braden & Bergstrom, 1994)	To assess the validity of a measure via known groups	Patients who developed pressure sores had lower Braden scores than those who did not ($t(100) = 5.18$, $p < .0001$)

cient when two groups are being compared in terms of multiple dependent variables (or multiple background characteristics, if the table is summarizing tests for bias).

By convention, researchers communicate four pieces of information when reporting the results of statistical tests, including *t*-tests and other tests described in this book: (1) the name of the test statistic, (2) the value of the computed statistic, (3) the degrees of freedom, and (4) the significance level. The value of the statistic is usually presented to two decimal places (e.g., $t = 1.54$). Degrees of freedom are either referenced directly (e.g., $df = 99$) or are indicated in parentheses just before the value of the test statistic [e.g., $t(99) = 1.54$]. The following are two examples of how the results for the fictitious study on the experimental preparation to alleviate children's preprocedure distress might be reported, depending on which set of hypotheses were tested:

1. A two-tailed *t*-test for independent groups was used to test for differences in measures of distress among children in the experimental and control groups. The *t*-test revealed that the mean preprocedure pulse rate of children in the experimental group (95.0) was not significantly differ-

ent from that of children in the control group (105.0), $t(18) = -1.85, p > .05$. The strength of the relationship between group status and the children's pulse rate, as indicated by a point biserial correlation coefficient, was .40.

2. A one-tailed t-test for independent groups was used to test the hypothesis that the experimental intervention would have a favorable effect on measures of the children's distress. The t-test revealed that the mean preprocedure pulse rate of children in the experimental group (95.0) was significantly lower than that of children in the control group (105.0), $t(18) = -1.85, p < .05$. The strength of the relationship between group status and the children's pulse rate, as indicated by a point biserial correlation coefficient, was .40.

In both examples, the test statistic is identified, and the means for the two groups are reported. The value of the t statistic is presented, with degrees of freedom shown in parentheses. Then the significance is reported, both in words ("not significantly different from" and "significantly lower than") and by the probability level ($p > .05$ or $p < .05$). The final sentence provides the reader with information about the magnitude of the relationship between the independent and dependent variables. In practice, researchers often fail to present this information, but its inclusion can be very informative.

When a power analysis has been performed, the results are often reported in the discussion section of a report rather than in the results section, because the primary utility of such an analysis is to facilitate interpretation of the findings. For example, the following might be included in the discussion section of a report if the two-tailed test had been used to test the nondirectional hypothesis:

> Although the two groups did not have significantly different preprocedure pulse rates, it is possible that the small sample size in the present study resulted in an inadequate test of the effectiveness of the intervention. The point biserial correlation coefficient suggests that the relationship between the intervention and the children's pulse rates was moderately strong. Moreover, a power analysis revealed that the effect size was fairly large (.78). Statistical power was found to be .42, which is substantially below the conventional standard of .80. It is recommended that the study be replicated with a larger sample of children, inasmuch as the present study is inconclusive.

When t-tests are presented in tables, the results are often reported in conjunction with information about means and standard deviations. Table 6–5 illustrates what a table might be like for a study in which there are multiple dependent variables. In this table, there are four different dependent variables, listed in the first column. For each dependent variable, the table presents the means and SDs for the two groups, followed by the value of the computed t statistic and its associated p level. The degrees of freedom for the four tests are noted in a footnote. It is usually unnecessary to specify that the pooled variance formula was used, since this is the standard formula. However, if the separate variance estimate was used because the homogeneity of variance assumption was untenable, this should be pointed out in the table. Note that Table 6–5 could be expanded to include an additional column to report the values of r_{pb}.

TABLE 6–5. EXAMPLE OF TABLE WITH TWO-TAILED INDEPENDENT GROUPS t-TESTS

Outcome Measure	Experimental ($n = 10$)		Control ($n = 10$)		t	p^*
	Mean	SD	Mean	SD		
Preprocedure Pulse (bpm)	95.0	12.4	105.0	11.8	−1.85	NS
Postprocedure Pulse (bpm)	92.3	11.9	97.5	12.7	−0.98	NS
Nurses' Preprocedure Rating of Distress**	7.9	2.1	8.8	1.5	−2.22	<.05
Nurses' Postprocedure Rating of Distress**	5.6	1.8	5.9	1.7	−0.78	NS

*Two-tailed p values, $df = 18$
**Distress was rated from 0 (no distress) to 10 (extreme distress).

Results of t-Tests Comparing Experimental and Control Groups on Four Outcomes

RESEARCH EXAMPLE

Examples of t-tests abound in nursing research journals. Below is a recent example of an interesting study in which t-tests were used for several purposes.

Roberts, Krouse, and Michaud (1995) examined differences in patient perceptions of two types of nurse-patient interactive styles. The investigators were interested in determining the effectiveness of negotiated approaches designed to equalize the provider-patient interaction and to foster patient participation in health care decisions. A sample of 98 university students with upper respiratory symptoms participated in either an actively negotiated process of decision making ($n = 53$) or a nonnegotiated process ($n = 45$) with a nurse. Seven nurses involved in the delivery of care were trained in both the negotiated and nonnegotiated approaches. Each nurse was assigned, on a random basis, to an approach for an entire day and all patients seen by a given nurse on a given day received the same approach.

To examine the possibility of selection biases, the investigators used t-tests to compare the age and grade level of patients in the two groups. There were no significant group differences in terms of these background characteristics. With respect to the substantive analyses, the two groups were compared in terms of scores on the Nurse-Patient Interactive Tool (N-PIT), a scale designed to assess patients' perceptions of the nurse-patient interaction with regard to four separately scored dimensions: Agreement with Plan, Control versus Powerlessness, Intent to Comply, and Feelings of Coercion. The group means and SDs and the t-test results are shown in Table 6–6. As this table indicates, there was a significant difference on the Control versus Powerlessness subscale of the N-PIT scale. Subjects in the negotiated group perceived greater control over decisions occurring within the interaction with the nurse than did subjects in the nonnegotiated condition. The researchers concluded that the results suggest that nurses can engage in an active negotiation process with patients and influence feelings of control in decision making.

TABLE 6–6.   MEANS, SDS AND *t*-TEST RESULTS FOR NURSE-PATIENT INTERACTION TOOL SCALES

N-PIT Scale	Negotiated Group (n = 53)		Nonnegotiated Group (n = 45)		t	p
	M	SD	M	SD		
Agreement with Plan	3.75	0.31	3.67	0.37	1.06	NS
Control vs. Powerlessness	3.42	0.41	3.07	0.51	3.57	<.001
Intent to Comply	3.70	0.31	3.69	0.39	0.18	NS
Feelings of Coercion	1.40	0.51	1.42	0.46	0.23	NS

Adapted from Table 2 of Roberts et al.'s (1995) report.

SUMMARY

The **two-sample *t*-test** is used to make inferences about the equality of two population means, based on two sample means. The basic null and alternative hypotheses being tested are H_0: $\mu_1 = \mu_2$ and H_1: $\mu_1 \neq \mu_2$.

The *t*-test is used when there are two levels of a nominal-level independent variable (e.g., experimental versus control), and when the dependent variable is measured on an interval or ratio scale. A *t*-test assumes that subjects are randomly sampled, that the dependent variable is normally distributed, and that there is **homogeneity of variances** of the two populations—i.e., that variability in the two populations is comparable. The last assumption is robust to violation when the two sample sizes are similar.

The basic formula for computing the *t* statistic has the differences between the two sample means in the numerator and the estimated **standard error of the difference** in the denominator. Computationally, there are different formulas for different situations. When the subjects in the two groups are independently sampled and are not connected to one another in any way, the **independent groups *t*-test** is appropriate. When the assumption of homogeneity of variances is valid in an independent groups *t*-test, the **pooled variance estimate** is used to estimate the standard error of the difference. When the variances are not equal and sample sizes are dissimilar, a **separate variance estimate** should be used. A third formula is used for the **dependent groups *t*-test,** which is appropriate when the subjects in the two groups are the same people or are paired in some systematic way (e.g., husbands in Group 1 and wives in Group 2). In all three cases, the computed value of *t* is compared to a tabled value to determine if the group means are significantly different from one another.

A *t*-test indicates the existence of a relationship between the independent (group) variable and the dependent variable. A statistic known as the **point biserial correlation**

coefficient (r_{pb}), which is readily computed from the value of t, can be used as an index of the magnitude of the relationship.

Power analysis, which yields an estimate of the probability of rejecting the null hypothesis, is a useful procedure when the results of a *t*-test are nonsignificant (and also in the determination of sample size requirements during the planning phase of a study). A power analysis uses information on the **effect size** (the magnitude of the effect of the independent variable on the dependent variable, or γ), sample size, and α to yield an estimate of the power of the statistical test. An acceptable risk for a Type II error, by convention, is .20 (i.e., power = .80).

Researchers use *t*-tests for directly addressing their research questions when the main questions involve the comparison of two group means. A *t*-test can also be used in two-group situations to test for **selection bias, attrition bias, nonresponse bias,** and **cohort bias,** and in some situations to assess the **construct validity** of an instrument via the **known groups technique.**

EXERCISES

The following exercises cover concepts presented in this chapter. Exercises indicated with a dagger (†) can be checked against answers appearing in Appendix A. Additionally, Chapter 6 of the accompanying *Applications Manual* offers supplementary exercises, including ones that require computer analysis of a data set on diskette.

† 1. For which of the following situations is the independent groups *t*-test appropriate (if inappropriate, indicate why):
   a. The independent variable (IV) is type of stimulation for premature infants (auditory versus visual versus tactile); the dependent variable (DV) is cardiac responsiveness.
   b. The IV is parental role (mother versus father); the DV is degree of bonding with the infant.
   c. The IV is infant birth weight (low birth weight versus normal birth weight); the DV is number of days absent from school in first grade.
   d. The IV is gender (men versus women); the DV is compliance versus noncompliance with a medication regimen.
   e. The IV is radiation treatments (before versus after treatment); the DV is cancer patients' perceived self-efficacy.

† 2. For which of the following situations is the dependent groups *t*-test appropriate (if inappropriate, indicate why):
   a. The independent variable (IV) is presence or absence of conversation directed to comatose patients; the dependent variable (DV) is the patients' intracranial pressure.
   b. The IV is role (patient versus nurse); the DV is perceived functional ability of the patient 48 hours after surgery.

    c. The IV is time since incarceration (1 month versus 3 months versus 6 months); the DV is body weight.

    d. The IV is menopausal status group (premenopausal versus postmenopausal); the DV is attitudes toward menopause.

    e. The IV is nap therapy for narcoleptics (before versus after treatment); the DV is unplanned naps the following week (had versus did not have an unplanned nap).

† 3. Suppose we wanted to test the hypothesis that a control group of cancer patients (Group 1) would report higher mean pain ratings than an experimental group receiving special massage treatments (Group 2). Using the following information, compute a t statistic for independent groups:

$$\overline{X}_1 = 78.5 \qquad s^2_1 = 42.1 \qquad n_1 = 25$$
$$\overline{X}_2 = 72.1 \qquad s^2_2 = 39.7 \qquad n_2 = 25$$

What are the degrees of freedom and the value of t? Using $\alpha = .05$ for a two-tailed test, is this t statistically significant?

† 4. What is the point biserial correlation coefficient for the t-test described in Exercise 3? How would you describe the strength of the relationship between the independent and dependent variables qualitatively?

5. Write one or two sentences that could be used to report the results obtained for the t-test in Exercise 3.

† 6. For Exercise 3, assume that the pooled SD for the two groups is 7.05. Perform a power analysis, indicating the value of γ' and δ. What is the power of the t-test for $\alpha = .05$ and conversely, what is the probability of a Type II error (β)?

† 7. For each of the following t values, indicate whether the t is statistically significant for a two-tailed test, at the specified alpha:

    a. $t = 2.40$, $df = 25$, $\alpha = .01$

    b. $t = 2.40$, $df = 25$, $\alpha = .05$

    c. $t = 5.52$, $df = 10$, $\alpha = .01$

    d. $t = 2.02$, $df = 150$, $\alpha = .05$

† 8. State the critical (tabled) value of t that would be used to reject the null hypothesis of equality of population means, for an independent groups t-test under each of the following conditions:

    a. $H_1: \mu_1 \neq \mu_2$; $n_1 = 20$, $n_2 = 20$; $\alpha = .05$

    b. $H_1: \mu_1 > \mu_2$; $n_1 = 30$, $n_2 = 30$; $\alpha = .01$

    c. $H_1: \mu_1 \neq \mu_2$; $n_1 = 10$, $n_2 = 10$; $\alpha = .01$

    d. $H_1: \mu_1 > \mu_2$; $n_1 = 60$, $n_2 = 60$; $\alpha = .05$

    e. $H_1: \mu_1 \neq \mu_2$; $n_1 = 15$, $n_2 = 10$; $\alpha = .01$

† 9. For a power analysis, assume that $\gamma = .50$, $\alpha = .05$ for a two-tailed test, and the number of subjects in each of two groups is 18. What is the value of δ and $(1 - \beta)$? For the same effect size (.50), approximately what n per group would be needed to achieve power $= .80$?

† 10. The following are data for subcutaneous oxygen tension ($PSCO_2$, measured in mm Hg) 12 hours after the start of two protocols, administered to the same 10 healthy subjects in random order—a bed rest protocol and a high-activity protocol:

Subject	Bed Rest	High Activity
1	67	63
2	68	62
3	70	69
4	66	64
5	68	67
6	62	60
7	71	66
8	65	65
9	67	63
10	65	62

Compute the t statistic for dependent groups and the df for these data. Using $\alpha = .05$ for a two-tailed test, is this t statistically significant?

11. Write one or two sentences that could be used to report the results obtained for the t-test in Exercise 10.

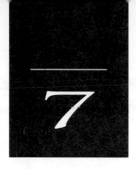

Analysis of Variance

Many research situations involve the comparison of the means of two groups—a situation in which the use of the two-sample t-test is appropriate, as discussed in Chapter 6. However, the t-test is not appropriate when the means of three or more groups are compared, or when the means for two groups are compared at two or more points in time in a single analysis (e.g., an experimental and control group being compared both before and after an intervention). In these and several other research situations, a technique known as **analysis of variance** (often abbreviated **ANOVA**) is used to draw inferences about population means.

BASIC CONCEPTS FOR ANOVA

Suppose we were interested in examining the effects of body position on cardiovascular responses during the Valsalva maneuver. One hundred healthy adults are randomly assigned to four position groups: Group 1, lying flat on back; Group 2, sitting partially upright in bed at a 45° angle; Group 3, lying on right side with legs slightly bent; and Group 4, sitting in a chair at a 90° angle. Various measures of cardiovascular functioning are taken during the strain phase of the maneuver. Suppose we found the following mean systolic blood pressure readings for the four groups:

- Group 1: 124.8 mm Hg
- Group 2: 119.6 mm Hg
- Group 3: 130.8 mm Hg
- Group 4, 125.4 mm Hg

Our research question is whether the observed group differences in systolic blood pressure (the dependent variable) reflect true effects of body position (the independent variable) in the four populations (a hypothetically infinite number of people in the different body positions), or whether the mean sample differences are the result of random fluctuations.

We cannot answer this question by merely looking at the means. The group means *are* different from one another, but such differences might have occurred simply by chance. We cannot use a *t*-test to test group differences in this example, because there are more than two groups. In such a situation, an analysis of variance is appropriate.

The Null and Alternative Hypotheses

The null hypothesis in an ANOVA situation is similar to that for a *t*-test; it posits the absence of a relationship between the independent and dependent variables. In other words, the null hypothesis is that the population means are equal. Stated formally, the null hypothesis for the example at hand[1] is:

$$H_0: \mu_1 = \mu_2 = \mu_3 = \mu_4$$

where μ_1 = population mean for Group 1 (those lying flat on back)
μ_2 = population mean for Group 2 (those sitting partially upright at a 45° angle)
μ_3 = population mean for Group 3 (those lying on side)
μ_4 = population mean for Group 4 (those sitting in a chair at a 90° angle)

The basic alternative hypothesis is:

$$H_1: \text{not } H_0$$

The alternative hypothesis simply states that H_0, taken as a whole, is not true. There are many alternative ways in which the null hypothesis might be false. For example, it might be that only $\mu_1 \neq \mu_2$, or that $\mu_3 \neq \mu_4$, or that all four population means are unequal, and so on. The alternative hypothesis does not distinguish among these various possibilities, but rather asserts that a relationship exists between the independent and dependent variables such that the population means are *not* all equal.

In an ANOVA situation, the null hypothesis is tested using procedures that are similar in principle to those discussed in the previous two chapters. That is, we begin by using sample data to compute a test statistic. The statistic is treated as a "score" in a sampling distribution that assumes the null hypothesis is true. If the statistic falls within the rejec-

---

[1]More generally, we can say that the null hypothesis for a multigroup situation is:

$$H_0: \mu_1 = \mu_2 = \ldots = \mu_k$$

where μ = means of each population
k = number of populations being compared

tion region of the sampling distribution (i.e., the "score" is improbable if the null is true), then we reject the null hypothesis and conclude that the group means are not equal.

Assumptions and Requirements for Analysis of Variance

Like the *t*-test, analysis of variance is appropriate when the dependent variable is measured on an interval or ratio scale, and when the independent variable is a nominal-level variable. The independent variable also could be an ordinal-level variable with a small number of levels—e.g., very low-birth-weight, low-birth-weight, or normal-birth-weight infants.

The assumptions for using ANOVA are also similar to those that applied to the *t*-test. First, it is assumed that the groups being compared are composed of randomly sampled subjects. Second, the dependent variable is assumed to be normally distributed in the population's. Third, the populations from which the groups are drawn are assumed to have equal variances, an assumption that allows the variability from each group to be pooled into a single estimate of the population variance. ANOVA is robust with regard to these last two assumptions. That is, ANOVA tends to yield accurate results even if the population distributions depart moderately from normality (especially if the number of cases in a group is large) and even if the population variances are not homogeneous (provided that the group sample sizes are not very small and are about equal).

One further assumption is relevant for between-subjects designs: it is assumed that the subjects in the groups have been independently sampled. In other words, for a simple analysis of variance it is assumed that the subjects in the groups are not the same people, nor are they matched with individuals who are in the other groups. However, if the same subjects are exposed to three or more different conditions, or measured at three or more points in time, a **repeated measures analysis of variance** (analogous to the dependent groups *t*-test) can be used.

Given the similarities between the *t*-test and ANOVA, you may wonder why researchers do not simply use a series of *t*-tests. For instance, in our example of body positions, we could use a *t*-test to compare Group 1 with Group 2, Group 2 with Group 3, and so on. One problem with this approach is that it is tedious. A total of six separate *t* statistics would have to be computed with four groups (10 would be required with five groups, and 15 would be needed with six groups). More importantly, the risk of a Type I error would increase; the more statistical tests you perform, the more likely it is that some will be significant simply by chance. When the level of significance is .05, there is a 1 in 20 chance that one *t*-test will yield a significant result even when the null hypothesis is true. If we performed six *t*-tests to compare all possible pairs of the four body position groups, the probability of committing a Type I error is much greater than the desired .05 (in fact, in this case, the probability would be .18). Thus, multiple *t*-tests should not be used to compare group means when there are more than two groups.

General Logic of Analysis of Variance

Computationally, an analysis of variance is more complex than a *t*-test. However, the underlying logic of ANOVA is not very difficult. It involves analyzing and sorting out differences in scores (i.e., variability) among the subjects in the sample.

A simple example will be used to illustrate this process. Suppose we had a sample of myocardial infarction patients in a music therapy group (Group 1), a relaxation therapy group (Group 2), or a control group (Group 3). Fifteen subjects are randomly assigned to the three groups and then their stress levels are measured to determine if the interventions were effective in minimizing stress. The stress scores can range from a low of 0 for no stress to 10 for extreme stress. Some fictitious data are shown in Table 7–1.

It is clear from inspecting this table that there is considerable intersubject variation. The scores cover the full range from 0 to 10. There is variation both within the groups (for example, in Group 1 the scores range from 0 to 6) and between the groups (the group means range from 2.0 to 7.0). In analysis of variance, **between-group variance** (differences between groups) is contrasted to **within-group variance** (differences between subjects within the groups). When the null hypothesis is true, between-group variation is about the same as within-group variation because all variation stems simply from random fluctuations. But when the groups are systematically different from one another, between-group variation tends to be large, relative to variation within the groups. The larger the between-group variance is in comparison to the within-group variance, the greater is the likelihood that the samples do not come from populations with equal means.

Together, the within-group and between-group variations are the two sources that contribute to total variation in a distribution of scores. We can illustrate the concept of **partitioning variance** into source components more clearly with a concrete example for one subject. Let us consider the score of the first person in Group 1. This person's stress score (0) deviates from the mean of Group 1 (3.0) by 3.0 points (within-group

TABLE 7–1. STRESS SCORES IN THREE GROUPS: EXAMPLE OF WITHIN-GROUP AND BETWEEN-GROUP VARIATION

Group 1 Music Therapy	Group 2 Relaxation Therapy	Group 3 Controls	
0	1	5	
6	4	6	
2	3	10	*Within-group variation*
4	2	8	
3	0	6	
$\Sigma X = 15$	10	35	
$\bar{X}_1 = 3.0$	$\bar{X}_2 = 2.0$	$\bar{X}_3 = 7.0$	Grand Mean $(\bar{X}_G) = 4.0$

←————————— *Between-group variation* —————————→

variation). The Group 1 mean (3.0) deviates from the overall sample **grand mean** $(\bar{X}_G)$ of 4.0 by 1.0 point (between-group variation). The first subject's score (0) deviates from the grand mean of 4.0 (total variation) by 4.0 points. In other words, for this subject:

$$
\begin{aligned}
\text{Within-group variation} &= 3.0 \\
\text{Between-group variation} &= \underline{1.0} \\
\text{Total variation} &= 4.0
\end{aligned}
$$

When deviations such as these are obtained for everyone in the sample, we can put the information together to construct a ratio of aggregate between-group variation to within-group variation. The value of this ratio—referred to as the ***F* ratio**[2]—constitutes the sample statistic that is tested in ANOVA. In other words:

$$
F = \frac{\text{Between-group variability}}{\text{Within-group variability}}
$$

If the group means are all equal, there is no between-group variability; the F will be zero and will lead to acceptance of the null hypothesis. But if the mean scores in the groups are different, the question is whether the differences are sufficiently large to justify the conclusion that the population means are different. When the group means in a sample are different, the differences can be attributable to two factors: (1) sampling error and (2) the effect of the independent variable. Thus, we can also portray the F ratio as follows:

$$
F = \frac{\text{Effect of independent variable} + \text{Sampling error}}{\text{Sampling error}}
$$

This equation illustrates that if the independent variable has no effect on the dependent variable, the between-group estimate of variance would reflect only sampling error—just as the within-group estimate of variance would reflect sampling error. The result would be a value of F that, over the long run, would be 1.0. By contrast, if the independent variable has an effect, the F ratio would, over the long run, be greater than 1.0.

Sampling Distribution of the *F* Ratio

Suppose we had three populations (1, 2, and 3), where the means of the three populations on a variable of interest were equal (i.e., $\mu_1 = \mu_2 = \mu_3$; the null hypothesis is true). If we selected a random sample of 50 individuals from each population and computed an F ratio (through computational procedures to be described subsequently), we would

---

[2]The statistic was named F in honor of Sir Ronald Fisher, who first described the analysis of variance procedure and the relevant sampling distributions.

expect the value of F to be about 1.0—but, because of sampling fluctuation, it would not always be exactly 1.0 (e.g., it might be .79 or 1.24). If we repeatedly sampled 50 subjects from the populations, we would have a large number of F ratios, which could be treated as "scores" in a sampling distribution. Such a distribution is called the **sampling distribution of the F ratio.** With this sampling distribution, we can determine which values of F are improbable when the null hypothesis is true.

Just as there are different sampling distributions of t for different degrees of freedom, there are also different F distributions depending on the number of groups and the number of subjects in each group. Thus, the sampling distribution of the F ratio can take on many different shapes, but in all cases F distributions are unimodal and positively skewed. Two examples of F distributions are shown in Figure 7–1. In both cases, the areas corresponding to 5% and 1% of the distributions are indicated. These would constitute the critical regions for rejecting the null hypothesis for $\alpha = .05$ and $.01$, respectively. As was true for the t statistic, researchers use prepared tables to determine the minimum value of F needed to reject the null hypothesis.

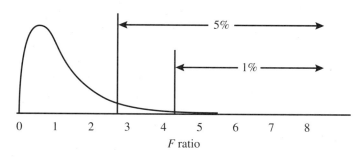

F Distribution: Number of groups = 5; Number of subjects per group = 5

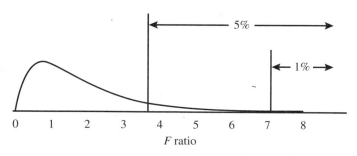

F Distribution: Number of groups = 7; Number of subjects per group = 2

FIGURE 7–1.   EXAMPLES OF *F*-RATIO SAMPLING DISTRIBUTIONS WITH DIFFERENT *N*s AND NUMBER OF GROUPS

PROCEDURES AND CALCULATIONS FOR ANOVA

There are several situations in which an analysis of variance can be used. While each requires somewhat different calculations, the underlying logic is similar to that presented in the previous section. Here, we present a detailed computational example for the simplest form of ANOVA, and subsequently we discuss on a more limited basis two other types of applications.

One-Way ANOVA

The simplest (and most common) ANOVA situation involves the comparison of group means for three or more independent groups,[3] such as in our examples of the effect of body positions on systolic blood pressure and of the effect of different therapies on stress scores. These situations call for a **one-way analysis of variance.** The phrase "one-way" signifies that there is a single independent variable whose effect on a dependent variable is under study.

The calculation of the F statistic for the one-way ANOVA involves computing several deviation scores that are then squared—similar to the procedures for computing the variance and SD. We will work through one computational example, using the data on stress scores from Table 7–1.

Table 7–2 shows all the computations required for the ANOVA. The computational formula for the F statistic involves a concept known as the **sum of squares,** which is the sum of the squared deviations around a mean. The **sum of squares within** or SS_W (shown in panel A of Table 7–2) captures the variation of each individual subject relative to the mean of his or her group—that is, the within-group variability. To find the value of SS_W, we first compute a group mean ($\overline{X}$), subtract this value from each individual score to obtain deviation scores (x), square the deviation scores (x^2), and then sum the squares within each group (Σx^2). In our example, the sum of the squared within-group deviation scores is 20.0 for Group 1, 10.0 for Group 2, and 16.0 for Group 3. Then, the summed, squared deviations for each group are themselves added, to yield the value for SS_W. Here, $SS_W = 46.0 \, (20.0 + 10.0 + 16.0).$[4]

---

[3]Actually, ANOVA can also be used when there are only two groups, although the t-test is generally used in a two-group situation. In fact, for two independent groups, the F distribution and the t distribution are mathematically related such that:

$$F = t^2$$

[4]A formula that can be used to compute SS_W is as follows:

$$SS_W = \Sigma x_1^2 + \Sigma x_2^2 + \ldots + \Sigma x_k^2$$

where x = deviation scores of each subject from the respective group mean
k = number of groups

TABLE 7–2. STRESS SCORES IN THREE GROUPS: COMPUTATION OF THE F STATISTIC

A. *Deviations from Group Means (Within-Group Variation)*

Group 1 Music Therapy			Group 2 Relaxation Therapy			Group 3 Controls		
X	$X - \bar{X}_1$	x_1^2	X	$X - \bar{X}_2$	x_2^2	X	$X - \bar{X}_3$	x_3^2
0	−3	9	1	−1	1	5	−2	4
6	3	9	4	2	4	6	−1	1
2	−1	1	3	1	1	10	3	9
4	1	1	2	0	0	8	1	1
3	0	0	0	−2	4	6	−1	1
$\bar{X} = 3.0$			2.0			7.0		Grand Mean $(\bar{X}_G) = 4.0$
$\Sigma x^2 =$		20.0			10.0		16.0	$SS_W = 46.0$

B. *Deviations from Grand Mean*
(Total Variation)

X	$X - \bar{X}_G$	x_G^2
0	−4	16
6	2	4
2	−2	4
4	0	0
3	−1	1
1	−3	9
4	0	0
3	−1	1
2	−2	4
0	−4	16
5	1	1
6	2	4
10	6	36
8	4	16
6	2	4
$\bar{X}_G = 4.0$		$SS_T = 116.0$

C. *Deviation of Group Means from Grand Mean*
(Between-Group Variation)

$\bar{X}$	$\bar{X} - \bar{X}_G$	x_G^2	n	$(x_G^2 \times n)$
3.0	−1	1	5	5.0
2.0	−2	4	5	20.0
7.0	3	9	5	45.0
$\bar{X}_G = 4.0$				$SS_B = 70.0$

D. *F Ratio*

$SS_B = 70.0$ $df_B = 2$ $MS_B = 35.0$

$SS_W = 46.0$ $df_W = 12$ $MS_W = 3.83$

$SS_T = 116.0$

$F = 9.13$

The **sum of squares between** or SS_B (shown in panel C of Table 7–2) captures the variation of the group means relative to the grand mean—that is, the between-group variability. The SS_B component is obtained by first subtracting the value of the grand mean $(\bar{X}_G)$ from each group mean $(\bar{X})$ and then squaring this deviation score (x_G^2). In our example, the mean of 3.0 for Group 1 is subtracted from the grand mean of 4.0, and then the deviation score (-1.0) is squared to yield 1.0. Since we need a between-group value for each subject, this value is multiplied by group size (here $n = 5$), to yield the value of 5.0. When the same process is carried out for each group, the values are added together to obtain the sum of squares between. In this example, $SS_B = 70.0\,(5.0 + 20.0 + 45.0)$.[5]

Although it is not necessary to calculate a **total sum of squares (SS_T)** to compute the F statistic, it is useful to see that SS_W and SS_B, when added, comprise the total variability in the distribution of sample scores. Panel B of Table 7–2 shows the calculation of SS_T, which captures the variation of all individual scores relative to the grand mean. The grand mean ($\overline{X}_G$) is first subtracted from each of the 15 scores, these deviation scores are squared, and then the sum across subjects is computed. In our example, $SS_T = 116.0$. It can be shown that total variability has been partitioned into a between component and a within component:

$$SS_W + SS_B = SS_T$$
$$46.0 + 70.0 = 116.0$$

We now have almost everything that is needed to compute the F statistic. The formula for F is:

$$F = \frac{SS_B\,/\,df_B}{SS_W\,/\,df_W}$$

where SS_B = sum of squares between
SS_W = sum of squares within
df_B = degrees of freedom between
df_W = degrees of freedom within

As this formula indicates, the two sums of squares are divided by their respective degrees of freedom. The formulas for computing degrees of freedom for a one-way ANOVA are:

$$df_B = k - 1$$
$$df_W = N - k$$

---

[5]An alternative formula that can be used to compute SS_B is:

$$SS_B = \left[\frac{(\Sigma X_1)^2}{n_1} + \frac{(\Sigma X_2)^2}{n_2} + \ldots + \frac{(\Sigma X_k)^2}{n_k} \right] - \frac{(\Sigma X_{Tot})^2}{N}$$

where $X_1, X_2, \ldots, X_k$ = individual scores in groups $1, 2, \ldots, k$
k = number of groups
X_{Tot} = individual scores for all subjects
n = number of subjects in each group
N = total number of subjects in sample

where k = number of groups
N = total number of subjects in the study

In the present example, then, we can compute F as follows:

$$F = \frac{70.0 / (3 - 1)}{46.0 / (15 - 3)} = \frac{35.0}{3.83} = 9.13$$

Before discussing the procedures for determining whether this F statistic is statistically significant, we should explain a special ANOVA term—**mean square.** By dividing the sum of the squared deviations by degrees of freedom, we are essentially computing an "average" (or mean) amount of variation—much as we do when we compute the variance for a variable. The specific name of the numerator for the F statistic is the **mean square between**—the average amount of between-group variation. The **mean square within,** the term in the denominator, is the average amount of within-group variation. Thus, the formula for computing F could also be presented as:

$$F = \frac{MS_B}{MS_W}$$

where MS_B = mean square between
MS_W = mean square within

In our example, the computed F of 9.13 is greater than 1.0—the value that would be expected if the null hypothesis were true. We must consult a table to determine if the computed F is sufficiently large to reject the null hypothesis. Table B–3 in Appendix B presents the critical values for the F distribution for various degrees of freedom and three values of α (.05, .01, and .001). To use this table, you first find the page corresponding to the desired significance level. Next, reading across the top row, find the column for the appropriate degrees of freedom between. Then, reading down the left-most column, find the row for the appropriate degrees of freedom within. The critical value is at the intersection of the column and row. In our example, let us assume that $\alpha = .05$. With $df_B = 2$ and $df_W = 12$, the critical value of F for $\alpha = .05$ is 3.88. Our computed value of F—9.13—is larger than the tabled value. Therefore, we can reject the null hypothesis that the three group means are equal. In fewer than 5 samples out of 100 would the F statistic be this large if the null hypothesis were true.

The rejection of the null hypothesis, based on the ANOVA procedure, tells us only that the population means are probably unequal. We cannot at this point conclude that each group differs significantly from every other group. For example, we cannot assert that $\mu_1 \neq \mu_2 \neq \mu_3$. Other procedures, discussed later in this chapter, are needed to help us determine the nature of the inequality between group means.

Two-Way ANOVA

One-way ANOVA is used to test the effect of a single independent variable on a dependent variable. When the effects of two or more independent variables on a dependent variable are being studied simultaneously, **multifactor ANOVA** can be used. Usually, a multifactor ANOVA is described as being of a specific number of factors (i.e., independent variables). The most common multifactor ANOVA is the **two-way ANOVA,** which involves two independent variables. Multifactor analysis of variance rarely involves more than three independent variables. For the purposes of simplicity, we will focus our discussion on the two-way ANOVA, although the concepts can be extended to more than two factors, as appropriate.

Two-way ANOVAs can be used with various research designs. For example, both of the independent variables could be experimentally manipulated by the researcher, with subjects assigned to different combinations of the two independent variables (a **factorial design**). Alternatively, one variable might be manipulated while the other is not, such as when males versus females are randomly assigned separately to treatment groups (a **randomized block design**). A two-way ANOVA could also be used when neither independent variable is experimentally manipulated (e.g., males versus females for the first independent variable, smokers versus nonsmokers for the second independent variable).[6] In general, then, a two-way ANOVA can be used when there are two nominal-level independent variables.

Because the calculations for a two-way ANOVA are cumbersome, we do not attempt to completely work through a computational example here. However, we will use a concrete example to highlight the logic and central features of the two-way ANOVA.

Suppose that we wanted to compare the relative efficacy of the two treatments for reducing stress in myocardial infarction patients—music therapy and relaxation therapy—without the control group. We will call the type-of-treatment variable Factor A, with two levels. At the same time, however, we want to know whether the treatments are more effective if they are administered in the morning or in the evening. The time-of-treatment variable, Factor B, also has two levels—which means that the design can be described as a 2×2 design (two levels of Factor A by two levels of Factor B). In this study, subjects will be randomly assigned to one of the four groups. Some fictitious data for this study for

---

[6]By tradition, data from an experimental study (i.e., a study in which the researcher manipulates the independent variable) are usually analyzed by analysis of variance, but data from a nonexperimental study are more likely to be analyzed by alternative statistical procedures that are discussed later in this book.

20 subjects—5 per group—are presented in Table 7–3. As this table indicates, the mean for the music therapy treatment (2.0) is lower than the mean for the relaxation therapy treatment (3.0). The means for the morning treatments and the evening treatments are identical (2.5). But the lowest mean stress score is observed among those who received the music therapy in the evening (1.0), while the highest mean is observed among those who received relaxation treatment in the evening (4.0).

In a factorial design such as this one, the researcher is testing three null hypotheses. The first concerns the equality of population means for the type-of-treatment factor, across both times of administration. That is, the null hypothesis is that the mean stress score for those in music therapy is the same as that for those in relaxation therapy. The second null hypothesis concerns the equality of population means for the time-of-treatment factor, across both types of treatment. This null hypothesis stipulates that the mean for morning treatment is the same as the mean for evening treatment.

The third null hypothesis, called an **interaction hypothesis,** is more complex. It concerns the joint effects, or interaction, of Factors A and B. Interaction concerns whether the effect of one independent variable is consistent for every level of a second independent variable. A major advantage of a two-way ANOVA is that researchers can directly examine such interaction effects. If each independent variable was examined separately in two different studies, it would not be possible to test for interactions. In our present example, the question is whether the two therapies have the same effects at different times of day. Perhaps music therapy is more effective in the morning and relaxation therapy is more effective in the evening, for example. For interactions, the null hypothesis is that the population means for each combination of factors are equal.

TABLE 7–3. STRESS SCORES IN A 2 × 2 DESIGN: EXAMPLE OF TWO-WAY ANOVA

Factor B—Time of Treatment	Factor A—Treatment		
	Music Therapy (1)	Relaxation Therapy (2)	
Morning (1)	0 6 Group 1 2 $\bar{X}_{11} = 3.0$ 4 3	1 4 Group 2 3 $\bar{X}_{21} = 2.0$ 2 0	Morning Subjects $\bar{X}_{B1} = 2.5$
Evening (2)	1 2 Group 3 1 $\bar{X}_{12} = 1.0$ 0 1	2 6 Group 4 5 $\bar{X}_{22} = 4.0$ 4 3	Evening Subjects $\bar{X}_{B2} = 2.5$
	Music Therapy Subjects $\bar{X}_{A1} = 2.0$	Relaxation Therapy Subjects $\bar{X}_{A2} = 3.0$	All Subjects $\bar{X}_{G} = 2.5$

The logic of the two-way ANOVA is similar to that for the one-way ANOVA; the total variation in the scores of the subjects is partitioned into different components, and between-group variation is contrasted with within-group variation. However, now there are four, rather than two, components contributing to variability, because there are three sources of between-group variation:

$$SS_T = SS_W + SS_A + SS_B + SS_{AB}$$

where SS_T = total variability
  SS_W = within-group variability
  SS_A = variability associated with Factor A
  SS_B = variability associated with Factor B
  SS_{AB} = variability associated with the interaction of Factors A and B

Because there are three hypotheses being tested, three F ratios must be computed. In each case, the sum of squares (i.e., the squared deviation around the relevant mean) is divided by its respective degrees of freedom to yield a mean square. Then, the mean square for the three "between" components is divided by the mean square within, to yield the values of F. As an example, the F ratio for the interaction term is:

$$F_{AB} = \frac{SS_{AB} / df_{AB}}{SS_W / df_W} = \frac{MS_{AB}}{MS_W}$$

Although computational formulas are not presented,[7] the three F values for the data presented in Table 7–3 are as follows:

$$F_A = 1.91 \qquad F_B = 0.00 \qquad F_{AB} = 7.62$$

The final step, as before, is to compare these computed values of F to tabled values for the F distribution. For the Fs corresponding to the two independent variables (called the **main effects**), the degrees of freedom equals the number of levels, minus 1. For both independent variables in our example there are two levels, so $df_A = 1$ and $df_B = 1$. The formula for degrees of freedom for the test of the interaction effects is:

$$df_{AB} = (k_A - 1)(k_B - 1)$$

where k_A = number of levels of Factor A
  k_B = number of levels of Factor B

---

[7]Those who might wish to perform a two-way ANOVA manually can find the appropriate formulas in such texts as Jaccard and Becker (1990), McCall (1990), or Welkowitz et al. (1991).

Thus, in the present example, the *df* for the interaction term is $(2 - 1)(2 - 1) = 1$. For the within-group term, the *df* is:

$$df_W = N - (df_A + df_B + df_{AB} + 1)$$

In the present example, then

$$df_W = 20 - (1 + 1 + 1 + 1) = 16$$

Let us assume that we are testing the three hypotheses using $\alpha = .05$. Consulting Table B–3, we find that with 1 and 16 degrees of freedom—which is the appropriate *df* for all three tests—the critical value of *F* is 4.49. For our three computed *F* values, only the *F* for the interaction term (7.62) is statistically significant. We must accept the null hypotheses that the population means for type of treatment are equal, and that the population means for the time of treatment are equal. However, we reject the null hypothesis that stipulates equality of population means across treatment type conjoined with treatment time.

Interaction is a concept that merits further discussion. The interaction effect of type and time of treatment refers to the effect of particular joint combinations of the two factors. It represents the joint effect over and above the sum of the separate effects. This concept can be readily demonstrated graphically.

Suppose, for the sake of illustration, that the means for the music therapy were 2.0 in the morning and 1.0 in the evening, and that the means for the relaxation therapy were 3.0 in the morning and 2.0 in the evening. These means are graphed in Figure 7–2 (A). This graph shows a situation in which there is no interaction; music and relaxation therapy have similar effects on stress relative to one another, regardless of time of day (i.e., the means are lower for music therapy than for relaxation therapy both in the morning and in the evening). Furthermore, the two time periods have similar effects on stress relative to one another, regardless of which therapy is used (i.e., stress is lower in the evening than in the morning for both music and relaxation therapy). There are no unique effects associated with a particular combination of the two factors.

The graph in Figure 7–2 (B) displays the means we obtained in our example (i.e., for the data shown in Table 7–3). The crossed lines illustrate the interaction; stress is lowest among those who got music therapy in the evening (but music therapy was *less* effective in the morning), while stress is highest among those who got relaxation therapy in the evening (but relaxation therapy was *more* effective in the morning).

Figure 7–2 (C) illustrates a different type of interaction. In this graph, the mean stress scores are 2.0 in the morning, regardless of which type of treatment is administered. In the evening, however, the mean for the relaxation therapy is 4.0, while that for the music therapy is 1.0. Thus, in this second interaction, type of treatment has a different effect on stress only in the evening. Of course, we cannot tell whether an interaction effect is statistically significant simply by plotting the means on a graph. Only a full sta-

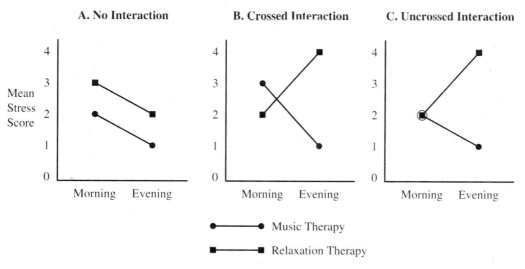

FIGURE 7–2. GRAPHS ILLUSTRATING INTERACTION EFFECTS

tistical analysis via the two-way ANOVA would enable us to draw conclusions about interactions in the population.

Repeated Measures ANOVA

Repeated measures analysis of variance (sometimes abbreviated **RANOVA**) is used for within-subjects designs. That is, it is used when means are computed for the same subjects at three or more points in time. A one-way repeated measures ANOVA is an extension of the dependent groups *t*-test, just as the simple one-way ANOVA is an extension of the independent groups *t*-test.

In some nonexperimental studies, multiple measures of the same subjects are taken to capture the effects of the passage of time (e.g., mean weight of low-birth-weight infants at 1 week, 2 weeks, and 3 weeks after birth). In other situations, multiple measures are obtained as a design feature in an experimental **repeated measures design,** which allows subjects to serve as their own controls. For instance, in an example we used earlier to illustrate a one-way ANOVA, we randomly assigned 100 subjects to four different body position groups (25 subjects per group), and then compared the groups with respect to systolic blood pressure readings during the Valsalva maneuver. This design is depicted in Table 7–4 (A). However, we could have designed the study so that the same subjects were used to assess blood pressure in all four body positions, thereby reducing the total number of subjects needed (Design B of Table 7–4). Ideally, the subjects would be randomly assigned to different *orderings* of body position to rule out systematic carryover and ordering effects.

TABLE 7–4. ILLUSTRATIONS OF DIFFERENT DESIGNS USING ANOVA AND RANOVA

A. Independent Groups One-Way ANOVA
Independent Variable: Body position—4 independent groups (between subjects)

	Group 1 Lying down $\bar{X}_1$	Group 2 Sitting at 45° $\bar{X}_2$	Group 3 Lying on side $\bar{X}_3$	Group 4 Sitting at 90° $\bar{X}_4$

B. One-Way Repeated Measures
Independent Variable: Body position—same subjects in 4 body positions (within subjects)

	Position 1 Lying down $\bar{X}_1$	Position 2 Sitting at 45° $\bar{X}_2$	Position 3 Lying on side $\bar{X}_3$	Position 4 Sitting at 90° $\bar{X}_4$

C. Two-Way Mixed Design
Independent Variable$_1$: Time of measurement—before vs. during Valsalva maneuver (within subjects)
Independent Variable$_2$: Body position—4 independent groups (between subjects)

	Group 1 Lying down	Group 2 Sitting at 45°	Group 3 Lying on side	Group 4 Sitting at 90°
Before	$\bar{X}_{1Before}$	$\bar{X}_{2Before}$	$\bar{X}_{3Before}$	$\bar{X}_{4Before}$
During	$\bar{X}_{1During}$	$\bar{X}_{2During}$	$\bar{X}_{3During}$	$\bar{X}_{4During}$

D. Two-Way Within Subjects Repeated Measures
Independent Variable$_1$: Time of measurement—before vs. during Valsalva maneuver (within subjects)
Independent Variable$_2$: Body position—same subjects in random ordering of 4 body positions (within subjects)

	Position 1 Lying down	Position 2 Sitting at 45°	Position 3 Lying on side	Position 4 Sitting at 90°
Before	$\bar{X}_{1Before}$	$\bar{X}_{2Before}$	$\bar{X}_{3Before}$	$\bar{X}_{4Before}$
During	$\bar{X}_{1During}$	$\bar{X}_{2During}$	$\bar{X}_{3During}$	$\bar{X}_{4During}$

Repeated measures ANOVA can also be used in a multifactor situation. We could have a two-way RANOVA in which one factor was within-subjects and the second factor was between-subjects—a design that is sometimes referred to as a **mixed design.** For example, we might want to have measures of blood pressure before versus during the Valsalva maneuver as the first factor (within-subjects) and body position for four independent groups as the second factor (between-subjects) as illustrated in Table 7–4 (C). Finally, both factors can be within-subjects—e.g., before and during measures of blood pressure for the same subjects in different orderings of body position, as in Table 7–4 (D).

For the sake of simplicity, we focus here on the one-way repeated measures situation—Table 7–4 (B). Suppose, for example, that we wanted to compare three interventions for preterm infants, with regard to effects on the infants' heart rates: (1) nonnutritive sucking, (2) nonnutritive sucking plus rocking, or (3) rocking alone. Using an

TABLE 7–5. HEART RATES FOR INFANTS IN THREE CONDITIONS: EXAMPLE OF ONE-WAY REPEATED MEASURES ANOVA

Subject	Condition 1 Nonnutritive Sucking	Condition 2 Nonnutritive Sucking Plus Rocking	Condition 3 Rocking	
1	152	155	170	
2	132	135	140	
3	175	180	202	
4	165	170	183	
5	143	149	152	
6	160	171	188	
7	150	148	161	
8	157	162	176	
9	138	143	152	
10	171	176	191	
11	148	151	157	
12	145	144	168	
	$\Sigma X = 1836$	1884	2040	
	$\bar{X}_1 = 153.0$	$\bar{X}_2 = 157.0$	$\bar{X}_3 = 170.0$	$\bar{X}_G = 160.0$

experimental repeated measures design, the 12 infants participating in the study are randomly assigned to six different orderings of the three treatments.[8] Heart rate measurements are taken on all 12 infants following each condition. The null hypothesis for this study is that type of intervention does not influence heart rate (i.e., $\mu_1 = \mu_2 = \mu_3$). The alternative hypothesis is that there is a relationship between type of intervention and heart rate (i.e., that the three population means are not all equal). Some fictitious heart rate data for the 12 infants are shown in Table 7–5. As these data indicate, there is variability in heart rates both across subjects within each condition, and across the three treatment conditions within subjects.

As was true with other ANOVA situations, the total variability in the dependent variable can be represented by the total sum of squares, which can be partitioned into different contributing components. In a repeated measures ANOVA, there are three sources of variation contributing to total variability:

$$SS_{total} = SS_{conditions} + SS_{subjects} + SS_{error}$$

Conceptually, the **sum of squares conditions** is equivalent to the sum of squares between in a between-subjects design; it represents the effect of the independent variable. The **sum of squares error** is conceptually similar to the sum of squares within in

---

[8]The six possible orderings are as follows: 123, 132, 213, 231, 312, and 321.

regular ANOVA, in that they both represent the effect of random fluctuations. The third component, **sum of squares subjects,** has no counterpart in a simple one-way ANOVA, because the subjects in the groups being compared in a regular ANOVA are not the same people. The $SS_{subjects}$ term captures individual differences, the effects of which are consistent across conditions. That is, regardless of conditions, some infants tend to have high heart rates (e.g., Subject 3) and others tend to have low heart rates (e.g., Subject 2). Because the effect of individual differences can be identified and statistically isolated from the error (random fluctuation) term, a repeated measure ANOVA results in a more sensitive test of the relationship between the independent and dependent variables than an ANOVA with independent groups. By statistical isolation, we mean that the variability attributable to individual differences is not part of the denominator in computing the F statistic. The formula for the F statistic that is used to estimate the equivalence of population means across conditions contrasts $SS_{conditions}$ with SS_{error}:

$$F = \frac{SS_{conditions} / df_{conditions}}{SS_{error} / df_{error}} = \frac{MS_{conditions}}{MS_{error}}$$

The degrees of freedom in a one-way RANOVA can be easily computed using the following formulas:

$$df_{conditions} = k - 1$$
$$df_{subjects} = N - 1$$
$$df_{error} = (k - 1)(N - 1)$$

Thus, in our present example, the degrees of freedom for conditions and error, which we need to calculate F, are:

$$df_{conditions} = 3 - 1 = 2$$
$$df_{error} = (3 - 1)(12 - 1) = 22$$

We do not show the actual formulas and calculations for the sums of squares,[9] but the values are $SS_{conditions} = 1896.0$ and $SS_{error} = 368.0$. We can compute the following F statistic for our current example:

$$F = \frac{1896.0 / 2}{368.0 / 22} = \frac{948.0}{16.73} = 56.67$$

As before, we must compare the computed F statistic to a tabled F value. Let us suppose that our significance criterion for this example is .001. With 2 and 22 degrees of freedom and $\alpha = .001$, the tabled value of F is 9.61. Thus, since the computed value

---

[9]Those wishing to perform the calculations for the RANOVA manually can consult such texts as Jaccard and Becker (1990).

of F is substantially larger than the critical value, we can conclude that the differences in the condition means are statistically significant. In fewer than 1 out of 1000 samples from the population of preterm infants subjected to the three conditions would we expect to find an F of 56.67 on the basis of chance alone, if the null hypothesis were really true.

OTHER STATISTICAL ISSUES RELATING TO ANOVA

As with t-tests, ANOVA addresses the very important question of whether or not a relationship exists between the independent and dependent variables. In this section we discuss other related analyses that address questions about the nature and strength of the relationship, and about the power of the statistical test.

The Nature of the Relationship

The F test for analysis of variance considers the null hypothesis of equality of means against the alternative that not all the population means are equal. The rejection of the null indicates the probability that there is a relationship between the independent and dependent variable—that is, that the population means are unequal. A significant F test does not, however, tell us which pairs of means are significantly different from one another. To determine the exact nature of the relationship between the independent and dependent variables, additional analyses are necessary.

A number of alternative tests—referred to as **multiple comparison procedures**—are available for comparing pairs of means.[10] These procedures are preferable to using multiple t-tests because they offer better protection against the risk of a Type I error (i.e., an incorrect inference that differences between pairs of means are significant). Among the most common multiple comparison tests are the **Scheffé test, Tukey's honestly significant difference (HSD) test, the Student-Newman-Keuls test, Duncan's test, and Fisher's least significant difference (LSD) test.** There is some controversy among statisticians regarding which of these tests has the greatest accuracy (see Kirk, 1968; Winer, 1971), but a full discussion of the alternatives and their merits and shortcomings is beyond the scope of this book.

One of the simplest multiple comparison methods is Fisher's LSD test, also known as the **protected t-test.** When an ANOVA F test is statistically significant, pairs of

---

[10]The multiple comparison procedures we discuss here sometimes are referred to as **post hoc tests** or **a posteriori comparisons,** which are comparisons completed *after* an ANOVA has produced a significant result. Occasionally, however, researchers decide in advance which specific pairs of means they want to compare. That is, they have a substantive interest in comparing certain groups, prior to learning what the data look like. In this situation, the researcher might use **a priori comparisons,** which are also referred to in some statistics books as **planned comparisons.** The advantage of planned comparisons is that they increase the power and precision of the data analysis. Planned comparisons are briefly discussed in Chapter 11, and are more fully described in Hays (1988); they can be performed in SPSS using the CONTRAST command within the ONEWAY procedure and through the REGRESSION procedure.

means can be compared by t-tests that use the MS_W term from ANOVA as the estimate of the population variance. We will use as an illustration our earlier example for the simple one-way ANOVA, which compared mean stress scores for three groups of subjects (a music therapy group, a relaxation therapy group, and a control group). In this example, we rejected the null hypothesis that all the population means were equal, so we can proceed to compare the three pairs of means using protected t-tests. The following are the three null and alternative hypotheses being tested via the multiple comparisons:

$$H_0: \mu_1 = \mu_2 \qquad H_1: \mu_1 \neq \mu_2$$
$$H_0: \mu_1 = \mu_3 \qquad H_1: \mu_1 \neq \mu_3$$
$$H_0: \mu_2 = \mu_3 \qquad H_1: \mu_2 \neq \mu_3$$

The formula for Fisher's LSD procedure (here, using notation for the first null hypothesis) is:

$$t = \frac{\overline{X}_1 - \overline{X}_2}{\sqrt{MS_W \left(\dfrac{1}{n_1} + \dfrac{1}{n_2} \right)}}$$

where $\overline{X}_1, \overline{X}_2$ = means for Groups 1 and 2
MS_W = mean square within from ANOVA
n_1, n_2 = number of cases for Groups 1 and 2

Table 7–6, which summarizes the calculation of the protected ts for the three pairs of means in our example, shows that the computed values are 0.81 ($\overline{X}_1$ versus $\overline{X}_2$), -3.23 ($\overline{X}_1$ versus $\overline{X}_3$), and -4.04 ($\overline{X}_2$ versus $\overline{X}_3$). To find the critical value in the t table, we need to compute the degrees of freedom as follows:

$$df = N - k = df_W$$

In our present example, then, $df = 15 - 3 = 12$. Consulting Table B–2 of Appendix B, we find that the critical value of t for $df = 12$ and $\alpha = .05$ is 2.18. Thus, the difference between the means of Groups 1 and 3 *and* the difference between the means of Groups 2 and 3 are statistically significant. Both therapies resulted in significantly lower stress scores than the absence of a therapy (i.e., the control condition). However, the means for Groups 1 and 2 were not significantly different.

When the group sample sizes are equal, as they are in the present example, it becomes possible to determine what least significant difference *(LSD)* between means is needed for significance, using the following formula:

$$LSD = t_{tabled} \sqrt{MS_W (2 \div n)}$$

TABLE 7–6. COMPUTATION OF FISHER'S *LSD* TEST FOR STRESS SCORE EXAMPLE

	Music Therapy	Relaxation Therapy	Controls
Means:	$\bar{X}_1 = 3.0$	$\bar{X}_2 = 2.0$	$\bar{X}_3 = 7.0$
ns:	$n_1 = 5$	$n_2 = 5$	$n_3 = 5$
	$MS_W = 3.83$		

Pairs	Calculation of protected t
$\bar{X}_1$ and $\bar{X}_2$	$t = \dfrac{3.0 - 2.0}{\sqrt{3.83\left(\dfrac{1}{5} + \dfrac{1}{5}\right)}} = \dfrac{1.0}{\sqrt{3.83\,(.40)}} = 0.81$
$\bar{X}_1$ and $\bar{X}_3$	$t = \dfrac{3.0 - 7.0}{\sqrt{3.83\left(\dfrac{1}{5} + \dfrac{1}{5}\right)}} = \dfrac{-4.0}{\sqrt{3.83\,(.40)}} = -3.23$
$\bar{X}_2$ and $\bar{X}_3$	$t = \dfrac{2.0 - 7.0}{\sqrt{3.83\left(\dfrac{1}{5} + \dfrac{1}{5}\right)}} = \dfrac{-5.0}{\sqrt{3.83\,(.40)}} = -4.04$

Thus, in our example:

$$LSD = 2.18\sqrt{3.83\,(.40)} = 2.70$$

All pairs of means differing by at least 2.70 points on the stress scale would be significantly different from one another at $\alpha = .05$.

Protected t-tests can also be used in factorial designs when there are significant F tests that require clarification. Of course, when the design is 2×2, as in the example we presented in this chapter (type of treatment $\times$ time of treatment), there is no need to clarify the nature of effect for the two factors; if the F test for a factor is significant, then the two levels of the factor are significantly different. However, a significant interaction (which we observed in our example) *does* require clarification. Here, our concern is determining significant differences between the *cells* (combinations of the two factors). We can use the previously presented formula to compute the *LSD*.[11] Although we do not show the computations, the value for MS_W is 2.63, and, for $df = 16$ (20 subjects minus 4 cells) and $\alpha = .05$, the critical (tabled) value of t is 2.12. Thus:

$$LSD = 2.12\sqrt{2.63\,(2 \div 5)} = 2.17$$

The *LSD* indicates that all differences between cell means that are greater than or equal to 2.17 are significant at the .05 level. Referring back to Table 7–3, we find that only one

---

[11]The *LSD* formula also can be used in multifactor ANOVA when one of the factors having three or more levels results in a significant F test, so long as the group ns are equal.

pair of cell means is significantly different; in the evening only, music therapy is signif-icantly different from relaxation therapy. The mean difference of 3.0 between these two cell means (4.0 − 1.0) exceeds the *LSD* of 2.17.

The Magnitude of the Relationship

As noted in Chapter 6, statistical significance does not necessarily mean a powerful re-lationship between the independent and dependent variables. When a researcher wishes to determine the magnitude of a relationship in the context of an ANOVA situation, the index that is sometimes used is **eta-squared** (eta^2). Eta^2 can be readily computed from the components for the F formula. For a one-way analysis of variance:

$$\text{eta}^2 = \frac{SS_B}{SS_T}$$

From this formula, we can see that eta^2 represents the proportion of the total vari-ability in a set of scores that is attributable to the independent variable (i.e., variability between groups). It may be recalled from Chapter 4 that the correlation coefficient r, when squared, represents the proportion of variability in the dependent variable ex-plained by the independent variable, and thus r^2 and eta^2 are conceptually equivalent.

For our example in which stress scores for three groups of subjects (music therapy, relaxation therapy, controls) were compared, we can compute the following:

$$\text{eta}^2 = \frac{70.0}{116.0} = .60$$

This is a powerful relationship: 60% of the variability in stress scores is attributable to the different treatments. It is unusual to find a value of eta^2 this high in actual interven-tion studies; our example was deliberately contrived to yield significant results. With a small N (again, deliberately small to minimize computational complexity), a very strong relationship was needed to achieve statistical significance.

The procedures for computing eta^2 for a multifactor ANOVA are analogous to those just described; the sum of squares attributable to the factor (or interaction) of in-terest is contrasted with the total sum of squares. For a one-way repeated measures ANOVA, the formula for computing eta^2 is:

$$\text{eta}^2 = \frac{SS_{\text{conditions}}}{SS_{\text{conditions}} + SS_{\text{error}}}$$

Eta^2 in the context of a one-way RANOVA represents the proportion of variability in the dependent variable attributable to the independent variable *after variability asso-ciated with individual differences has been removed*. In our example of the one-way

RANOVA, which involved assigning infants to different orderings of three different interventions (Table 7–5), we find that:

$$\text{eta}^2 = \frac{1896.0}{1896.0 + 368.0} = .84$$

This tells us that 84% of the variability in the infants' heart rates is attributable to the different conditions, after the influence of individual differences in heart rates is removed. Such information about the magnitude of the relationship greatly enhances our ability to interpret the results of the ANOVA.

Power and ANOVA

As discussed in Chapter 6, power analysis is used to estimate the probability of rejecting the null hypothesis. When used during the design phase of a study, power analysis helps the researcher to make decisions about an appropriate sample size to minimize the risk of a Type II error. When applied after a study is completed, power analysis helps with the interpretation of results, particularly when group differences are not statistically significant.

There are alternative methods of doing a power analysis in an ANOVA context. The simplest approach involves estimation of the population eta^2, which can be used directly as the estimate of effect size. When a power analysis is performed to obtain sample size requirements, eta^2 must be *estimated* from other sources, such as a similar prior study or the researcher's own pilot work. However, when power analysis is performed following an ANOVA for interpretive purposes, the eta^2 from the study itself can be used as the population estimate of the effect size.

To illustrate a power analysis for a one-way ANOVA, let us use our now-familiar example of stress scores in three treatment groups. The eta^2 (effect size) for the data shown in Table 7–2 was found to be .60. To determine the power of the ANOVA, we also need the significance criterion ($\alpha = .05$) and group size ($n = 5$). Table 7–7, which is appropriate when $\alpha = .05$ and the number of groups is 3, allows us to determine the power in this example. The top row presents estimates of the population eta^2. Reading down in the column headed by .60, we look for the group size of 5, and then read across to the left to find the estimate of power. Although the group size of 5 does not appear in the table, we can interpolate; 5 falls between 4 and 6, so power is between the corresponding power values of .95 and .99. The power analysis indicates, then, that the risk of having committed a Type II error in this study was under 5%—well below the standard acceptable risk of 20%.

To use Table 7–7 to estimate sample size requirements, you would enter the table at the row for the desired power (usually .80) and the column for the estimated value of eta^2. The value at the intersection indicates the needed sample size *per group*. For ex-

TABLE 7–7. POWER TABLE FOR ANOVA, FOR THREE GROUPS WITH $\alpha = .05$*

	POPULATION ETA²													
POWER	.01	.03	.05	.07	.10	.15	.20	.25	.30	.40	.50	.60	.70	.80
.10	22	8	5	4	3	2	2	2	—	—	—	—	—	—
.25	76	26	16	9	7	5	4	3	—	—	—	—	—	—
.50	165	55	32	23	16	10	8	6	5	3	3	2	2	—
.70	255	84	50	35	24	16	11	9	7	5	4	3	2	2
.80	319	105	62	44	30	19	14	11	9	6	4	3	2	2
.90	417	137	81	57	39	25	18	14	11	7	5	4	3	2
.95	511	168	99	69	47	30	22	16	13	9	6	4	3	2
.99	708	232	137	96	65	41	29	22	18	12	8	6	4	3

*Entries in body of table are for *n*, the number of subjects *per group.*

ample, if the estimated eta² were .10, 30 subjects per group would be needed to achieve a power of .80.

As was true in the *t*-test situation, Cohen (1977) has established some criteria for describing effect sizes in an ANOVA context. Cohen's conventional values for small, medium, and large effects correspond to values of eta² of .01, .06, and .14, respectively. Thus, it is clear that the eta² of .60 that we obtained in our example is very large, indeed. When a researcher uses power analysis to estimate sample size requirements and cannot find specific information for estimating the population effect size, the researcher can, as a last resort, use Cohen's conventions if there is evidence supporting an assumption that effects will be small, medium, or large.

When there are four, five, or six groups or when alpha is .01, the power tables in Table C–2 in Appendix C should be used in lieu of Table 7–7. When the number of groups is larger than 6, or when the design calls for a repeated measures ANOVA, the power tables in Cohen (1977) or Jaccard and Becker (1990) can be consulted.

THE COMPUTER AND ANOVA

With the widespread availability of computers, analyses of variance are rarely done by hand. In this section, we present several printouts for ANOVAs that were performed by a computer.

One-Way ANOVA

For a simple (between-subjects) one-way ANOVA, statistical software packages often have several alternative programs.[12] Figure 7–3 presents the computer printout for

[12]For example, in SPSS, one-way ANOVAs can be performed using the ONEWAY, MEANS, and ANOVA commands.

```
          - - - - - - - - - - O N E W A Y - -     - - - - - -
```

A
```
      Variable  STRESS      STRESS SCORES
   By Variable  TYPE        TYPE OF THERAPY
```

Analysis of Variance

Source	D.F.	Sum of Squares	Mean Squares	F Ratio	F Prob.
Between Groups	2	70.0000	35.0000	9.1304	.0039
Within Groups	12	46.0000	3.8333		
Total	14	116.0000			

B

Group	Count	Mean	Standard Deviation	Standard Error	95 Pct Conf Int for Mean		
MUSIC	5	3.0000	2.2361	1.0000	.2236	To	5.7764
RELAX	5	2.0000	1.5811	.7071	.0368	To	3.9632
CONTROL	5	7.0000	2.0000	.8944	4.5167	To	9.4833
Total	15	4.0000	2.8785	.7432	2.4059	To	5.5941

Group	Minimum	Maximum
MUSIC	.0000	6.0000
RELAX	.0000	4.0000
CONTROL	5.0000	10.0000
Total	.0000	10.0000

C   Levene Test for Homogeneity of Variances

Statistic	df1	df2	2-tail Sig.
.2424	2	12	.788

D   Multiple Range Test

LSD Procedure
Ranges for the   .050 level -

```
        3.08    3.08
```

The ranges above are table ranges.
The value actually compared with Mean(J)-Mean(I) is..
        1.3844 * Range * Sqrt(1/N(I) + 1/N(J))

(*) Denotes pairs of groups significantly different at the .050 level

```
                          R M C
                          E U O
                          L S N
                          A I T
                          X C R
                              O
                              L

        Mean      Group

        2.0000    RELAX
        3.0000    MUSIC
        7.0000    CONTROL    * *
```

FIGURE 7-3. COMPUTER PRINTOUT OF A ONE-WAY ANOVA

analysis of the stress score data presented in Table 7–2. This program was chosen because it is the one that performs multiple comparison procedures (although the other SPSS/PC alternatives provide information on eta^2, while this one does not).[13] Panel A of the printout presents a summary of the ANOVA for stress scores by treatment group; it shows the *df*s, sums of squares, mean squares, value of the computed F statistic, and the actual probability value for F. The computed F shown here, 9.1304, is essentially the same as the F we computed manually, to a greater degree of precision. The probability level (.0039) indicates that in only about 4 samples out of 1000 (more precisely, 39 out of 10,000) would an F this large be found by chance alone.

Panel B shows descriptive information for the three groups, as well as for the total sample. The descriptive statistics include the number of cases (count), mean, *SD,* standard error, the 95% confidence interval around each mean, and the range of score values (minimum and maximum).

Panel C shows the results of the Levene test for the homogeneity of the group variances. This statistic tests the null hypothesis that the variances of the three populations are equal—one of the assumptions of the ANOVA procedure. Since the test statistic (.2424) is not significant ($p = .788$), we can conclude that the three populations have equal variances.

The last panel (D) shows the results of the *LSD* multiple comparison procedure.[14] This panel does not show the actual value of the protected *t* or *LSD,*[15] but it does show (via the asterisks at the intersection of the row labeled CONTROL and the columns la-

---

[13]The SPSS/PC command that produced the printout for Figure 7–3 is as follows:

```
ONEWAY VARIABLES=STRESS BY TYPE (1,3)
    /RANGES=LSD
    /OPTIONS = 6
    /STATISTICS=1,3.
```

[14]SPSS/PC offers seven different multiple comparison options. In the present example, all seven procedures resulted in the same conclusion—i.e., that the control group was significantly different from both treatment groups, but that music therapy was not significantly different from relaxation therapy.

[15]However, the value of *LSD* can be computed from the information displayed. The printout indicates that the tabled range is 3.08 and that the value actually compared with Mean(J) − Mean (I) is:

$$1.3844 \times \text{Range} \times \sqrt{1/N(I) + 1/N(J)}$$

Thus,

$$1.3844 \times 3.08 \times \sqrt{1/5 + 1/5} = 2.70$$

This is the same value for the *LSD* that we computed manually.

beled RELAX and MUSIC) that both therapy groups are significantly different from controls, at the .05 level.

Two-Way ANOVA

Figure 7–4 presents the computer printout for the two-way analysis of variance applied to the data in Table 7–3.[16] The top panel displays all the means, i.e., the mean stress scores for the total sample, for the two levels of TIME (collapsed across type of treatment), for the two levels of TYPE (collapsed across time), and for the four individual cells of TYPE $\times$ TIME. The numbers in parentheses indicate the number of subjects contributing to the respective means.

Panel B summarizes the analysis of variance. It shows the sum of squares, *df*, mean square, *F*, and significance of *F* for the various components of total variability in stress scores. The first line, labeled "Main Effects," captures all variation attributable to *either* of the two factors. The next two lines decompose the main effects into the separate TIME and TYPE factors. Since there was no variability in the two levels of the TIME factor (both means were 2.50), the sum of squares, mean square, and value of *F* are 0.00. The probability of obtaining these group means if the null hypothesis was true is 1.00. For the TYPE factor, the probability of obtaining an *F* of 1.905 is .187; in about 19 samples out of 100, we could expect to find an F this large simply on the basis of chance. This is an unacceptably high risk of a Type I error, so we accept the null hypothesis that the two types of treatment are equivalent. Next, we find information relating to the interaction of the two factors. The *F* of 7.619 has a significance of .014. Thus, with $\alpha = .05$, we can reject the null hypothesis that the cell means are equal. All of the variability attributable to the main effects *and* the interaction effect is shown on the line labeled "Explained," and all of the variability attributable to other factors (i.e., within-group variability) is shown on the line labeled "Residual." The mean square within, against which all other mean squares are compared, is 2.625.

To conserve space, we do not show in Figure 7–4 a third panel from the printout that provided various other pieces of information, including information on eta^2 for the two main effects. The value of eta^2 for the time-of-treatment factor was 0.00 (which is not surprising, given that the morning and evening means are identical), and the value of eta^2 for the type-of-treatment factor was $.27^2$, or .07. This indicates a modest relationship between stress scores and type of treatment; only 7% of the variability in stress scores can be attributed to treatment type.

---

[16]The following SPSS/PC command produced the printout for Figure 7–4:

```
ANOVA VARIABLES=STRESS BY TIME (1,2) TYPE (1,2)
    /STATISTICS = 3.
```

```
              * * *  C E L L   M E A N S  * * *

                 STRESS    STRESS SCORES
A          BY TIME         TIME OF TREATMENT
                 TYPE      TYPE OF THERAPY


   TOTAL POPULATION

       2.50
   (    20)


   TIME
           1            2

       2.50         2.50
   (    10) (       10)


   TYPE
           1            2

       2.00         3.00
   (    10) (       10)



           TYPE
                 1            2
   TIME
       1         3.00         2.00
               (    5) (       5)

       2         1.00         4.00
               (    5) (       5)
```

B   * * * A N A L Y S I S   O F   V A R I A N C E * * *

```
                 STRESS    STRESS SCORES
           BY    TIME      TIME OF TREATMENT
                 TYPE      TYPE OF THERAPY
```

Source of Variation	Sum of Squares	DF	Mean Square	F	Signif of F
Main Effects	5.000	2	2.500	.952	.407
TIME	.000	1	.000	.000	1.000
TYPE	5.000	1	5.000	1.905	.187
2-way Interactions	20.000	1	20.000	7.619	.014
TIME TYPE	20.000	1	20.000	7.619	.014
Explained	25.000	3	8.333	3.175	.053
Residual	42.000	16	2.625		
Total	67.000	19	3.526		

FIGURE 7–4.   COMPUTER PRINTOUT OF A TWO-WAY ANOVA

A - - - - - - - - - -
Cell Means and Standard Deviations
Variable .. NNS   HEART RATE FOR NONNUTRITIVE SUCKING

	Mean	Std. Dev.	N
For entire sample	153.000	13.080	12

- - - - - - - - - -
Variable .. NNSROCK   HEART RATE FOR NNS PLUS ROCKING

	Mean	Std. Dev.	N
For entire sample	157.000	14.504	12

- - - - - - - - - -
Variable .. ROCKING   HEART RATE FOR ROCKING ONLY

	Mean	Std. Dev.	N
For entire sample	170.000	18.577	12

B * * ANALYSIS OF VARIANCE -- DESIGN 1 * *

Tests involving 'CONDITON' Within-Subject Effect.

AVERAGED Tests of Significance for MEAS.1 using UNIQUE sums of squares

Source of Variation	SS	DF	MS	F	Sig of F
WITHIN CELLS	368.00	22	16.73		
CONDITON	1896.00	2	948.00	56.67	.000

- - - - - - - - - -

FIGURE 7–5.   COMPUTER PRINTOUT OF A ONE-WAY REPEATED MEASURES ANOVA

Repeated Measures ANOVA

Figure 7–5 presents a portion of a printout for a one-way repeated measures ANOVA applied to the data in Table 7–5.[17] (The full printout contains many peripheral statistics that we explain in a subsequent chapter.)

Panel A shows the mean, standard deviation, and number of subjects for the three conditions to which the infants were exposed. The mean heart rate for the NNS condition (nonnutritive sucking) is 153.0, the mean for NNSROCK (nonnutritive sucking plus rocking) is 157.0, and the mean for ROCKING (rocking only) is 170.0.

The bottom panel summarizes the analysis of variance for the within-subjects effect. It shows the sum of squares (SS), degrees of freedom (DF), and the mean square (MS) for "within cells" (which we referred to as the error component) and for the con-

---

[17]The SPSS/PC command that produced the printout for Figure 7–5 is as follows:

```
MANOVA NNS NNSROCK ROCKING
  /WSFACTORS = CONDITION (3)
  /PRINT=CELLINFO (MEANS) SIGNIF (AVERF) HOMOGENEITY.
```

dition component (i.e., the three treatments). When the mean square condition is divided by the mean square within cells, the resulting F of 56.67 has a probability of .000. We cannot tell from this information exactly what the probability level is; we know only that it is less than .0005, which would have rounded to .001.

RESEARCH APPLICATIONS OF ANOVA

Analysis of variance is a widely used statistical technique among researchers in many fields. This section briefly reviews some of the major applications of ANOVA, and presents methods of reporting on the results of ANOVA in research reports.

The Uses of ANOVA

As we have suggested throughout this chapter, analysis of variance is a versatile statistical technique that is appropriate in a variety of situations. It can be used to make inferences about population means for both nonexperimental and experimental designs, for both within-subjects and between-subjects designs, and for mixed designs in which there

TABLE 7–8. EXAMPLES OF STUDIES THAT HAVE USED ANOVA TO ADDRESS RESEARCH QUESTIONS

Research Question	Type of Research Design	Type of ANOVA	Multiple Comparison
What is the mean recovery rating after hip fracture among three groups of women discharged home, to short-term nursing home stay, or to longer-term nursing home stay? (Williams, Oberst, & Bjorklund, 1994)	Nonexperimental	Simple one-way ANOVA	Tukey HSD
What is the effect of ovarian hormone cessation and supplementation (five groups) on body weight in rats? (Bond, Heitkemper, & Jarrett, 1994)	Experimental	Simple one-way ANOVA	Tukey B test
What is the magnitude of social support among persons with multiple sclerosis in relation to illness duration, gender, and presence/absence of spouse? (Gulick, 1994)	Nonexperimental	Multifactor, between subjects, $(3 \times 2 \times 2)$	—
What is the effect of two separate informational interventions on maternal coping with unplanned childhood hospitalization? (Melnyk, 1994)	Experimental	Multifactor, between subjects, (2×2)	Duncan's test
What is the effect of topical nitroglycerin ointment (versus a placebo) to facilitate venous cannulation on vein size? (Griffith, James, & Cropp, 1994)	Experimental	Within subjects (before/after) $\times$ between subjects (experimental/control)	Scheffé's test

arc both nonexperimental and experimental factors—or both between-subjects and within-subjects factors. It can be used with as few as two levels per factor, or with many levels.

The main uses of ANOVA are, not surprisingly, comparable to those of the *t*-test, as reviewed in the previous chapter. We briefly illustrate these applications here.

1. *Answering Research Questions.* Many substantive research questions can be directly answered using ANOVA. Table 7–8 illustrates some of the research questions that have been addressed in recent years using analysis of variance. As this table shows, the research applications for ANOVA are diverse both substantively and methodologically.

2. *Testing Biases.* As noted in Chapter 6, researchers often make group comparisons to determine the existence and extent of any biases that could affect the interpretation of the results. Selection biases—group differences resulting from extraneous characteristics rather than from the effect of the independent variable—are among the most worrisome and most frequently tested. For example, Tappen (1994) used an experimental design to study the effect of (1) skill training, (2) a traditional stimulation approach, and (3) regular care on the ability to perform basic activities of daily living among nursing home residents with dementia. Although the researcher was able to randomly assign patients to the three groups, she tested for selection bias by comparing the three groups on age, mental status, and pretreatment functional ability, using one-way ANOVAs. Whenever there are more than two groups to compare, ANOVA can also be used to test for other biases discussed in Chapter 6.

3. *Establishing the Validity of Instruments.* Sometimes ANOVA is used in conjunction with the known-groups technique to examine the construct validity of newly developed instruments. For example, Hagerty and Patusky (1995), in their study to develop a measure of sense of belonging (described as the research example in Chapter 4), used ANOVA to contrast the SOBI scale scores of their three groups: students, depressed patients, and nuns. The researchers also used the *LSD* post hoc comparison tests and determined that all three groups had significantly different scores from each other on both scales of the instrument.

The Presentation of ANOVAs in Research Reports

As with *t*-tests, the results of ANOVA are usually reported in the text alone if there are only one or two *F* tests. However, if there are numerous tests—or if the test is for a complex multifactor design—a table is an efficient way to summarize the results. The text can then be used to highlight the most important features of the table.

Two alternative table styles are frequently used for reporting ANOVAs. One approach is similar to the table style used for *t*-tests; the table reports the means, *SD*s, and *n*s for the groups being compared, as well as the value of *F* for each group comparison with the associated probability level. An example of an ANOVA table with this format is presented in Table 7–9. This table summarizes the results of an experimental study in which three treatment groups are compared with respect to pain control procedures and pain ratings following coronary surgery. The table shows the means and *SD*s for the three groups, the *F* statistics, and the *p* values for four separate dependent variables. According to this

TABLE 7-9. EXAMPLE OF A TABLE FOR ANALYSIS OF VARIANCE RESULTS

Pain-Related Outcomes	Air Mattress Group (n = 50)		Mattress Plus Exercise Group (n = 50)		Control Group (n = 50)		F	p
	M	SD	M	SD	M	SD		
Number of Turns	7.0	3.2	5.9	3.9	6.9	3.4	1.96	NS
Number of Times Acetaminophen Given	1.6	1.1	0.7	0.6	1.5	1.4	5.01	<.01
Number of Times Other Medications Given	0.6	1.6	0.6	1.1	1.4	1.7	3.27	<.05
Pain Rating 48 Hours Postsurgery	39.5	41.2	16.2	18.5	34.6	30.2	7.99	<.001

Pain Control Procedures and Pain Ratings for Coronary Surgical Patients, by Treatment Group: ANOVA Results

table, three of the four ANOVAs were statistically significant at or beyond the .05 level, but the F value for the first outcome (number of turns) was not significant.

An alternative is to present a full ANOVA summary table such as the one in Table 7–10, which summarizes the results of our 2×2 ANOVA example on stress scores. We have added a second outcome measure (Coping Scale scores) to illustrate how information for two dependent variables can be presented in the same table. The summary table shows the values for the sums of squares, degrees of freedom, mean squares, and the F statistics for main effects and interactions for both dependent variables. This approach is

TABLE 7-10. EXAMPLE OF AN ANOVA SUMMARY TABLE FOR A MULTIFACTOR ANOVA

Outcome and Source of Variation	Sum of Squares	df	Mean Square	F	p
Stress Scale Scores					
Between					
Type of Treatment	5.00	1	5.00	1.91	NS
Time of Treatment	0.00	1	0.00	0.00	NS
Type × Time Interaction	20.00	1	20.00	7.62	<.05
Within	42.00	16	2.63		
Total	67.00	19	3.53		
Coping Scale Scores					
Between					
Type of Treatment	54.00	1	54.00	6.08	<.05
Time of Treatment	27.00	1	27.00	3.04	NS
Type × Time Interaction	35.00	1	35.00	3.94	NS
Within	142.00	16	8.88		
Total	258.00	19	13.58		

ANOVA Summary Table for Stress and Coping Scales, by Type and Time of Treatment

especially likely to be used in a multifactor ANOVA or in a mixed design because it allows for a convenient presentation of the F tests for all factors and interactions. However, when such a table is used to summarize ANOVAs, there usually needs to be a separate table showing the means and SDs. In Table 7–10, for example, there is a significant group difference for the type-of-treatment factor on the Coping Scale, but we cannot tell from the table whether the coping scores were better in the music therapy or in the relaxation therapy group.

When ANOVA information is presented in tables, the text can be used to emphasize the main features. Here is an example of how the results from Table 7–10 could be presented in the body of the report (we have added some information about the direction of differences for the Coping Scale):

> A two-way ANOVA was used to examine differences in the effectiveness of the two treatments and two times of administration with respect to patients' self-reported stress levels and ability to cope. The ANOVA summary table (Table 7–10) indicates that the time factor had no effect on scores on the Stress or Coping scales. However, there was a significant type-by-time of treatment interaction for the Stress Scale; in the evening only, music therapy resulted in significantly lower stress scores than relaxation therapy, $F(1, 16) = 7.62$, p $< .05$. Type of treatment, in and of itself, had no significant effect on stress scores. With respect to the Coping Scale, it was found that, across both time periods, patients in the music therapy group scored significantly more favorably than those in the relaxation therapy group, $F(1,16) = 6.08$, p $< .05$. Type of treatment was unrelated to coping scores.

The text can also be used to expand on information that is less conveniently presented in tables. For example, the results of multiple comparison tests that isolate the group comparisons responsible for a significant F are often presented in the text, although tables may also be used. Information on eta^2, if this statistic has been calculated, can be presented either in a table (e.g., in an additional final column in Table 7–9) or in the text. If a power analysis has been performed to help interpret nonsignificant results, information on the estimated power (or beta) usually is reported in the discussion section of the report.

RESEARCH EXAMPLE

The results of a recent investigation that used ANOVAs and multiple comparison procedures are summarized here to further illustrate the use of ANOVA to address research questions.

> Shelledy, Rau, and Thomas-Goodfellow (1995) studied the ventilatory efficiency of three modes of mechanical ventilation used for ventilatory support in a sample of 10 healthy volunteer subjects. The modes being compared were assist-control, synchronized intermittent mandatory ventilation (SIMV), and SIMV with 10 cm H_2O (0.98 kPa) of pressure support (SIMV+PS). The five outcome measures were minute volume, respiratory rate, average tidal volume, oxygen consumption, and ventilatory equivalent. The 10 subjects, serving as their own controls, were subjected to

all three conditions in a random order. One-way repeated measures ANOVAs were used to analyze mean differences in the conditions.

The researchers presented ANOVA results in the text and in graphs. With 2 and 18 *df*, there were significant condition differences with respect to average tidal volume ($F = 4.79$, $p = .02$), minute volume ($F = 5.13$, $p = .02$), oxygen consumption ($F = 4.11$, $p = .04$), and ventilatory equivalent ($F = 5.87$, $p = .01$). The differences with respect to respiratory rate were not statistically significant ($F = 0.43$, $p = .66$).

The four ANOVAs resulting in a significant *F* value were followed by Tukey multiple comparison tests to determine which specific pairs of conditions were significantly different. The results were presented in a table, which is reproduced in adapted form here as Table 7–11. As shown in this table, the post hoc tests revealed that SIMV with pressure support produced significantly greater values than SIMV alone for all four measures of ventilatory efficiency for which there was a significant *F* test. Moreover, the SIMV+PS mode produced significantly greater minute volume and ventilatory equivalent than the assist-control mode. There were no significant differences between assist-control and SIMV alone on any of the outcomes measures.

SUMMARY

Analysis of Variance (ANOVA) is used to draw inferences about population means when there are more than two means being compared. ANOVA tests the null hypothesis that the population means are equal against the alternative hypothesis that an inequality of population means exists.

ANOVA involves the **partitioning of variance** of the dependent variable into the components that contribute to score variability. In its most basic form, ANOVA contrasts **between-group variance** (variability arising from group differences) to **within-group variance** (variability between subjects within groups). The ratio of the two sources of variation yields a statistic—the **F ratio**—that can be compared to tabled val-

TABLE 7–11 MEANS, SDS, AND PAIRWISE MULTIPLE COMPARISONS FOR VARIABLES COMPARED BY MODE OF VENTILATORY SUPPORT

Outcome	Means (*SD*)			Pair Diffs.
	Assist-Control	SIMV	SIMV + PS	
Total Respiratory Rate (breaths/min)	15 (3.4)	15 (3.3)	16 (4.5)	
Average Tidal Volume (ml)	624 (54)	583 (35)	708 (34)	*
Minute Ventilation (L/min)	8.9 (1.8)	8.7 (1.6)	11.3 (3.4)	*†
O_2 Consumption (ml/min)	296 (41.4)	282 (43.5)	321 (61.2)	*
Ventilatory Equivalent (VE/VO$_2$-L/L VO$_2$)	30 (3.6)	31 (3.5)	35 (5.7)	*†
Tukey Multiple Comparison Tests:	*SIMV + PS different from SIMV mode, $p < .05$			
	†SIMV + PS different from assist-control mode, $p < .05$			

Adapted from Table II of Shelledy et al.'s (1995) report.

ues for F distributions. To actually compute the F ratio statistic, the **sum of squares** (sum of squared deviations about a mean) for each source of variation is divided by its respective degrees of freedom, to yield a **mean square**—which is essentially a variance. Then, the mean square between (MS_B) is divided by the mean square within (MS_W) to arrive at a value for the F ratio.

Analysis of variance can be used in a variety of circumstances. A **one-way ANOVA** is used to compare means for three or more independent groups. A **multifactor ANOVA** is used when there are two or more nominal-level independent variables, called **factors** in this context. The most common multifactor ANOVA is a **two-way ANOVA.** Multifactor ANOVA tests for both **main effects** (i.e., the effects of the independent variables on the dependent variable) and **interaction effects** (i.e., the effects of the independent variables in combination). **Repeated measures ANOVA (RANOVA)** is used for within-subjects designs, when means are computed for the *same* subjects three or more times.

If an ANOVA yields a significant F, **multiple comparison procedures (post hoc tests)** must be performed to determine the *nature* of the relationship between the independent and dependent variables. There are several alternative procedures, such as **Fisher's *LSD* test** (the **protected *t*-test**), that help to identify the group differences that contributed to the significant F statistic. A statistic known as **eta² (eta-squared)** can be computed directly from the components used to compute the F statistic to determine the strength of the relationship between the independent and dependent variables. Eta² is also used as the estimate of the effect size in power analyses for an ANOVA situation.

EXERCISES

The following exercises cover concepts presented in this chapter. Exercises indicated with a dagger (†) can be checked against answers appearing in Appendix A. Additionally, Chapter 7 of the accompanying *Applications Manual* offers supplementary exercises, including ones that require computer analysis of a data set on diskette.

† 1. For each of the following situations, indicate whether ANOVA is appropriate; if not appropriate, the reason why not; and, if appropriate, the type of ANOVA that would be used (i.e., one-way, repeated measures, etc.):

    a. The independent variable (IV) is age group—people in their 60s, 70s, and 80s; the dependent variable (DV) is health-related hardiness, as measured on a 20-item scale.

    b. The IVs are ethnicity (white, African American, Hispanic) and birth weight (<2500 grams vs. ≥ 2500 grams); the DV is serum bilirubin levels.

    c. The IV is maternal breastfeeding status (breastfeeds versus does not breastfeed); the DV is maternal bonding with infant, as measured on a 10-item self-report scale.

   d. The IV is treatment group for patients with drug-induced shivering (extremity wraps versus high room temperature vs. normal room temperature without wraps); the DV is myocardial oxygen consumption, measured before and after treatment.
   e. The IV is length of gestation (preterm versus term versus postterm birth); the DV is epidural anesthesia during labor (yes versus no).
   f. The IV is time since diagnosis of multiple sclerosis (measured 1 month, 6 months, and 2 years after diagnosis); the DV is psychological adaptation to the disease, as measured by the Purpose-in-Life test.
† 2. Suppose we wanted to compare the somatic complaints (as measured on a scale known as the Physical Symptom Survey or PSS) of three groups of people: non-smokers, smokers, and people who recently quit smoking. Using the following data for PSS scores, do a one-way ANOVA to test the hypothesis that the population means are equal:

Nonsmokers	Smokers	Quitters
19	26	37
23	29	32
17	22	27
20	30	41
26	23	38

   What are the means for the three groups? Compute the sums of squares, degrees of freedom, and mean squares for these data. What is the value of F? Using an alpha of .05, is the F statistically significant?
† 3. Using the data from Exercise 2, compute three protected t-tests to compare all possible pairs of means. Also, for $\alpha = .05$, what is the value of LSD? Which pairs are significantly different from one another at $\alpha = .05$, using this multiple comparison procedure?
† 4. For the data in Exercise 2, what is the value of eta²? What is the *approximate* estimated power for this ANOVA? Explain what the eta-squared and estimated power indicate.
  5. Write a few sentences that could be used to describe the results of the analyses from Exercises 2 to 4.
† 6. For each of the following F values, indicate whether the F is statistically significant, at the specified α level:
   a. $F = 2.80$, $df = 4, 40$, $\alpha = .01$
   b. $F = 5.02$, $df = 3, 60$, $\alpha = .001$
   c. $F = 3.45$, $df = 3, 27$, $\alpha = .05$
   d. $F = 4.99$, $df = 2, 150$, $\alpha = .01$
   e. $F = 2.09$, $df = 2, 250$, $\alpha = .05$
† 7. Suppose that we were interested in studying the self-esteem of men versus women (Factor A) in two exercise status groups—nonexercisers versus exercisers (Factor B)—with 20 subjects in each of the four groups. Use the following information to

compute three F tests, and determine which, if any, is statistically significant at the .05 level:

Means: Male Exercisers: 39.0   Male Nonexercisers: 37.0
         Female Exercisers: 34.0   Female Nonexercisers: 29.0
         All Exercisers: 36.5   All Nonexercisers: 33.0
         All Males: 38.0   All Females: 31.5

Sums of Squares: $SS_T = 1{,}190.50$ $SS_W = 1{,}025.0$
                   $SS_A = 74.50$ $SS_B = 37.0$ $SS_{AB} = 54.00$

8. Interpret the meaning of the F tests from Exercise 7 (assume that higher scores on the self-esteem scale mean higher self-esteem). Write a few sentences summarizing the results.

† 9. Suppose we used a repeated measures design to test for differences in bruising from subcutaneous sodium heparin injections at three sites (arm, leg, and abdomen) in a sample of 15 medical/surgical patients. Surface area of the bruises (in mm^2) is measured 72 hours after each injection, which are administered to sites in random order at 8-hour intervals. Use the following information to compute the F statistic to determine if there were significant differences in bruising by site, at the .05 level:

Means: Arm: 212.0 mm^2 Leg: 99.0 mm^2 Abdomen: 93.0 mm^2
Sums of Squares: $SS_{site} = 17{,}993.00$ $SS_{error} = 48{,}349.00$

† 10. Estimate the approximate power of the statistical test for each of the following situations:
   a. $eta^2 = .25$, $\alpha = .05$, $n = 10$ per group
   b. $eta^2 = .10$, $\alpha = .05$, $n = 15$ per group
   c. $eta^2 = .04$, $\alpha = .05$, $n = 70$ per group
   d. $eta^2 = .15$, $\alpha = .05$, $n = 15$ per group
   e. $eta^2 = .40$, $\alpha = .05$, $n = 8$ per group

Chi-Square and Other Nonparametric Tests

Thus far, we have discussed inferential statistical tests that are parametric. In this chapter we examine several nonparametric tests.

THE CHI-SQUARE TEST

The nonparametric test that is most frequently used by researchers is, without question, **chi-square.** The chi-square statistic is used in several different types of applications, but in this section we focus primarily on the most widely used application, known as the **chi-square test of independence.**[1] This test is designed to make inferences about the existence of a relationship between two categorical variables.[2] The chi-square test of independence is a method of testing the significance of the relationship between two variables that are crosstabulated in a contingency table (see Chapter 4).

Suppose that we wanted to examine whether there were differences in the rate of complications for patients receiving intravenous medications with a heparin lock in place, without changing it, for 72 hours versus 96 hours. Patients are randomly assigned to the two groups, and then the incidence of any complication (e.g., blocking, leaking, purulence, phlebitis, etc.) is recorded. Table 8–1 presents hypothetical data for 100 patients (50 in each group), arrayed descriptively in a 2 × 2 contingency table. As this

---

[1]Although widely referred to as the chi-square test, the test is sometimes called chi-square*d*, which is actually a more appropriate term since the symbolic representation for the test is the Greek letter chi, squared.

[2]It is possible to analyze the relationships among three or more categorical variables by a technique known as **log-linear analysis,** sometimes referred to as **multiway frequency analysis.** For a discussion of log-linear analysis, see Tabachnick and Fidell (1989).

TABLE 8–1. HYPOTHETICAL DATA FOR HEPARIN LOCK CHI-SQUARE EXAMPLE

Complication Incidence	Heparin Lock Placement Time Group		
	72 Hours	96 Hours	Total
Had Complications	9 (18.0%)	11 (22.0%)	20 (20.0%)
Had No Complications	41 (82.0%)	39 (78.0%)	80 (80.0%)
Total	50	50	100

table shows, there was a higher rate of complications in the 96-hour group (22%) than in the 72-hour group (18%). The research question is whether the observed group differences in the rate of complications (the dependent variable) reflects the effect of the length of time the heparin locks were in place (the independent variable), or whether the differences reflect random sampling fluctuations. The chi-square test would be used to address this question.

The Null and Alternative Hypotheses for the Chi-Square Test

The null hypothesis for the chi-square test, as for other tests, stipulates the absence of a relationship between the independent and dependent variables. The null hypothesis is stated in terms of the independence of the two variables. For our current example, the null and alternative hypotheses may be stated as follows:

H_0: Complication incidence and length of heparin lock placement are independent (not related)

H_1: Complication incidence and length of heparin lock placement are *not* independent (they *are* related)

General Logic of the Chi-Square Test

The chi-square test contrasts the **observed frequencies** in each cell of a contingency table (i.e., the frequencies observed within the actual data) with expected frequencies. The **expected frequencies** represent the number of cases that would be found in each cell if the null hypothesis were true—that is, if the two variables were totally unrelated. In our example, if the length of heparin lock placement had no effect on the rate of complications, the percentages should be identical in the two groups. Since 20% of the overall sample of patients had complications, we would expect that 20% in both groups (20% × 50 = 10 patients) would experience complications if the null hypothesis were true. Similarly, 80% of the patients did not have complications, so the expected frequency for the two bottom cells of Table 8–1 would be 40 (80% × 50).

If the actual, observed frequencies in a contingency table are *identical* to the expected frequencies, the value of the chi-square statistic will equal 0, which is also the population value of chi-square when the two variables are unrelated. However, a chi-square based on sample data will often not equal exactly 0, even when the variables are not related, because of sampling error. Thus, as with other statistics we have discussed, the computed value of the chi-square statistic must be compared to a critical value in a table, to determine if the value of the statistic is "improbable" at a specified level of probability. The critical tabled values are based on **sampling distributions of the chi-square statistic.**

There are different chi-square distributions depending on the degrees of freedom, which in turn depend on the number of categories for each variable. (We discuss the calculation of degrees of freedom subsequently.) Figure 8–1 presents examples of two chi-square distributions, for tests involving a 2 × 2 (4-cell) contingency table and a 5 × 3 (15-cell) contingency table. The areas corresponding to 5% and 1% of these distributions are shown on this figure. These areas constitute the critical regions for the rejection of the null hypothesis with $\alpha = .05$ and $.01$, respectively.

Assumptions and Requirements for the Chi-Square Test

The chi-square test is used when both the independent and the dependent variables are measured on a nominal scale—that is, when the variables can best be described through

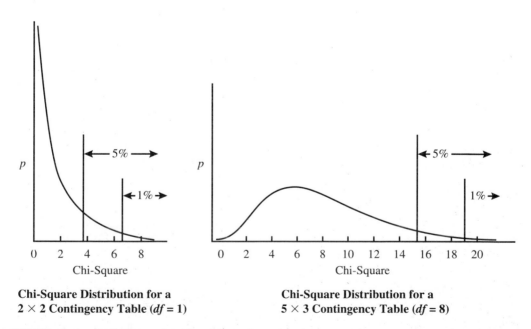

**Chi-Square Distribution for a
2 × 2 Contingency Table ($df = 1$)**

**Chi-Square Distribution for a
5 × 3 Contingency Table ($df = 8$)**

FIGURE 8–1. EXAMPLE OF CHI-SQUARE DISTRIBUTIONS WITH DIFFERENT DEGREES OF FREEDOM

frequencies, rather than means. Chi-square can also be used for ordinal-level variables if there are only a few categories (e.g., assistant professor, associate professor, full professor). The chi-square test can also be applied to interval or ratio data that have been classified into a small number of groups. For example, the variable age (a ratio-level variable) could be classified as an ordinal-level variable with four categories: under 20, 20 to 29, 30 to 39, and 40 or older. However, if a researcher has interval-level or ratio-level data, it is usually preferable to use a more powerful parametric procedure, such as ANOVA or a t-test, with the raw (ungrouped) data.

Like parametric tests for between-subjects designs, the chi-square test assumes that the observations are randomly and independently sampled from the population of interest. Each subject must qualify for one and only one cell of the contingency table.

Unlike the tests we have discussed in preceding chapters, the chi-square test does *not* make any assumptions about the shape of the distribution of values in the population, nor about the homogeneity of group variances. However, there is one further assumption that concerns sample size: chi-square requires that the *expected frequency* of each cell be greater than 0. In fact, it is often recommended that the expected frequency of each cell be at least 5, especially if the number of cells is small, as in a 2×2 contingency table.[3] When there are a large number of cells, chi-square will yield valid results if no more than 20% of the cells have expected frequencies under 5—so long as all cells have an expected frequency greater than 0. For example, in a 5×4 contingency table, four cells (20% $\times$ 20) could have expected frequencies between 1 and 4. Note that the cell size requirement involves *expected* frequencies, not observed ones. However, as the size of the overall sample increases, so do expected frequencies.

Calculation of the Chi-Square Statistic

The chi-square statistic is relatively easy to compute manually. The first step is to calculate the expected frequencies for each cell of the contingency table. The following formula can be used:

$$E = \frac{R_f C_f}{N}$$

where E = expected frequency for a cell
      R_f = observed frequency for the entire row the cell is in
      C_f = observed frequency for the entire column the cell is in
      N = total sample size

---

[3]If chi-square is invalid for a 2×2 table because of low expected frequencies, an alternative test known as **Fisher's exact test** can be used. The computations for the Fisher exact test are complex but, fortunately, most computer programs for chi-square analysis compute Fisher's exact test automatically if the expected cell value for a 2×2 table is less than 5.

Let us apply this formula to the first cell in our example of heparin lock placement groups (Table 8–1):

$$E = \frac{(50)(20)}{100} = \frac{1000}{100} = 10$$

This is consistent with our earlier discussion, in which we noted that 20% of the sample had complications, so 20% of each group ($n = 10$) would be expected to have complications if the null hypothesis were true. Thus, the expected frequency for the two upper cells is 10, while that for the two bottom cells is 40.[4]

We can now compute the chi-square statistic, which involves comparing expected and observed frequencies in each cell. The formula for chi-square is:

$$\chi^2 = \Sigma \, \frac{(O - E)^2}{E}$$

where χ^2 = chi-square
O = observed frequency for a cell
E = expected frequency for a cell
Σ = the sum of the $(O - E)^2/E$ ratios for all cells

To compute χ^2, the expected frequency for each cell is subtracted from the observed frequency, the result is squared, and then this value is divided by the cell's expected frequency. When these calculations are performed for each cell, all the values are added together to yield a value of χ^2 (chi-square). Table 8–2 works through the computations for our heparin lock example. In this example, the computed value of χ^2 is 0.25.

The computed value of χ^2 must now be compared to a tabled value for the established level of significance, which we will set at .05. To use the chi-square table (Table B–4 of Appendix B), we must first compute the degrees of freedom. For the chi-square test, the formula is:

$$df = (R - 1)(C - 1)$$

where R = number of rows
C = number of columns

4Note that in a 2 3 2 table, we need only use the formula to compute one E. Thereafter, we can subtract the computed value of that E from the marginal frequencies to obtain the Es for all other cells, because the marginal frequencies are fixed (i.e., expected marginal frequencies are the same as observed marginal frequencies). Thus, once we have the E of 10 for the first cell, we can subtract this value from the row frequency of 20 to obtain the expected frequency for the upper right cell (20 2 10 5 10). We can obtain the bottom left E by subtracting 10 from the column total (50 2 10 5 40). The remaining cell can be computed by subtracting 40 from the corresponding row total (80 2 40 5 40).

TABLE 8–2. CALCULATION OF THE CHI-SQUARE STATISTIC FOR HEPARIN LOCK DATA

Cell	Observed Frequency O	Expected Frequency E	$(O - E)$	$(O - E)^2$	$(O - E)^2/E$
Complication, 72 Hr.	9	10	−1	1	0.100
Complication, 96 Hr.	11	10	1	1	0.100
No Complication, 72 Hr.	41	40	1	1	0.025
No Complication, 96 Hr.	39	40	−1	1	0.025
					$\chi^2 = \overline{0.250}$

In our present example, both R and C are equal to 2, so the number of degrees of freedom is $(2 - 1)(2 - 1)$, which equals 1. We find in Table B–4 that with $\alpha = .05$ and $df = 1$, the tabled value of χ^2 is 3.84. Since our calculated value of chi-square is considerably less that 3.84, we must accept the null hypothesis that the complication rate is unrelated to heparin lock placement time.

Yates' Correction

When both variables in the contingency table have only two levels—that is, when we have a 2 × 2 table—a correction factor known as **Yates' correction for continuity** is sometimes used in computing chi-square. There is some disagreement regarding the use of Yates' correction (see Jaccard & Becker, 1990), but it is widely used in situations in which the expected frequency for any cell in a 2 × 2 table is less than 10.

The correction involves subtracting 0.5 from the absolute value of $O - E$ for each cell before this value is squared. In other words, the formula for chi-square with Yates' correction is:

$$\chi^2 = \Sigma \frac{(|O - E| - .5)^2}{E}$$

One of the reasons this correction factor is controversial is that it reduces the power of the chi-square test to detect significant differences. If the formula were applied to the data in our heparin lock example, the value of χ^2 would be reduced from 0.25 to 0.0625. In both cases, the null hypothesis would be accepted. However, in some situations, the application of Yates' correction alters the researcher's decision from rejection to acceptance of the null. If expected frequencies are large, the correction factor should probably not be applied, but if they are small and if a conservative decision is considered desirable, the Yates' correction may be appropriate.

Strength of the Relationship in Two-Variable Contingency Tables

The chi-square statistic provides information about the existence of a relationship between two nominal-level variables, but not about the magnitude of the relationship. To facilitate interpretation of the results—especially when a significant chi-square value has been obtained—it may be useful to have a measure of the strength of the association.

There are a number of alternative indexes that have been proposed. In a 2 × 2 table, the most widely reported index is the **phi coefficient** (ϕ). The formula for ϕ is based directly on the computed chi-square statistic:

$$\phi = \sqrt{\frac{\chi^2}{N}}$$

In our heparin lock example, the phi coefficient would be:

$$\phi = \sqrt{\frac{0.25}{100}} = \sqrt{.0025} = .05$$

The phi coefficient can range from 0 to 1, and can be interpreted as a Pearson r.[5] The larger the value of ϕ, the stronger is the relationship between the variables. Thus, a ϕ of .05 indicates a weak relationship between placement time groups and incidence of complications.

When the table is larger than 2 × 2, a different index must be used to measure the strength of the relationship between the variables. One such index is **Cramér's V**. The formula for the V statistic is as follows:

$$V = \sqrt{\frac{\chi^2}{N(k-1)}}$$

In this formula, k is the smaller of either R (number of rows) or C (number of columns). It can be seen that in our heparin lock example, k would equal 2, so that the formula for V in this case is identical to the formula for ϕ. As with ϕ, the V statistic can range from 0 to 1, and larger values indicate a stronger relationship between the variables. For tables that are bigger than 2 × 2, a large value for the V statistic means that there is a tendency for particular categories of the independent variable to be associated with particular categories of the dependent variable.

---

[5]In fact, ϕ *is a Pearson r.* We would obtain the same value of .05 if we used the codes of 0 and 1 to designate the two heparin lock groups, and the codes of 0 and 1 for the two complication conditions, and then calculated a Pearson's correlation coefficient using the formula presented in Chapter 4.

Nature of the Relationship

When the contingency table is 2×2 and a chi-square test has led to the rejection of the null hypothesis, the direction of the relationship between the two variables can be determined by inspecting the relative frequencies. For instance, if our heparin lock example *had* yielded a significant chi-square value, we would conclude that complications are greater when the heparin locks are left in place for 96 hours than when they are in place only 72 hours because the complication rate was higher in the 96-hour group.

Like ANOVA, the chi-square test applies to the data for the two variables taken as a whole. For a table larger than 2×2, a significant chi-square provides no information regarding which cells are responsible for rejecting the null hypothesis. There are post hoc procedures for chi-square tests just as for ANOVA (see, for example, Cohen, 1967; Goodman, 1964), but the mathematics are relatively complex and these procedures generally are unavailable in routine statistical software packages. However, we can gain descriptive insights into the nature of the relationship by examining the components contributing to the value of χ^2—i.e., the values shown in the last column of Table 8–2. In a 4×2 table, for example, there would be eight such components, and those with the greatest values are the ones disproportionately contributing to a high χ^2. These components would help us to better understand which cells are most responsible for the rejection of the null hypothesis.

Power in the Context of Chi-Square

Cramér's *V* statistic can be used to determine the power of a chi-square test. As we have noted in earlier chapters, a power estimate is often extremely useful in interpreting results when a statistical test is nonsignificant. Power analysis can also be used prior to an investigation to estimate the needed sample size, but in this situation the researcher would need to have an estimate of Cramér's *V*.

Tables for estimating power within a chi-square context are presented in Table C–3 of Appendix C. Because different tables are needed for contingency tables of different dimensions and for different levels of α, this appendix covers only the most common situations—that is, for $\alpha = .05$, and for contingency tables no greater than 4×4. For power estimates when $\alpha = .01$, the reader should consult Jaccard and Becker (1990) or Cohen (1977).

For the sake of convenience, the power table for a 2×2 design is reproduced here as Table 8–3. The left-hand column of the table presents different power levels, and the top row presents the population values for Cramér's statistic. In the example we have discussed throughout this chapter, the value of *V* was .05, which is not represented in the table. However, we can see that with a sample of 100 patients and a *V* less than .10 (the lowest *V* shown in the table), the power of the test would be substantially less than .25. In other words, the risk of a Type II error is greater than 75%. Thinking in terms of sample size requirements, if we wanted to achieve a power of .80 when the strength of the

TABLE 8–3. POWER TABLE FOR A 2 × 2 CONTINGENCY TABLE FOR α = .05 AS A FUNCTION OF POPULATION VALUES OF CRAMÉR'S V*

Power	Population Value of Cramér's V Statistic								
	.10	.20	.30	.40	.50	.60	.70	.80	.90
.25	165	41	18	10	7	5	3	3	2
.50	385	96	43	24	15	11	8	6	5
.60	490	122	54	31	20	14	10	8	6
.70	617	154	69	39	25	17	13	10	8
.80	785	196	87	49	31	22	16	12	10
.85	898	224	100	56	36	25	18	14	11
.90	1051	263	117	66	42	29	21	16	13
.95	1300	325	144	81	52	36	27	20	16
.99	1837	459	204	115	73	51	37	29	23

*The entries are sample size requirements to achieve the specified power, at a given value of Cramér's V (for a 2 × 2 contingency table, Cramér's $V = \phi$).

relationship between the two variables in the population yielded a V of .05, we would need a sample size substantially greater than 785 (the sample size if V were .10 rather than .05).[6]

Since the estimated power in our example is so low, we would probably want to be cautious in recommending that heparin locks be left in place for 96 hours. Even small effects that are not statistically significant *could* be clinically important, and thus a replication of the study with a larger sample of patients would be advisable.

Chi-Square Goodness-of-Fit Test

Although the chi-square test we have discussed thus far is the most commonly used application of the chi-square statistic, we briefly mention here another application. The **chi-square goodness-of-fit test** is used to draw inferences when there is only *one* nominal-level variable.

Suppose that we had a random sample of 500 lung cancer patients. The data reveal that there are 285 men and 215 women in the sample. The research question is whether the gender split represents population differences in the rate of contracting the disease, or whether the different proportions reflect sampling error. The null hypothesis is that in the population of lung cancer patients the proportion of men and women is equivalent.

As with the chi-square test of independence, the goodness-of-fit test contrasts expected and observed frequencies. With a sample of 500 patients, we would expect to

---

[6]In fact, although it is not shown in the table, the sample size would need to be around 2000 subjects.

find 250 men and 250 women if the null hypothesis were true. Applying the chi-square formula presented earlier, we would obtain the following:

$$\chi^2 = \frac{(285-250)^2}{250} + \frac{(215-250)^2}{250}$$

$$\chi^2 = \frac{(35)^2}{250} + \frac{(-35)^2}{250} = \frac{1225}{250} + \frac{1225}{250} = 9.80$$

The degrees of freedom for the goodness-of-fit test are $k-1$, where k is the number of categories of the single variable. In our example, then, since $k = 2$, there is 1 degree of freedom. From Table B–4, the critical value of chi-square with 1 df and $\alpha = .05$ is 3.84. Since our computed value of chi-square (9.80) is larger than the tabled value, we reject the null hypothesis and conclude that the sample was drawn from a population in which men are more likely than women to contract lung cancer.

OTHER NONPARAMETRIC TESTS

Nonparametric tests are generally used either when the dependent variable is measured on a nominal or ordinal scale or when the assumptions for more powerful parametric tests cannot be met, especially if the sample size is small. There are dozens of nonparametric tests for different situations, only a handful of which are covered here. Those interested in a more comprehensive coverage of nonparametric procedures should consult Siegel (1956), Marascuilo and McSweeney (1977), or Gibbons (1993).

Table 8–4 summarizes the tests covered in this chapter, and indicates the situations in which these tests are appropriate. For situations in which a parametric test such as the t-test or ANOVA cannot be used because the underlying assumptions are presumed to be

TABLE 8–4. REQUIREMENTS FOR SELECTED NONPARAMETRIC AND PARAMETRIC TESTS

Number of Groups	Between or Within Subjects*	Level of Measurement of Dependent Variable		
		Nominal	Ordinal	Interval or Ratio
2	Between	Chi-square test	Mann-Whitney U-test	t-test
3+	Between	Chi-square test	Kruskal-Wallis test	ANOVA
2	Within	McNemar test	Wilcoxon signed-ranks test	Paired t-test
3 +	Within	Cochran's Q test	Friedman test	RANOVA

*Between-subjects tests are for independent groups designs. Within-subjects tests are for repeated measures/dependent groups designs.

violated, the nonparametric ordinal-level test in the same row as the parametric test (listed in the last column of this table) would ordinarily be used. For example, if an independent groups t-test is inappropriate because the distribution of the dependent variable is markedly nonnormal, the Mann-Whitney U-test would probably be used to test group differences.

Most of the nonparametric procedures described in this section are called **rank tests.** While parametric tests focus on differences in population means, rank tests deal with differences in *location* (score distributions) between populations, based on ranks. Significance tests based on ranks are used either when the original data are in the form of rankings or, more typically, when a set of scores have been converted into ranks for the purpose of performing the test. To illustrate the basic ranking process, consider the following five heart rate values and their corresponding ranks:

Heart Rate	Rank
130	5
93	2
112	4
89	1
101	3

In this example, the person with the lowest heart rate is ranked 1, and the person with the highest heart rate is ranked 5.[7] We easily could have reversed the ranking so that the lowest heart rate had the highest ranking, and so on—the computational procedures for rank tests would be the same either way. However, it is somewhat easier to interpret the results if low ranks are associated with low data values and high ranks are associated with high values.

The Mann-Whitney *U*-Test

The **Mann-Whitney *U*-test** is a popular nonparametric analog of the independent groups t-test. This statistic tests the null hypothesis that two population distributions are identical against the alternative hypothesis that the distributions are *not* identical.

Suppose we had two groups of burn patients (Group A and Group B) who obtained the following scores on a scale measuring positive body image:

Group A: 14,   19,   11,   22,   17
Group B: 10,   16,   15,   18,   13

To perform the Mann-Whitney U-test, we must arrange all the scores in order and rank them, while maintaining information about group affiliation:

---

[7]When a tie occurs, the scores are assigned the average of the ranks. Thus, if the fifth person in the above example had a heart rate of 112, both scores of 112 (subjects 3 and 5) would be ranked 3.5.

Score:	10	11	13	14	15	16	17	18	19	22
Group:	B	A	B	A	B	B	A	B	A	A
Rank:	1	2	3	4	5	6	7	8	9	10

The ranks associated with each group are then separately summed to yield R_A and R_B:

$$R_A = 2 + 4 + 7 + 9 + 10 = 32$$
$$R_B = 1 + 3 + 5 + 6 + 8 = 23$$

The formula for computing the U statistic for group A is:

$$U_A = n_A n_B + \left[\frac{n_A (n_A + 1)}{2} \right] - R_A$$

where n_A = number of observations in Group A
n_B = number of observations in Group B
R_A = summed ranks for Group A

The formula for computing U_B would be analogous, except that the n for group B would be used in the numerator of the second term, and the R for group B would be used in the third term of the above formula. Using the formula, we would obtain the following:

$$U_A = (5) (5) + \left[\frac{(5) (6)}{2} \right] - 32 = 8$$

$$U_B = (5) (5) + \left[\frac{(5) (6)}{2} \right] - 23 = 17$$

The U value that is used as the test statistic is the *smaller* of the two Us, which in this case is $U_A = 8$. The critical values for U (for $\alpha = .05$) are presented in Table B–5 of Appendix B.[8] To use the table, we look for the number at the intersection of the appropriate row and column for n_A and n_B. In our present example, with $n_A = 5$ and $n_B = 5$, the critical value is 4. One must be very careful in using this table, because it is different from other tables of critical values we have described thus far; to be statistically significant, *the observed U must be equal to or less than the tabled value*. Since our obtained value of 8 is greater than the tabled value of 4, we must *retain* the null hypothesis that the two distributions are identical.

---

[8]The values in Table B–5 are for a nondirectional test with $\alpha = .05$. If the researcher is testing a directional hypothesis, or if a more stringent significance level is sought, more detailed tables of U must be used (for example, see Jaccard and Becker, 1990).

Note that Table B–5 is appropriate only when the sample size of both groups is 20 or less. When the n for either group is greater than 20, the value of U approaches a normal distribution. The following transformation formula can be applied to the obtained U statistic to yield a z statistic,[9] which can then be compared to the critical values for the normal distribution in Table B–1:

$$z = \frac{U - n_A n_B / 2}{\sqrt{\dfrac{(n_A)(n_B)(n_A + n_B + 1)}{12}}}$$

The Kruskal-Wallis Test

The **Kruskal-Wallis test** is the nonparametric counterpart of the simple one-way ANOVA. It is used to analyze the relationship between a dependent variable that is ordinal in nature and a categorical independent variable that has three or more levels (i.e., when there are three or more groups). The Kruskal-Wallis procedure tests the null hypothesis that the population distributions for the three (or more) independent groups are identical against the alternative that there are differences in the distributions. This test should be used only if there are five or more cases per group.

Suppose that we compared the life satisfaction of patients in three nursing homes, using a six-item scale, and obtained the following scores:

```
Home A:    6,   12,   18,   14,   17
Home B:   15,   19,   16,   20,   10
Home C:   30,   27,   24,   25,   22
```

As for the Mann-Whitney U-test, the scores must be ranked for the sample as a whole, and then the ranks must be summed separately for each group:

Score:	6	10	12	14	15	16	17	18	19	20	22	24	25	27	30
Group:	A	B	A	A	B	B	A	A	B	B	C	C	C	C	C
Rank:	1	2	3	4	5	6	7	8	9	10	11	12	13	14	15

$$R_A = 1 + 3 + 4 + 7 + 8 \qquad = 23$$
$$R_B = 2 + 5 + 6 + 9 + 10 \qquad = 32$$
$$R_C = 11 + 12 + 13 + 14 + 15 = 65$$

Kruskal and Wallis proposed the following formula for the test statistic, the **H statistic:**

---

[9]The U statistic transformed to a z statistic using this formula is equivalent to another test known as the **Wilcoxon rank sum test.**

$$H = \left[\frac{12}{N(N+1)} \right] \left[\Sigma \frac{R^2}{n} \right] - 3(N+1)$$

where N = total sample size
R = summed ranks for a group
n = number of observations in a group
Σ = sum of the R^2/n ratios for all groups

For the data in our present example of three groups of nursing home patients, the value of H is:

$$H = \left[\frac{12}{15(16)} \right] \left[\frac{23^2}{5} + \frac{32^2}{6} + \frac{65^2}{5} \right] - 3(16)$$

$$H = (0.05)(105.8 + 204.8 + 845.0) - 48 = 9.78$$

The H statistic has a sampling distribution that approximates a chi-square distribution with $k - 1$ degrees of freedom, where k is the number of groups. For $\alpha = .05$ with 2 degrees of freedom, the critical value of H from the chi-square table in Table B–4 of Appendix B is 5.99. Since the calculated value of H (9.78) is greater than this critical value, we reject the null hypothesis that the distribution of life satisfaction scores in the three nursing homes is identical.

As with ANOVA, a significant result does not mean that all groups are significantly different from one another. Post hoc tests are needed to determine the nature of the relationship between nursing homes and life satisfaction. Various procedures have been proposed, but the one that is most often recommended is the **Dunn procedure.** This procedure involves using the Mann-Whitney U-test to compare the ranks for all possible pairs of groups. However, to avoid a higher-than-desired risk of a Type I error, a correction factor (sometimes referred to as a **Bonferroni correction**) is used. The correction involves revising the significance level such that the desired α is divided by the number of pairs being compared. Thus, in the present example, to test for differences between the three pairs at the .05 significance level, the α would be .05 ÷ 3, or .017. This means that for a difference between pairs to be significant at $\alpha = .05$, the computed value for the U statistic would be compared to the critical value for $\alpha = .017$. If we were to apply the Dunn procedure to our current example, we would find that Home C was significantly different from the other two nursing homes, but that Home A and Home B were not statistically different from each other.[10]

---

[10]According to a computer analysis of these data, the actual significance levels were .42 (Home A versus Home B), .009 (Home A versus Home C), and .009 (Home B versus Home C).

McNemar Test

The **McNemar test** is used to test differences in proportions for dependent groups in a 2×2 within-subjects design. For example, if 50 subjects were asked before and after a special educational program whether or not they practiced breast self-examination (BSE), the McNemar test could be used to test changes in the rates of BSE. The null hypothesis is that there are no pretreatment to posttreatment changes in BSE, and the alternative hypothesis is that there are changes. Suppose that 30% of the women ($n = 15$) practiced BSE before the intervention, while 40% of the women ($n = 20$) did so after the intervention—that is, five women who previously did not practice BSE began to do so. What is the likelihood that the 10-percentage-point increase reflects a true difference in BSE practice?

The data for our example must first be arranged in a table that distributes the women based on whether they did or did not practice BSE at both points in time, such as we have done in Table 8–5. This table shows that 15 women practiced BSE both before and after the intervention (cell A), 30 women did not practice BSE at either point (cell D), and 5 women who originally did not practice BSE did so after the intervention (cell C). No woman who originally practiced BSE ceased to do so after the intervention (cell B).

It is possible to determine exact probabilities in this situation through the use of a distribution known as the **binomial distribution.** However, unless the sample size is quite small, it is more convenient to use the chi-square distribution. The following formula can be applied:

$$\chi^2 = \frac{(|C - B| - 1)^2}{C + B}$$

where C = number in cell C (changed from no to yes)
B = number in cell B (changed from yes to no)
$|\ |$ = the absolute value of the difference

TABLE 8–5. DISTRIBUTION OF BSE PRACTICE FOR MCNEMAR TEST EXAMPLE

		BSE After Intervention	
		Yes	No
	Yes	A 15	B 0
BSE Before Intervention	No	C 5	D 30

If we applied this formula to the data at hand, we would find:

$$\chi^2 = \frac{(|5 - 0| - 1)^2}{5 + 0} = \frac{16}{5} = 3.20$$

For the McNemar test, there is always 1 degree of freedom. If we set $\alpha = .05$, we find in the chi-square table (Table B–4) that the critical value of chi-square is 3.84. Thus, we must retain the null hypothesis. The change in the percentage of women who practiced BSE is not statistically significant at the .05 level.

The Wilcoxon Signed-Ranks Test

The **Wilcoxon signed-ranks test** is the nonparametric counterpart of the paired (dependent groups) t-test. It is used to test for group differences when there are two paired groups or a within-subjects design, and when the measurement of the dependent variable is ordinal. The Wilcoxon signed-ranks procedure tests the null hypothesis that the population distributions for the two sets of observations are identical, against the alternative hypothesis that they are not identical.

Suppose that we had 10 married couples whose child had undergone surgery. Both the husband and wife have completed a scale that is designed to measure the parents' anxiety about the operation. The scores shown in the first two columns of Table 8–6 were obtained. To perform the signed-ranks test, the score from one set must be subtracted from the corresponding scores in the other set, as shown in column 3 of the table. Next, the absolute values of the differences (column 4) are ranked, with the rank of 1 assigned for the smallest difference (column 5). Then, the ranks for the positive differences are separately summed, as are the ranks for the negative differences, as shown in the last two columns of Table 8–6. The table indicates that the positive ranks (which are associated with higher anxiety scores among the wives) totaled 30, while the negative ranks (associated with higher scores for the husbands) totaled 25.

If the null hypothesis that the husbands' and wives' anxiety scores are similarly distributed were true, the sum of the ranks for the negative differences should be about the same as the sum of ranks for positive differences. That is, in our example, the expected value of the ranks for both groups (R_E) is 27.5 $((R_+ + R_-)/2)$ under the assumption that the null hypothesis is true. Tables for the Wilcoxon signed-ranks test statistic, usually referred to as the **T statistic**, are available[11] and are precise when the number of pairs is 50 or fewer. However, when the number of pairs is 10 or greater, the sampling distribution of T approximates a normal distribution, and the following formula[12] can be used to compute a z statistic:

---

[11] The T statistic is equal to the smaller value of R_+ and R_-, which in this case would be 25. A table of values for T may be found in Jaccard and Becker (1990), Table L.

[12] It does not matter whether R_+ or R_- is used in the numerator of the formula, since both are equal distances from R_E. The only effect of the substitution would be to change the sign of z.

TABLE 8–6. WILCOXON SIGNED-RANKS TEST EXAMPLE: WIVES' VERSUS HUSBANDS' ANXIETY

(1) Wife	(2) Husband	(3) Difference	(4) |Difference|	(5) Rank	(6) R_+	(7) R_-
17	16	1	1	1	1	
19	14	5	5	5	5	
16	20	−4	4	4		4
18	12	6	6	6	6	
22	24	−2	2	2		2
18	21	−3	3	3		3
15	24	−9	9	9		9
22	11	11	11	10	10	
14	21	−7	7	7		7
23	15	8	8	8	8	
					$R_+ = 30$	$R_- = 25$

$$z = \frac{R_+ - R_E}{\sqrt{\frac{(2n + 1) R_E}{6}}}$$

Using the data from our present example, we would compute z as follows:

$$z = \frac{30 - 27.5}{\sqrt{\frac{(20 + 1) \, 27.5}{6}}} = \frac{2.5}{\sqrt{\frac{577.5}{6}}} = \frac{2.5}{9.811} = 0.255$$

Using the values for the normal distribution (Table B–1), the critical value for rejecting the null hypothesis with $\alpha = .05$ is 1.96. Thus, the null hypothesis is accepted. The data do not justify the conclusion that husbands and wives in the population differ in their anxiety in relation to their child's surgery.

Cochran's Q-Test

Cochran's Q-test can be used to test for population differences in proportions when the dependent variable is dichotomous and when there are three or more repeated observations or correlated groups. For example, suppose a sample of 10 elderly patients with constipation problems was put on a special fiber-rich diet, and bowel movements were recorded for three consecutive days, beginning with the day the treatment was initiated. Table 8–7 presents some hypothetical data for this example, with 0 used as the code for

TABLE 8–7. COCHRAN'S Q-TEST EXAMPLE: BOWEL MOVEMENTS FOLLOWING FIBER-RICH DIET

Patient	Day 1	Day 2	Day 3	Row Sum	Row Sum²
1	1	0	1	2	4
2	0	1	1	2	4
3	0	1	0	1	1
4	0	1	1	2	4
5	1	1	1	3	9
6	0	0	1	1	1
7	0	1	0	1	1
8	1	0	1	2	4
9	0	1	1	2	4
10	0	1	1	2	4
	$S_{C_1} = 3$	$S_{C_2} = 7$	$S_{C_3} = 8$	$S_R = 18$	$S_R^2 = 36$
				Mean $(M_R) = 18/3 = 6$	

Codes: 0 = no bowel movement
1 = bowel movement

no bowel movement, and 1 as the code for a bowel movement. According to this table, a total of three patients had bowel movements on Day 1, while seven and eight patients had bowel movements on Days 2 and 3, respectively. The research question is whether the differences reflect true population changes or are the result of sampling fluctuation.

To compute the Q statistic, the number of cases coded 1 must be summed across both columns (S_C) and rows (S_R), as shown in Table 8–7. Then, each summed row value must be squared (S_R^2), and these squared values must be summed. The Q statistic can then be computed using the following formula:

$$Q = \frac{k(k-1)\, \Sigma(S_C - M_R)^2}{k(S_R) - S_R^2}$$

where k = number of groups/times of observation
S_C = sum for each column (i.e., for each k)
S_R = sum of all summed rows
M_R = mean of the summed rows (S_R/k)
Σ = sum of the $(S_C - M_R)^2$ values for the k columns

Although the formula looks complex, it boils down to the insertion of various sums and squares, and the computation is not difficult. In our example, we find:

$$Q = \frac{3\,(2)\,[(3-6)^2 + (7-6)^2 + (8-6)^2]}{(3)\,(18) - 36}$$

$$Q = \frac{(6)\,(9 + 1 + 4)}{54 - 36} = \frac{(6)\,(14)}{18} = 4.67$$

When the number of observations per group is 10 or greater, the Q statistic is distributed approximately as chi-square with k − 1 degrees of freedom. In our example, with $df = 2$ and $\alpha = .05$, the critical value of Q from the chi-square distribution (Table B–4 of Appendix B) is 5.99. Since our obtained value of Q is less than the tabled value, we accept the null hypothesis. The differences in the proportions for the three days of observation are not statistically significant.

The Friedman Test

Like Cochran's Q, the **Friedman test** is used when there are three or more correlated groups, or three or more sets of observations for the same subjects. However, the Friedman test is used when the dependent variable is measured on an ordinal scale. The Friedman test is the nonparametric counterpart of the one-way repeated measures ANOVA, and is sometimes referred to as a nonparametric ANOVA, although the procedure does not, in fact, analyze variance.

Suppose that nine nurses are asked to read descriptions of three patients with Do-Not-Resuscitate orders—an AIDS patient, a cancer patient, and a patient with Alzheimer's disease. The descriptions are presented to the nurses in a random order. For each patient, the nurse is asked a series of questions about the care that he or she thinks should be provided, and the responses are used to create an index of the nurses' aggressiveness of nursing care. Fictitious data for this hypothetical study are presented in Table 8–8. The null hypothesis is that the nurses' scores on aggressiveness of nursing care are unrelated to the type of the patient's illness.

The Friedman test involves ranking the scores for each subject across the different conditions. For example, the first nurse had a score of 15 for the Alzheimer patient description, which is assigned the rank of 1 because it is the lowest score for that nurse. The ranks of 2 and 3 are assigned to the AIDS and cancer patient conditions, respectively, for the first nurse. The ranks for each condition are then summed. For example, the sum of the ranks for the AIDS patient description is 17. If the null hypothesis were true, we would expect the sum of the ranks for each condition to be about equal; any differences in the rankings across subjects would simply reflect sampling error. The formula for the Friedman test, which follows a chi-square distribution, is as follows:

$$\chi^2 = \left[\frac{12\,(\Sigma R^2)}{Nk\,(k + 1)} \right] - 3N\,(k + 1)$$

where k = number of conditions or groups
R = sum of the ranks for each k condition/group
Σ = sum of the squared sum of ranks (R^2) for the k conditions
N = number of subjects

TABLE 8–8. FRIEDMAN'S TEST EXAMPLE: NURSES' AGGRESSIVENESS OF NURSING CARE FOR DNR PATIENTS WITH DIFFERENT ILLNESSES

Nurse	Score (Rank)		
	AIDS	Cancer	Alzheimer
1	17 (2)	18 (3)	15 (1)
2	15 (2)	20 (3)	11 (1)
3	14 (3)	12 (1)	13 (2)
4	11 (1)	19 (3)	18 (2)
5	18 (2)	20 (3)	17 (1)
6	16 (3)	14 (1)	15 (2)
7	12 (1)	14 (3)	13 (2)
8	9 (1)	13 (3)	12 (2)
9	16 (2)	17 (3)	15 (1)
	$R_1 = 17$	$R_2 = 23$	$R_3 = 14$

Using the data from the example presented in Table 8–8, we would calculate the Friedman test as follows:

$$\chi^2 = \left[\frac{12 \left(17^2 + 23^2 + 14^2 \right)}{(9)(3)(3+1)} \right] - (3)(9)(3+1)$$

$$\chi^2 = \left[\frac{(12)(289 + 529 + 196)}{108} \right] - 108 = 112.67 - 108 = 4.67$$

With an alpha level of .05 and $k - 1 = 2$ degrees of freedom, the critical value from the chi-square table (Table B–4) is 5.99. Since the computed value does not exceed the tabled value of chi-square, the null hypothesis is retained. The nurses' scores for aggressiveness of nursing care are not significantly different for the three patient descriptions.

If we *had* rejected the null hypothesis in this example, it would have been necessary to conduct additional analyses to determine which comparisons were driving the results. The Dunn procedure with the Bonferroni correction, described earlier, could be used to isolate the pairs of conditions that were significantly different from one another.

Strength of Association Indexes

Each of the nonparametric tests we have described in this section provides a means of testing the existence of a relationship between an independent and dependent variable.

TABLE 8–9. TABLE OF INDEXES OF MAGNITUDE OF RELATIONSHIP ASSOCIATED WITH SELECTED NONPARAMETRIC STATISTICS

Nonparametric Test	Index of Magnitude of Relationship
Chi-square	Phi coefficient, ϕ (2 × 2)
	Cramér's V
McNemar	Phi coefficient
Mann-Whitney U	Glass rank biserial correlation coefficient
Wilcoxon signed-ranks	Matched-pairs rank biserial coefficient
Kruskal-Wallis	Epsilon-squared
Friedman	Epsilon-squared

While it is beyond the scope of this book to describe indexes for measuring the *strength* of the relationship for the situations in which these nonparametric tests would be used, such indexes do exist, although they are not often reported in the literature. Table 8–9 summarizes indexes that are associated with most of the nonparametric procedures we have described. Formulas for calculating these indexes may be found in Jaccard and Becker (1990) and Welkowitz et al. (1991).

THE COMPUTER AND NONPARAMETRIC TESTS

Compared to parametric tests, nonparametric tests are easy to compute with a hand calculator. When the sample size is small (as it often is when nonparametric procedures are used), manual calculation actually may be faster than entering data onto a computer file and then using a computer program to perform the analyses. However, almost all statistical software packages do offer a variety of nonparametric tests. In this section we review some printouts for several of the statistics discussed in this chapter.

Computer Example of the Chi-Square Test

Figure 8–2 presents the computer printout for the chi-square analysis of the heparin lock data that were shown in Table 8–1.[13] Panel A of this printout shows the descriptive crosstabulation. Each cell of the 2 × 2 table contains information on the frequency (count) and column percentage for that cell. (A more detailed discussion of how to read contingency tables was presented in Chapter 4.) Here, we also instructed the computer to print the expected frequency for each cell. Thus, for the first cell there were nine pa-

---

[13]The SPSS/PC command that created the printout in Figure 8–2 is as follows:

```
CROSSTABS TABLES=COMPLICS BY HEPGROUP
    /CELLS=COUNT COLUMN EXPECTED
    /STATISTICS=CHISQ PHI.
```

A   COMPLICS COMPLICATIONS by HEPGROUP PLACEMENT TIME GROUP

```
                        HEPGROUP        Page 1 of 1
                Count  |
                Exp Val|72 HRS    96 HRS
                Col Pct|                      Row
                       |    1    |    2   | Total
COMPLICS     ----------+---------+--------+
               1       |    9    |   11   |    20
   HAD COMPLICATION    |  10.0   |  10.0  |  20.0%
                       |  18.0%  |  22.0% |
                       +---------+--------+
               2       |   41    |   39   |    80
   NO COMPLICATIONS    |  40.0   |  40.0  |  80.0%
                       |  82.0%  |  78.0% |
                       +---------+--------+
               Column      50        50       100
               Total     50.0%     50.0%   100.0%
```

B

Chi-Square	Value	DF	Significance
Pearson	.25000	1	.61707
Continuity Correction	.06250	1	.80259
Likelihood Ratio	.25034	1	.61684
Mantel-Haenszel test for linear association	.24750	1	.61884

Minimum Expected Frequency -   10.000

C

Statistic	Value	ASE1	T-value	Approximate Significance
Phi	.05000			.61707 *1
Cramer's V	.05000			.61707 *1

*1 Pearson chi-square probability

Number of Missing Observations: 0

FIGURE 8–2.   COMPUTER PRINTOUT OF A CHI-SQUARE ANALYSIS

tients (Count) with complications in the 72-hour heparin lock group; the expected frequency was 10 (Exp Val), and the percentage with complications in the 72-hour group was 18% (Col Pct).

Panel B of Figure 8–2 presents the results of the chi-square test. The basic chi-square statistic is shown in the first row, labeled Pearson (after the statistician who developed the test). The computed value of chi-square is .25000, which is the value we obtained when we performed the calculation manually. With 1 *df,* the probability of obtaining this value of chi-square is .61707, which is not statistically significant. The next row shows the chi-square value after applying Yates' correction for continuity. Again, the value of .0625 corresponds to the value we obtained when we did the com-

```
- - - - - Mann-Whitney U - Wilcoxon Rank Sum W Test

    BODYIMAG   POSITIVE BODY IMAGE SCORE
  by GROUP


    Mean Rank     Cases

        6.40         5   GROUP = 1.00   GROUP A
        4.60         5   GROUP = 2.00   GROUP B
                    ---
                     10   Total

                                EXACT              Corrected for Ties
        U             W       2-tailed P           Z        2-tailed P
        8.0          32.0       .4206            -.9400        .3472
```

FIGURE 8–3.   COMPUTER PRINTOUT OF A MANN-WHITNEY *U*-TEST

putation by hand. The next two values of chi-square are automatically produced by the computer when a chi-square test is requested, but it is beyond the scope of this book to explain them.[14] In any event, it can be seen that the value of the basic chi-square statistic is quite similar to the values shown for "Likelihood Ratio" and "Mantel-Haenszel test for linear association."

The bottom panel of Figure 8–2 presents the values of the two measures of the strength of association that we described earlier. Consistent with our earlier calculations, the value of both the phi coefficient and Cramér's *V* statistic is .05.

Computer Examples of Other Nonparametric Tests

The computer printouts for other nonparametric tests we have discussed in this chapter are generally simple to produce and easy to read. Therefore, only a few illustrative examples will be shown here.

Figure 8–3 shows the printout for a Mann-Whitney *U*-test, using the data in which two groups of burn patients were compared in terms of body image scores.[15] The printout shows that the mean rank for Group A was 6.40, while that for Group B was 4.60. The value of the *U* statistic is 8.0. *W* is the sum of ranks for the group with the smallest *n*. In this case, since both groups had $n = 5$, the value of $W = 32.0$, which is the sum of ranks for the group with the smallest *U* value. Using the binomial distribution, the exact

---

[14]A discussion may be found in the SPSS/PC manual (Norusis, 1990).

[15]The SPSS/PC command that produced the printout in Figure 8–3 is as follows:

NPAR TESTS M-W=BODYIMAG BY GROUP (1,2).

```
- - - - - Kruskal-Wallis 1-way ANOVA

     LIFESAT    LIFE SATISFACTION SCORE
  by HOME

     Mean Rank    Cases

         4.60         5    HOME =    1    NURSING HOME A
         6.40         5    HOME =    2    NURSING HOME B
        13.00         5    HOME =    3    NURSING HOME C
                     ---
                      15    Total


                                               Corrected for Ties
      CASES    Chi-Square  Significance   Chi-Square  Significance
       15        9.7800         .0075        9.7800         .0075
```

FIGURE 8–4.   COMPUTER PRINTOUT OF A KRUSKAL-WALLIS TEST

probability value for a U of 8.0 is .4206, which is nonsignificant. The value for z was also computed $(-.9400)$, and the associated probability is shown (.3472). In this example, since the n for both groups was under 20, the exact probability rather than the probability based on the normal distribution should be used. In either case, however, the group differences are not statistically significant.

Figure 8–4 presents the printout for a Kruskal-Wallis test that analyzed the data on life satisfaction scores among the residents of three nursing homes.[16] The printout shows that the mean ranks for the scores in the three nursing homes were 4.60, 6.40, and 13.00, respectively. The value of the test statistic (under "Chi Square") is shown to be 9.7800, the same value we obtained manually. The actual significance level is .0075, indicating a statistically significant difference in the ranks. The printout recomputes the statistic when there are tied ranks, but in this case there were no ties, so that the value of the corrected test statistic is the same as the original value.

Finally, Figure 8–5 shows the printout for the Friedman test based on data presented in Table 8–8, which involved nine nurses' scores for aggressiveness of nursing care for three conditions.[17] The printout shows that the mean ranks were 1.89, 2.56, and 1.56 for the AIDS, cancer, and Alzheimer disease patient, respectively. The computed

---

[16]The SPSS/PC command that created the printout in Figure 8–4 is as follows:

NPAR TESTS K-W=LIFESAT BY HOME (1,3).

[17]The SPSS/PC command that created the printout in Figure 8–5 is as follows:

NPAR TESTS FRIEDMAN= AIDS CANCER ALZHEIMR.

```
- - - Friedman Two-way ANOVA

Mean Rank    Variable

     1.89    AIDS
     2.56    CANCER
     1.56    ALZHEIMR

     Cases           Chi-Square          D.F.    Significance
       9               4.6667              2         .0970
```

FIGURE 8–5. COMPUTER PRINTOUT OF A FRIEDMAN TEST

value of the test statistic is 4.6667 which, with $df = 2$, has a significance of .0970. For $\alpha = .05$, this value is not statistically significant.

RESEARCH APPLICATIONS OF NONPARAMETRIC TESTS

Except for the chi-square test for independence, nonparametric tests are not widely used in nursing research. In large part, this reflects the fact that parametric tests are more powerful than their nonparametric counterparts, and parametric tests are fairly robust to the violation of many underlying assumptions. Moreover, although psychosocial scales yield data that are—strictly speaking—ordinal, data from such scales are generally treated as interval-level. Nevertheless, nonparametric tests are often the most appropriate analytic procedures, especially when there is evidence that the assumptions for parametric tests cannot possibly be met (e.g., a markedly skewed distribution of the dependent variable).

This section examines some of the major applications of nonparametric tests and discusses methods of effectively displaying results from these tests in a research report.

The Uses of Nonparametric Tests

The nonparametric tests we have discussed in this chapter are, for the most part, used in much the same applications as those we discussed for *t*-tests and ANOVA in the previous two chapters. Therefore, we provide only a few illustrations.

1. *Answering Research Questions.* As with most inferential statistics, the primary use of nonparametric tests is substantive—that is, they are used mainly to test hypotheses and to answer research questions. Table 8–10 illustrates research questions that have been addressed using some of the nonparametric procedures described in this chapter.
2. *Testing Biases.* Nonparametric tests are also used in a methodological capacity to test for the nature and extent of any biases that need to be considered in interpreting

TABLE 8–10. EXAMPLES OF STUDIES USING NONPARAMETRIC TESTS TO ADDRESS SUBSTANTIVE RESEARCH QUESTIONS

Research Question	Nonparametric Test	Result
Does an intervention such as rocking or a pacifier reduce bouts of persistent crying in infants following the heelstick procedure? (Campos, 1994)	Chi-square test	$\chi^2 = 11.87$, $df = 2$, $p < .01$
Is participation in a medication discharge planning program related to rates of readmission to the hospital? (Schneider, Hornberger, Booker, Davis, & Kralicek, 1993)	Fisher's exact test	$p = .05$
Is there a relationship between nipple pain ratings and the presence or absence of (1) inflammation, (2) blisters, and (3) pus in the nipples of women in the first week of lactation? (Ziemer & Pigeon, 1993)	Mann-Whitney U-test	*(1) $p = .02$; (2) $p = .07$; (3) $p = .10$
Do dementia caregivers participating in different types of support groups differ with regard to (1) length of time as care-giver and (2) patient's level of impairment? (Farran & Keane-Hagerty, 1994)	Kruskal-Wallis test	* (1) $p = .06$; (2) $p = .0007$
Are infants with premature rupture of the membrane (PROM) at higher risk of neonatal sepsis than a matched sample of infants without PROM? (Levine, 1991)	McNemar's test	$\chi^2 = 4.54$, $df = 1$, $p = .038$
Is facilitated tucking effective in reducing (1) crying time, (2) sleep disruption time, and (3) sleep state changes after heelstick in premature neonates? (Corff, Seideman, Venkataraman, Lutes, & Yates, 1995)	Wilcoxon signed-ranks test	*(1) $p < .001$; (2) $p < .001$ (3) $p < .003$

*The value of the test statistic was not reported.

substantive results. For example, Daly and her colleagues (1994) studied the effectiveness of two different interventions aimed at meeting the needs of family members of ICU patients. First, however, they examined whether there were selection biases by using chi-square tests to determine if there were differences between the groups with respect to the family members' gender and relationship to the patient (i.e., spouse, daughter, etc.). As another example, Campos (1994) compared two interventions (rocking and pacifiers) against routine care to determine the effectiveness of interventions to comfort infants following a neonatal screening heelstick. Although infants were randomly assigned to the three conditions, Campos evaluated the success of the randomization by using chi-square tests to determine if the groups differed in terms of race, birth order, and maternal feeding method.

3. *Evaluating Representativeness.* The chi-square goodness-of-fit test can be used to test whether a sample of subjects is representative of the population from which it

has been drawn. For example, suppose a sample of teenage mothers were drawn from a hospital clinic and the researcher wanted to known whether the sample adequately represented teenage mothers statewide. Since there is published demographic information on many specific subgroups of the population (often at the local, state, and national level), it would be possible to use the goodness-of-fit test to examine whether the researcher's sample was representative in terms of such characteristics as marital status, race/ethnicity, educational attainment, receipt of public assistance, and so on. The goodness-of-fit procedure would test the null hypothesis that the sample does not differ from the population in the distribution of the characteristics for which there is relevant information.

The Presentation of Nonparametric Tests in Research Reports

As with other statistical information, nonparametric tests usually are presented in the text of a report when there are only one or two tests, but are usually reported in a table if there are more. The standard convention is to provide information about the value of the test statistic, the degrees of freedom, the sample size, and the significance level.

For tests that deal with a nominal-level dependent variable, such as the chi-square test of independence, multiple tests can be reported in a table in much the same fashion as a table for t-tests, except that the descriptive information reported is group percentages rather than group means. Table 8–11 presents an example of such a table that elaborates on our earlier example of heparin lock placement time groups. For four separate complication outcomes, the table shows the percentage in each group with the complication, the value of the chi-quare statistic, and the p value. The table also illustrates how the use of Yates' continuity correction was indicated in a footnote for those tests in which the expected frequency for one or more cell was less than 10. It also illustrates how Fisher's exact test was reported for an outcome for which the expected frequency for some cells was less than 5. It might also be noted that the table presents the actual

TABLE 8–11. EXAMPLE OF A TABLE FOR CHI-SQUARE TEST RESULTS

| Complication | Heparin Lock Placement Time Group | | χ^2 | p |
	72 hours (N = 50)	96 Hours (N = 50)		
Phlebitis	12.0%	16.0%	.08[a]	.77
Blocking/Leaking	8.0%	12.0%	.11[a]	.74
Purulence/Septicaemia	0.0%	2.0%	[b]	1.00
Any Complication	18.0%	22.0%	0.25	.62

NOTES: [a]Chi-square value after Yates' continuity correction
[b]Fisher's exact test

Percentage of Patients with Various Complications, by Length of Time Heparin Lock was in Place

probability values rather than the simpler NS designation, suggesting that the analyses were done on the computer rather than manually.

When a table is presented, the text is used to highlight and summarize results. Here is an example of how the text corresponding to this table might read:

> The table shows that the rates of various complications in the two heparin lock placement time groups were comparable for every type of complication considered. Overall, 18.0% of the 72-hour group, compared to 22.0% of the 96-hour group, had any type of complication, a difference that was not statistically significant. However, although none of the differences was significant, there was a modestly higher rate of complications in the 96-hour group for every complication. A post hoc power analysis revealed that the power of the statistical tests was quite low, and therefore a replication with a larger sample of subjects should be undertaken before any clinical changes are implemented.

When a chi-square test is applied to a contingency table of a fairly large dimensionality—for example, for a 3×4 design—it may be more informative to present all the contingency information in a table, particularly if there is a complex pattern of results for individual cells. When a full contingency table is presented, the results of the statistical table can be placed off to the side or in a footnote. For example, referring back to Table 4–7 in Chapter 4, the first crosstabulation (Acid Inhibitors Absent) from Metheny et al.'s (1993) study could have the following footnote: $\chi^2 = 228.35$, $df = 2$, $p < .00001$. The second crosstabulation (Acid Inhibitors Present) could have the following footnote: $\chi^2 = 202.73$, $df = 2$, $p < .00001$.

When the dependent variables are measured on an ordinal scale—for example, when Mann-Whitney U-tests or Kruskal-Wallis tests have been performed—a common strategy for table presentation is to present the medians for the different groups being compared for each dependent variable, followed by information on the statistical test results. However, group means are sometimes presented in tables in lieu of medians when it is sensible to compute a mean.

RESEARCH EXAMPLE

In this section we briefly summarize a study that used multiple chi-square tests of independence.

> Hamilton and Seidman (1993) conducted a study that examined the differences between men's and women's recovery from an acute myocardial infarction (AMI). Recovery from AMI was examined with respect to three outcome areas: employment behavior and household chores, participation in cardiac rehabilitation, and sexual activity. The sample for the study consisted of 62 AMI patients (42 men and 20 women) who had been hospitalized in a coronary care unit of a tertiary care medical center.
>
>   Chi-square tests were used first to test for demographic and medical differences between the men and women. The two groups were found to be similar in some respects (e.g., education, type

TABLE 8–12. GENDER DIFFERENCES IN TYPES OF ACTIVITIES ENGAGED IN 4 TO 6 WEEKS AFTER ACUTE MYOCARDIAL INFARCTION

Activity	Women $n = 20$ (%)	Men $n = 41$ (%)	χ^2	p
Cooking	80	37	15.4	.000
Washing dishes	80	37	10.1	.001
Bedmaking	63	24	9.4	.002
Doing laundry	55	17	9.3	.002
Sweeping	40	12	6.2	.013
Doing outdoor work	10	29	2.8	NS
Vacuuming	25	15	1.0	NS

Adapted from Table II of Hamilton and Seidman's (1993) report.

of AMI, presence of one or more additional disease at the time of infarction), but there were significant differences for a few background characteristics (e.g., men were more likely than women to be currently married).

With regard to the substantive analyses, the researchers found a great many gender differences in activities during the recovery from an AMI. Men and women were equally likely to return to work, but women reported that they received less counseling from health care workers about work decisions than men. With regard to household chores, 75% of the women, compared to 33% of the men, said they assumed responsibility for household management within 4 to 6 weeks after the AMI ($\chi^2 = 14.3$, $p = .002$). Women were significantly more likely to have responsibility for a wide range of household chores, as shown in Table 8–12—an abbreviated version of the researcher's Table II. There were no gender differences with regard to participation in a cardiac rehabilitation program. However, women were significantly more likely than men to decrease the frequency of sexual activity following the AMI ($\chi^2 = 9.0$, $p = .012$).

SUMMARY

The **chi-square test of independence,** the most widely used nonparametric procedure, is designed to make inferences about population differences in proportions between two or more groups. It is used when both the independent and dependent variable are measured on the nominal scale. The chi-square statistic is computed by contrasting **expected frequencies** (frequencies expected if the null hypothesis of no relationship between variables were true) and **observed frequencies** for each cell in a contingency table. In a 2×2 table in which the expected frequency is less than 10, it is often recommended that **Yates' correction for continuity** be applied, and when the expected frequency is less than 5, an alternative test known as **Fisher's exact test** is often used. The index used to measure the strength of the relationship is the **phi coefficient** for a 2×2 table and **Cramér's V** for a larger table. Cramér's V can be used as the effect size in a power analysis in the context of a chi-square situation. The **chi-square goodness-of-fit test** is used to draw inferences when there is only one nominal level variable about which inferences are to be made.

There are numerous other nonparametric tests, only a few of which are covered in this chapter. For between-subjects, independent groups designs with an ordinal-level dependent variable, the **Mann-Whitney U-test** can be used to test differences in ranks between two groups, and the **Kruskal-Wallis test** can be used to compare ranks when there are three or more groups. These tests are the nonparametric counterparts of the t-test and ANOVA, respectively. For dependent groups (within-subjects designs) and a dichotomous dependent variable, the **McNemar test** can be used for two paired groups or sets of observations, and **Cochran's Q test** is appropriate for three or more groups or observations. For two dependent groups with ordinal data, the **Wilcoxon signed-ranks test** may be used, and when there are more than two groups or observations, the **Friedman test** is appropriate. These tests are the nonparametric analogs of the paired t-test and repeated measures ANOVA, respectively. When either the Kruskal-Wallis or Friedman test is statistically significant, the **Dunn procedure** (ideally with a **Bonferroni correction** to reduce the risk of a Type I error) can be used to determine the nature of the relationship between the independent and dependent variables (i.e., to isolate the pairs of groups or observations responsible for a significant overall test).

EXERCISES

The following exercises cover concepts presented in this chapter. Exercises indicated with a dagger (†) can be checked against answers appearing in Appendix A. Additionally, Chapter 8 of the accompanying *Applications Manual* offers supplementary exercises, including ones that require computer analysis of a data set on diskette.

† 1. Calculate the chi-square statistic and degrees of freedom for the following set of data for 300 people:

	Group A	Group B	Group C	Total
Had a Flu Shot	20	45	25	90
Did Not Have a Flu Shot	80	55	75	210
Total	100	100	100	300

Is the value of chi-square statistically significant at the .05 level? Based on the $(O - E)^2/E$ components contributing to chi-square, comment on the nature of the relationship between groups and flu shot status.

† 2. For the data presented in Exercise 1, compute Cramér's V statistic. Then estimate the approximate power of the chi-square test, using Table C–3 in Appendix C.

3. Using the statistical information obtained in the first two exercises, write a paragraph summarizing the results of the analyses.

† 4. Given each of the following circumstances, determine whether the calculated values of chi-square are statistically significant:
   a. $\chi^2 = 3.72$, $df = 1$, $\alpha = .05$
   b. $\chi^2 = 9.59$, $df = 4$, $\alpha = .05$
   c. $\chi^2 = 10.67$, $df = 3$, $\alpha = .01$
   d. $\chi^2 = 9.88$, $df = 2$, $\alpha = .01$

† 5. In a pilot test involving an experimental and control group and a dichotomous dependent variable, a researcher obtains a value for the phi coefficient of .19. *Approximately* how many subjects should the researcher use in a full-blown study of the effectiveness of the intervention to achieve a power of .80?

† 6. Match each of the nonparametric tests in Column A with its parametric counterpart in Column B:

A. *Nonparametric Test*	B. *Parametric Test*
1. Mann-Whitney U-test	a. Paired t-test
2. Friedman test	b. One-way ANOVA
3. Kruskal-Wallis test	c. Independent groups t-test
4. Wilcoxon signed-ranks test	d. Repeated measures ANOVA

† 7. Using the information provided, indicate which test you think should be used for each of the following situations:
   a. Independent variable: normal birth-weight versus low birth-weight infants; dependent variable: 1-minute Apgar scores (0 to 10 scale); sample size: 8 infants per group; skewness index $= -0.45$.
   b. Independent variable: time of measurement (before, during, and after surgery); dependent variable: heart rate; sample size: 30; skewness index $= 0.09$.
   c. Independent variable: time of measurement (before, during, and after intervention); dependent variable: did versus did not exercise daily; sample size: 30.
   d. Independent variable: infertility treatment A versus infertility treatment B versus control condition; dependent variable: did versus did not become pregnant; sample size: 60.
   e. Independent variable: drug A versus drug B versus placebo; dependent variable: scores on a depression scale; sample size: 9 per group; skewness index $= -0.36$.
   f. Independent variable: source of information (patient report versus hospital records); dependent variable: patient kept versus did not keep appointment for contraceptive counseling; sample size: 100 patients.

† 8. Below are three sets of *expected* frequencies for the four cells of 2 × 2 contingency tables. Comment on which statistical procedure would be appropriate for each, using the most conservative approach.

a.	4	4	b.	35	35	c.	9	9
	21	21		65	65		91	91

† 9. Compute the Mann-Whitney U statistic for the following scores on a coping ability scale:

Men:	21	25	31	16	19	29	27
Women:	24	18	28	17	22	23	20

Are the men significantly different from the women in terms of coping ability scores ($\alpha = .05$)?

† 10. Below are scores on a self-care agency scale for 10 patients before and after an intervention:

Before: 12 15 11 18 17 20 13 15 10 14
After: 15 17 17 17 22 27 21 11 20 23

Compute the appropriate nonparametric test statistic and determine whether there is a significant change in scores ($\alpha = .05$).

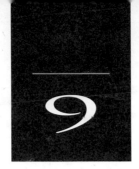

Correlation and Simple Regression

In Chapter 4, we discussed Pearson's r, a descriptive index that summarizes the magnitude and direction of a relationship between two variables. Correlation procedures are also used to draw inferences about relationships in populations based on sample data. This chapter discusses the inferential aspects of correlation coefficients, and also introduces the closely related topic of linear regression.

PEARSON'S r AND INFERENTIAL STATISTICS

Suppose that we were interested in examining the relationship between a widowed person's grief resolution following the death of a spouse (the dependent variable) and the length of the spouse's illness prior to death (the independent variable). We find that, for a sample of 50 widows and widowers, the Pearson r between scores on a grief resolution scale and length of spouse's illness is .26, indicating a modest tendency for longer illnesses to be associated with more favorable grief resolution.[1] However, the observed correlation in the sample does not in itself tell us whether the relationship is likely to exist in the corresponding population. A correlation of .26 could be the result of sampling error. We need to apply inferential statistics to determine the probability that there is a population correlation.

The Null and Alternative Hypotheses

As we discuss later in this chapter, there are several null hypotheses that can be tested in the context of Pearson's r. However, the basic and most widely tested null hypothesis is

[1]The computational formula for calculating Pearson's r is presented in Chapter 4.

that there is no relationship between the independent and dependent variables. When there is no relationship, the correlation is zero. Therefore, we can formally state the null hypothesis as follows:

$H_0: \rho = .00$

The population correlation coefficient is usually symbolized as ρ—rho, the lowercase Greek r. Thus, the null hypothesis stipulates that the correlation coefficient for the two variables in the population equals zero.

   The alternative hypothesis is that there *is* a relationship between the independent and dependent variables. The nondirectional alternative hypothesis can be stated as follows:

$H_0: \rho \neq .00$

   This alternative hypothesis does not predict the nature of the relationship between the two variables. If we had an *a priori* reason for hypothesizing the direction of the relationship, the alternative hypothesis could specify that direction. That is, we could test the hypothesis that ρ is greater than zero (if we had reason to believe that the variables were positively correlated) or that ρ is less than zero (if we believed that the variables were negatively correlated).

Sampling Distribution of a Correlation Coefficient

Sample data are used to test the probability that the null hypothesis is true against the appropriate alternative hypothesis. The sample correlation coefficient r is used as the estimate of ρ, and the statistic can be compared to a sampling distribution to determine whether the obtained value of r is "improbable" if the null hypothesis is true.

   A theoretical sampling distribution of a correlation coefficient can be constructed in much the same fashion as other sampling distributions. That is, one has to imagine drawing an infinite number of samples of a specified size and plotting the values of the correlation coefficients in a frequency distribution. The mean of the sampling distribution of the correlation coefficient is approximately ρ, the true population correlation. When $\rho = 0$ (i.e., when the null hypothesis is true), the sampling distribution is essentially normal with the mean centered on .00.

   Distributions of t are used as the statistical model to test the null hypothesis that two variables are not correlated. A t value can be computed with a formula that uses the value of r and the sample size, and then the resulting statistic can be compared to a t distribution with $N - 2$ degrees of freedom.[2] However, it is unnecessary to compute a t sta-

---

[2]The formula for computing t is:

$$t = \frac{r \sqrt{N - 2}}{\sqrt{1 - r^2}}$$

tistic, because statisticians have developed tabled values of r specifically to test the null hypothesis that a population correlation is zero, as we discuss subsequently.

Assumptions and Requirements for Pearson's r

Pearson's r is appropriate when both the independent and dependent variables are measured on approximately an interval level or on a ratio level. As discussed in Chapter 4, Pearson's r is suitable for detecting *linear* relationships between two variables, but is not appropriate as an index of curvilinear relationships.[3]

The test of the null hypothesis that $\rho = .00$ is based on several assumptions. First, as with other tests, it is assumed that the subjects have been randomly and independently sampled from the population of interest. Second, the variables being correlated (X and Y) are assumed to have an underlying distribution that is **bivariate normal**—that is, the scores on variable X are normally distributed *for each value of variable Y,* and vice versa. Finally, the scores must be **homoscedastic**—that is, for each value of X, the variability of the Y scores must be about the same, and vice versa. Failure to meet the last two assumptions generally has only a small effect on the validity of the statistical test, however, particularly when the sample size is at least 25 to 30.

Testing the Significance of Pearson's r

Earlier in this chapter, we presented an example in which the correlation between a widowed person's score on a grief resolution scale and the spouse's length of illness in a sample of 50 subjects was .26. Is this value large enough for us to conclude that a correlation exists in the population, or is it likely that the correlation of .26 in the sample was simply due to sampling error? We can proceed to test the null hypothesis that the population correlation is zero against the alternative hypothesis that it is not.

As usual, we perform the test by comparing the calculated test statistic against a critical value for the statistic from the appropriate table (Table B–6 of Appendix B). First, however, we must calculate degrees of freedom. For Pearson's r, the formula is:

$$df = N - 2$$

In our present example, then, there are 48 degrees of freedom ($50 - 2 = 48$). For a nondirectional (two-tailed) test with $\alpha = .05$, we find in column 3 of the table that the critical value of r with $df = 48$ is between .273 and .288 (i.e., between the values for 45 and 50 degrees of freedom). Since the obtained value of r is .26, we must accept the null hypothesis that the population correlation is zero. There is a greater than 5% probability that a correlation coefficient of .26 is the result of sampling error, and so we cannot conclude that the length of a spouse's illness is related to the widowed partner's grief resolution in the population.

---

[3]The existence and extent of a curvilinear relationship can be determined using a statistical technique known as **curvilinear regression.** The interested reader can consult Pedhazur (1982).

It might be noted that, had we tested a directional hypothesis, the outcome would have been different. If theory or prior research had led us to hypothesize in advance that grief resolution would be greater among those whose spouses were ill for a longer period prior to death, we would find in column 2 of Table B–6 that the critical value for a directional (one-tailed) test with $\alpha = .05$ would be about .233. Therefore, since the computed value of r is greater than the critical value, the null hypothesis would be rejected. Of course, it is inappropriate to use the critical values for a directional test *after* the correlation coefficient has been computed if a directional hypothesis was not specified in advance.

Note that when we accept a null hypothesis, we *cannot* conclude that there is no relationship between the two variables in the population. The possibility of a Type II error—the incorrect acceptance of the null hypothesis—still remains. Moreover, there is also a possibility that the variables are related in the population, but in a nonlinear fashion. The acceptance of the null hypothesis must, as always, be treated conservatively, especially if a power analysis (described subsequently) has not been performed.

Testing Differences Between Two Correlations

Although researchers are most often interested in testing the null hypothesis that the population correlation between two variables is zero, there are other hypotheses that can be tested. The most common alternative involves a test of the equivalence of two correlations. For example, suppose that in our example of grief resolution among widowed people, all of the subjects were widows. Let us suppose that we did another study with a sample of 50 widowers, using the same measure of grief resolution, and obtained a correlation coefficient of .45. The research question here is whether the difference in observed correlations for the men versus the women occurred simply as a function of sampling error, or whether there is a population difference between men and women in the relationship between grief resolution and length of spouse's illness. In this situation, the null hypothesis being tested is:

$H_0: \rho_A = \rho_B$

where ρ_A = population correlation for group A (widows)
ρ_B = population correlation for group B (widowers)

When ρ is not equal to zero—which this null hypothesis assumes—the sampling distribution of the correlation coefficient is skewed rather than approximately normal, and therefore the same table that was used to test the basic hypothesis of no relationship between variables cannot be used. However, the statistician Fisher developed a logarithmic transformation of r (usually referred to as the **r-to-z transformation**) that makes it possible to use the normal distribution for comparing two correlation coefficients.

Table B–7 of Appendix B presents the values for transforming correlation coefficients into values of z. To use this table, we must first find the value of r, and then read directly to the right the corresponding value of z. From this table we find that for widows, $r = .26$ so $z_A = .266$; for widowers, $r = .45$ so $z_B = .485$. With these transformed z values, the following formula can be used to compute a test statistic (z_{obs}) for the significance of the difference between the two[4]:

$$z_{obs} = \frac{|z_A - z_B|}{\sqrt{\dfrac{1}{n_A - 3} + \dfrac{1}{n_B - 3}}}$$

In our present example, the computed statistic would be:

$$z_{obs} = \frac{|.266 - .485|}{\sqrt{\dfrac{1}{50 - 3} + \dfrac{1}{50 - 3}}} = \frac{.219}{\sqrt{\dfrac{2}{47}}} = \frac{.219}{.206} = 1.06$$

The calculated z_{obs} statistic must now be compared to the critical value from the normal distribution (Table B–1). For $\alpha = .05$ for a nondirectional test, that critical value is 1.96. Since our value of z_{obs} is less than the critical value, the null hypothesis is retained. We cannot conclude that the correlation between grief resolution and length of spouse's illness is different for widows and widowers in the population.

The Strength and Nature of the Relationship

Unlike most other inferential statistics, Pearson's r directly conveys information about the strength and nature of the relationship between the two variables under consideration. The nature of the relationship is indicated by the sign of the correlation coefficient. A negative sign, it will be recalled, indicates that high values on one variable are associated with low values on the second. A positive sign (or a coefficient without a sign, which by convention is assumed to indicate a positive correlation) indicates that high values on X are associated with high values on Y.

The strength of the relationship between the variables is directly indicated by the absolute value of Pearson's r. The higher the absolute value of the correlation coefficient, the stronger the relationship. However, as discussed in Chapter 4, the magnitude of a correlation is often expressed in terms of r^2, which is formally known as the **coefficient of determination.**

---

[4]The test for the difference between the two correlations is based on the assumption that the two samples being compared are independent—i.e., that the correlations are based on different subjects. Procedures for testing the equivalence of correlations computed for the same subjects (e.g., comparing correlations for the same two variables measured at two points in time) may be found in Ferguson (1981).

It can be shown that r^2 is directly equivalent to eta-squared. As we saw in the chapter on ANOVA, eta^2 is the ratio of explained variance ($SS_{Explained}$) to total variance (SS_{Total}). Thus:

$$r^2 = eta^2 = \frac{SS_{Explained}}{SS_{Total}}$$

The coefficient of determination, then, tells us the proportion of variance in variable Y that is associated with variable X—the proportion of variance that is *shared* by the two variables. Thus, in the example we have used in this chapter where $r = .26$, we could say that about 7% of the variability in grief resolution is shared by (explained by) the variability in spouse's length of illness ($.26^2 = .068$).

When comparing two different correlations, it is more appropriate to use r^2 than r. For example, suppose that the correlation between grief resolution and spouse's age at death was .13—half the value of the correlation between grief resolution and spouse's length of illness. However, length of illness explains *four* times as much of the variance in grief resolution scores as spouse's age—.068 versus .017($.13^2$)—and this is the more informative and meaningful comparison.

Power and Pearson's r

As with other statistical tests we have discussed, there are two primary reasons for performing a power analysis in the context of a study involving Pearson's r. The first is to facilitate interpretation of the results, particularly when the correlation is not statistically significant. The second is to help in planning an investigation, to maximize the potential for significant results by having a sufficiently large sample size.

The effect size for the power analysis is, in this situation, the estimated value of ρ. Thus, we can use the sample correlation coefficient as the estimate of γ, the effect size. As in Chapter 6 where we discussed power analysis for comparing two group means (i.e., the t-test situation), we must first compute delta (δ) to make use of the appropriate power table (Table C–1 of Appendix C). The formula is:

$$\delta = \gamma \sqrt{N - 1}, \quad \text{or} \quad \delta = r \sqrt{N - 1}$$

In our example of grief resolution and spouse's length of illness, the value of δ would be:

$$\delta = .26 \sqrt{50 - 1} = .26 (7) = 1.82$$

With $\alpha = .05$, we find in Table C–1 that the power for a two-tailed test with $\delta = 1.82$ is approximately .45 (i.e., between .44 and .48, the values when $\delta = 1.8$ and 1.9, respectively). For a one-tailed, directional test, power would increase to approximately .57. In both cases, then, there is about a 50-50 risk of committing a Type II error. Thus, if we wanted to replicate the study, we would be well advised to use a larger sample size.

Table C–1 can also be used for sample size determinations. We see in this table that δ would need to be 2.8 to achieve a power of .80—the conventional standard— when $\alpha = .05$ for a two-tailed test. For a replication, then, if we assume that our original correlation coefficient is a reasonable estimate of ρ, we would arrive at the following equation:

$$2.8 = .26 \sqrt{N - 1}$$
$$N - 1 = (2.8/.26)^2 = 10.769^2 = 116$$
$$N = 116 + 1 = 117$$

Thus, we would need a sample size of about 117 subjects to reduce the risk of a Type II error to .20, given an estimated population correlation of .26.

By using the formula to compute δ and then turning to Table C–1 in Appendix C, a researcher can make rather fine determinations of power and sample size. For the sake of convenience, however, we offer a simpler but cruder table, shown here as Table 9–1. This table is appropriate only when $\alpha = .05$ and the test is two-tailed (nondirectional). To use the table to estimate power, you must find the estimate of the population correlation coefficient along the top row, and then find the closest value for the sample size in that column. The estimate of power is the value in the first column of that same row. Thus, in our example, we would use the column for .25. Since the sample size of 50 is between the values of 46 and 61 in the column headed by the correlation coefficient of .25, we can see that power lies between .40 and .50. And, to achieve a power of .80 with

TABLE 9–1. POWER AS A FUNCTION OF THE POPULATION CORRELATION COEFFICIENT, FOR $\alpha = .05$, NONDIRECTIONAL TEST

POWER	POPULATION CORRELATION COEFFICIENT										
	.05	.10	.15	.20	.25	.30	.40	.50	.60	.70	.80
.20	484*	121	54	30	19	13	8	5	3	2	2
.30	818	204	91	51	33	23	13	8	6	4	3
.40	1156	289	128	72	46	32	18	12	8	6	5
.50	1521	380	169	95	61	42	24	15	11	8	6
.60	1980	490	218	123	79	55	32	21	15	11	8
.70	2460	616	274	155	99	69	39	26	18	14	10
.80	3136	785	349	197	126	88	50	32	23	17	12
.90	4225	1050	468	263	169	118	67	43	30	22	17
.95	5184	1297	577	325	208	145	82	53	37	27	21
.99	7056	1841	819	461	296	205	116	75	50	36	28

*The entries in the table indicate the sample size required to achieve the specified power for the given correlation coefficient.

r = .26, Table 9–1 indicates that we would need a sample size of about 126. These values are close approximations to what we achieved using Table C–1.

Factors Affecting Pearson's *r*

There are several factors that have an effect on the magnitude of Pearson's *r*. These factors should be kept in mind in designing a correlational study, and in interpreting the results of correlational analyses. One of these factors is the existence of a curvilinear, rather than linear, relationship between the two variables, an issue discussed in Chapter 4. Several other issues are discussed here.

The Effect of a Restricted Range. If two variables are linearly related, the magnitude of the correlation coefficient is usually reduced when the range of values on one of the variables is restricted. It may be recalled that the formula for the correlation coefficient involves deviation scores—that is, deviations from the means of the two variables. When the range is restricted, the deviations are smaller and thus the magnitude of *r* is reduced.

This principle can best be illustrated graphically. Suppose we had a sample of smokers and nonsmokers and plotted their weekly number of packs of cigarettes smoked against a measure of pulmonary function, as shown in Figure 9–1. For the overall sample, the scatterplot suggests a strong negative correlation between weekly packs of cigarettes and pulmonary function. In fact, the computed correlation coefficient is −.81, a correlation that is significantly different from zero at the .001 level. Now suppose that instead of using the entire group, we restricted the sample to those people who

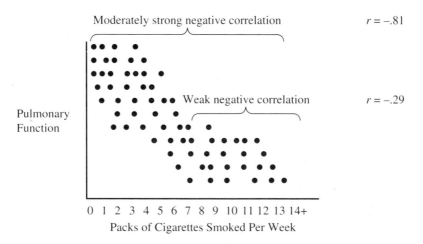

FIGURE 9–1. ILLUSTRATION OF THE EFFECT OF A RESTRICTED RANGE ON THE CORRELATION COEFFICIENT

smoked at least one pack of cigarettes per day—i.e., at least seven packs per week. As shown in the figure, the relationship between cigarette consumption and pulmonary function is now much less clear-cut. Although the scatterplot suggests a negative correlation among the regular smokers, it is fairly weak. Indeed, the computed correlation coefficient is −.29, which is not statistically significant from zero for $N = 25$. Note that a similar reduction in the correlation would occur if the range for the pulmonary function variable were restricted (e.g., if only those with very high or very low function were included in the sample).

The Effect of Extreme Groups. When only extreme groups are included in a sample, the magnitude of the correlation coefficient is often *increased*. To continue with our example of the correlation between smoking and pulmonary function, suppose we included in our sample only nonsmokers on the one hand, and people who smoked 10 or more packs of cigarettes per week on the other. In this situation, illustrated in Figure 9–2, the *range* of values on both variables is the same as it was originally, but the deviations from the mean are exaggerated because there are no subjects who are close to the mean on either variable. With this extreme-group sample, the correlation is markedly negative. The computed value of the correlation coefficient in this instance is −.96. Thus, when extreme groups from a population are sampled, care must be taken not to interpret the correlation coefficients as reflecting relationships for the entire population.

The Effect of an Outlier. When a sample of subjects is relatively small, a subject with an extreme value on one or both of the variables being correlated can have a dramatic effect on the magnitude of the correlation coefficient. An exaggerated illustration is graphed in

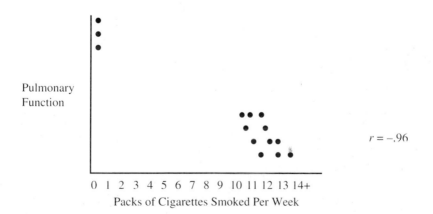

FIGURE 9–2.   ILLUSTRATION OF THE EFFECT OF USING EXTREME GROUPS ON THE CORRELATION COEFFICIENT

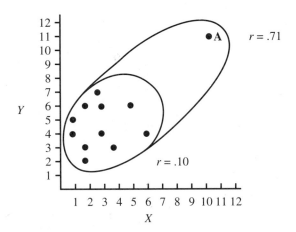

FIGURE 9–3.   ILLUSTRATION OF THE EFFECT OF AN OUTLIER ON THE CORRELATION COEFFI-CIENT

Figure 9–3. In this example, 11 of the 12 subjects in the sample had values for both the X and Y variables that were 7 or less. The twelfth subject, labeled A on the scatterplot, had extremely high values on both variables. The smaller ellipse surrounding the values without the outlier suggests a modest correlation—in fact, the actual value of Pearson's r for these 11 cases is .10. However, when the outlier is included, the shape of the outer ellipse is indicative of a much stronger relationship. The actual calculated value of r when the outlier is included is .71—a dramatically higher, and misleading, correlation coefficient.

When outliers represent legitimate score values rather than data entry or coding errors, care must be taken in using them in the analysis. Researchers sometimes analyze their data both ways—with and without outliers—and present both sets of results when the disparity is sufficiently great. Barnett and Lewis (1985) suggest alternative strategies for handling outliers.

The Effect of Unreliable Measures. Virtually all quantitative measures of variables contain some measurement error. Psychometricians generally refer to this error as **unreliability,** and they have developed methods of assessing how reliable measures are. In general, measures of psychosocial traits tend to be less reliable than measures of physiological attributes. While it is beyond the scope of this book to discuss measurement error in detail,[5] it should be noted that measurement error reduces the magnitude of correlation coefficients. Such an effect is referred to as **attenuation.** Thus, in interpreting modest cor-

---

[5]Information on measurement error can be obtained in research methods textbooks (e.g., Polit and Hungler, 1995) or in books on psychometric methods (e.g., Nunnally, 1978).

relation coefficients, it may be important to consider whether the magnitude might have been diminished by the use of relatively weak instruments.[6]

OTHER MEASURES OF ASSOCIATION

In addition to Pearson's r, there are other statistical indexes that are designed to describe relationships between two variables and to permit inferences about relationships in the population. Indeed, we have already discussed several of these in earlier chapters. For example, in Chapter 6 we described the point-biserial correlation coefficient, and in Chapter 8 we discussed the phi coefficient and Cramér's V. In this section we examine several other measures of bivariate relationships.

Spearman's Rank-Order Correlation

A statistic known as **Spearman's rank-order correlation** is a nonparametric analog of Pearson's r. A Spearman correlation is typically used when the dependent variable is measured on the ordinal scale, or when one or both variables being correlated is severely skewed or has an outlier. It is also preferred by some researchers when the number of cases is less than 30.

Suppose that we wanted to examine the correlation between nursing students' class rank at graduation and the students' rating of how likely it is that they would pursue a graduate degree, on a scale from 0 (totally unlikely) to 10 (totally probable). A Spearman's correlation coefficient (sometimes symbolized as r_S)[7] could be computed in such a situation. Some hypothetical data for ten students are presented in Table 9–2.

To compute Spearman's correlation coefficient, both variables must be rank ordered. The class rank variable is inherently rank ordered, but we must also rank order the students' ratings of the likelihood of going to graduate school. The rankings for this variable are shown in column 3 of Table 9–2. It may be noted that there was one tie: two students had a rating of 8. When ties occur, the two adjacent ranks (here, the ranks of 3 and 4) are averaged, and the average rank (here, 3.5) is assigned to both subjects. In the next step, the difference between the ranks for the two variables (D) is taken (column 5), and then the difference is squared (column 6). The sum of the squared differences is then used in the following formula:

$$r_S = 1 - \frac{6\,(\Sigma D^2)}{N\,(N^2 - 1)}$$

---

[6] Psychometricians have developed a formula for correcting attenuated correlation coefficients. The correction takes the reliability coefficients for one or both variables into account (see, for example, Nunnally, 1978, p. 218).

[7] The Spearman rank-order correlation coefficient is sometimes referred to as Spearman's rho (Spearman's ρ). However, to avoid any confusion between this statistic and the population parameter for Pearson's correlation coefficient, also symbolized as ρ, we use r_S for the Spearman coefficient.

TABLE 9–2. EXAMPLE OF SPEARMAN'S RANK-ORDER CORRELATION CALCULATION

(1) Student	(2) Grad School Rating*	(3) Grad School Rank (X)	(4) Class Rank (Y)	(5) D (X − Y)	(6) D² (X − Y)²
1	8	3.5	1	2.5	6.25
2	9	2	2	0	0.00
3	10	1	3	−2	4.00
4	5	7	4	3	9.00
5	7	5	5	0	0.00
6	8	3.5	6	−2.5	6.25
7	6	6	7	−1	1.00
8	4	8	8	0	0.00
9	2	10	9	1	1.00
10	3	9	10	−1	1.00
					$\Sigma D^2 = 28.50$

*Student's rating of likelihood of pursuing a graduate degree, from 0 (extremely unlikely) to 10 (extremely probable).

For the data presented in Table 9–2, we find that the Spearman correlation is:

$$r_S = 1 - \frac{6\,(28.5)}{10\,(10^2 - 1)} = 1 - \frac{171.0}{10\,(99)} = .83$$

Like Pearson's r, Spearman's r_S can range between -1.00 through 0.00 to $+1.00$. A high positive value, such as we obtained in our example, indicates a strong tendency for the paired ranks to be similar, while a negative value indicates a tendency for low ranks on one variable to be associated with high ranks on the other.

The null hypothesis when using Spearman's correlation is that there is no linear relationship between the two sets of ranks, i.e., that the population correlation (ρ) is zero. To test the hypothesis, the computed value of r_S can be compared to critical values that are presented in Table B–8 of Appendix B. With a sample size of 10, the critical value for $\alpha = .05$ (for a two-tailed test) is .648. Since the computed value is greater than the critical value, we can reject the null hypothesis and conclude that there is a population correlation between a student's rank in class and his or her projected probability of going to graduate school.

Note that the table of critical values for the Spearman correlation can only be used when $N \leq 30$ and ≥ 5. When there are more than 30 cases, a reasonably good approximation of the significance test can be obtained by using the table of critical values for Pearson's r (Table B–6) with $N - 2$ degrees of freedom.[8]

It might be noted that most of the measures of association we have presented thus far, including Spearman's rank-order correlation, are basically variants of the Pearson product-moment formula. For this reason, the methods discussed earlier in this chapter on power analysis are also appropriate for Spearman's rho, as well as for the phi coefficient and the point-biserial coefficient.

Kendall's Tau

The Spearman rank-order correlation approach is somewhat less accurate than might be desired because the approximations to theoretical sampling distributions are imperfect, especially for samples of intermediate size. For this reason, some researchers and statisticians prefer another index of rank-order correlations, known as **Kendall's tau** (symbolized as τ). While Kendall's tau has advantageous statistical properties, it is somewhat more complicated to compute, and will not be fully presented here. Most statistical software packages have a program that computes Kendall's tau, and the interested reader can consult Siegel (1956) or Glass and Stanley (1970) for computational procedures.

SIMPLE LINEAR REGRESSION

The term **regression** refers to a variety of techniques that are used to analyze relationships between variables and to make predictions about the values of variables. Regression-based procedures, which are based on correlational techniques, are the foundation of many complex statistics that we describe in later chapters of this book. In this chapter, we introduce regression concepts and describe the link between correlation and regression.

Equation for a Straight Line

When a relationship between two variables is linear and perfect, knowledge of the value of one variable allows you to know or predict the value of the second variable with complete accuracy. This is because the relationship can be characterized by a straight line, for which there is a simple equation. Let us consider the example we presented in Chapter 4 concerning the sponsor that donated $1 to a school's athletic fund

---

[8]A more precise method is to convert the Spearman correlation coefficient to a t statistic, which can then be compared to critical values of t (Table B–2) with $N - 2$ degrees of freedom, using the following formula:

$$t = \frac{r_\mathrm{s} \sqrt{N - 2}}{\sqrt{1 - r_\mathrm{s}^2}}$$

for every hour that students volunteered to work at the school's health clinic. As shown in Figure 9–4(A), the value of X (hours volunteered) is always equal to Y (dollars donated). The relationship between the two variables is linear and perfect, and so the relationship can be characterized by the following formula:

$$Y = X$$

Based on this equation, we would be able to predict perfectly the amount of the sponsor's donation if we knew the number of hours students volunteered. For 98 hours of volunteer time, for example, the donation would be $98.

Now suppose that the donor agreed to pay *$2.00* for every one hour volunteered. The relationship between hours and dollars for this arrangement, which again is perfect and linear, is shown in Figure 9–4(B). Formally, this relationship between X and Y can be stated as:

$$Y = 2X$$

Now, for 98 hours of volunteer time, the donation would be $196 (2 × $98). If you compare the graphs for the two equations [Figures 9–4 (A) and (B)], you can see that the

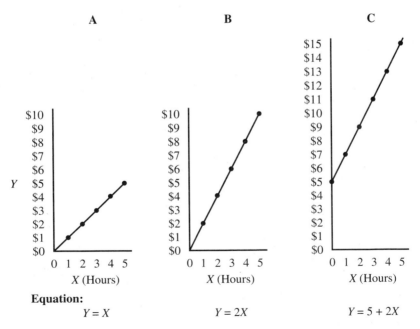

FIGURE 9–4.   EXAMPLES OF LINEAR RELATIONSHIPS WITH DIFFERENT SLOPES AND INTERCEPTS

lines have different angles: the **slope** of the line is greater in the second graph. Thus, relationships can be linear and perfect and yet differ with regard to the slopes of the lines that characterize them.

In both of these situations, if there were no student volunteers, there would be no donation. Suppose, however, that the donor decided to start with a flat $5 donation, and then *added* $2.00 for every hour worked. This relationship—which is again perfect and linear—is graphed in Figure 9–4(C). The slope of the line is identical to the slope shown in Figure 9–4(B), but the point at which the line crosses the Y axis—known as the **intercept**—is 5 in graph C rather than 0. The relationship shown in graph C can be stated as:

$$Y = 5 + 2X$$

Using this equation, we would find that for 98 hours worked, the amount of the donation would be $201 [$5 + (2 × $98)]. Thus, we can see with the three situations graphed in Figure 9–4 that linear relationships can differ in terms of the values of both slopes and intercepts.

Any straight line can be described in terms of its slope and intercept. The general equation for a straight line, sometimes referred to as the **linear model,** is:

$$Y = a + bX$$

where a = intercept constant
b = slope of the line

In the first situation shown in graph A, the value of the intercept constant a is 0 and the value of the slope b is 1; in graph B, $a = 0$, and $b = 2$; and in graph C, $a = 5$, and $b = 2$.

When plotted on Cartesian coordinates with an X and Y axis, there is always a slope and an intercept that describe the relationship between two perfectly correlated variables. When the variables are negatively correlated, the slope of the line—the value of b—is also negative. For example, suppose a professor gave students a 10-question test, with each question worth 10 points. The relationship between the number of questions wrong on the test and the test grade, shown in Figure 9–5, can be stated as:

$$Y = 100 - 10X$$

where Y = test grade
X = number of items wrong

A student with four questions wrong would have a grade of 60; a student with no questions wrong would have a grade of 100.

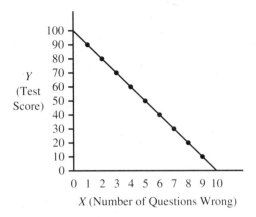

Equation: Y = 100 − 10X

FIGURE 9–5.   EXAMPLE OF A NEGATIVE LINEAR RELATIONSHIP

Thus, the usefulness of having an equation that characterizes a linear relationship is that for any value of X, we can determine or predict the value of Y. This ability for the linear model to make predictions makes it an attractive model for the research community.

The Basic Regression Equation

In research studies, relationships between variables are often linear, but they are almost never perfect. When a correlation between two variables is not perfect, the statistical technique of regression can be used to identify the straight line that runs through the data points with the best possible fit, as determined by a statistical criterion known as **least squares.** (We discuss this criterion at greater length below.)

To explain regression procedures, we will return to the example we presented in Chapter 4 regarding the correlation between nursing students' scores on a midterm and final statistics exam. Data for this example (originally shown in Table 4–4 and graphed in a scatterplot in Figure 4–2) are presented in Table 9–3. The midterm scores (X) are shown in column 1, and the final exam scores (Y) are shown in column 4. Applying the Pearson r formula to these data, we found that the correlation coefficient between the two sets of test scores is .955, an extremely high—but not perfect—correlation.

The **regression equation** is the formula for the best-fitting straight line to characterize the linear relationship between X and Y. The basic linear regression equation is:

$$Y' = a + bX$$

TABLE 9–3. CALCULATIONS FOR SIMPLE LINEAR REGRESSION EXAMPLE

(1) X Midterm	(2) x $(X - \bar{X})$	(3) x^2	(4) Y Final	(5) y $(Y - \bar{Y})$	(6) y^2	(7) xy	(8) Y'	(9) e $(Y - Y')$	(10) e^2
2	−3	9	3	−3	9	9	3.3	−0.3	0.09
6	1	1	7	1	1	1	6.9	0.1	0.01
5	0	0	6	0	0	0	6.0	0.0	0.00
9	4	16	8	2	4	8	9.6	−1.6	2.56
7	2	4	9	3	9	6	7.8	1.2	1.44
9	4	16	10	4	16	16	9.6	0.4	0.16
3	−2	4	4	−2	4	4	4.2	−0.2	0.04
4	−1	1	6	0	0	0	5.1	0.9	0.81
1	−4	16	2	−4	16	16	2.4	−0.4	0.16
4	−1	1	5	−1	1	1	5.1	−0.1	0.01
$\Sigma X = 50$	0	68	$\Sigma Y = 60$	0	60	61	$\Sigma Y' = 60$	0.0	5.28
$\bar{X} = 5.0$			$\bar{Y} = 6.0$				$\bar{Y}' = 6.0$		

$r = .955$

$b = \dfrac{\Sigma xy}{\Sigma x^2} = \dfrac{61}{68} = .90$

$a = \bar{Y} - b\bar{X} = 6.0 - .90(5.0) = 1.5$

$Y' = a + bX = 1.5 + .90X$

where Y' = predicted value of variable Y
$\quad a$ = intercept constant
$\quad b$ = slope of the line
$\quad X$ = actual value of variable X

The regression equation is identical to the equation for a straight line, except that it is an equation that *predicts* values of the variable Y (Y' , called **Y predicted**) rather than being based on actual values. This is the equation for the regression of Y (the dependent variable) on X (the independent or predictor variable).

To use the regression equation, we must solve for a, the intercept constant and b, the slope, which is usually referred to as the **regression coefficient** in the context of a regression equation. The formula for the regression coefficient is:

$$b = \frac{\Sigma xy}{\Sigma x^2}$$

where b = regression coefficient
$\quad x$ = deviations of X from $\bar{X}$
$\quad y$ = deviations of Y from $\bar{Y}$

In the numerator of this equation, deviation scores for the two variables are obtained, and then the cross products for all pairs of deviation scores are summed. In our example, this value is 61, shown in column 7 of Table 9–3. The denominator of the equation is the sum of the squared deviations for the independent variable X, which in our example is 68, shown in column 3. Thus, the regression coefficient is 61 ÷ 68, or .90.

Next, we must solve for the intercept constant. The formula is:

$$a = \bar{Y} - b\bar{X}$$

where a = intercept constant
   $\bar{Y}$ = mean of variable Y
   $\bar{X}$ = mean of variable X
   b = regression coefficient

In our example, the intercept constant would therefore be:

$$a = 6.0 - .90 (5.0) = 6.0 - 4.5 = 1.5$$

Thus, the regression equation for the data shown in Table 9–3 is:

$$Y' = 1.5 + .90X$$

You might be wondering, what is the point of solving this equation? The utility of regression is that allows us to make *predictions* about the values of one variable, based on the values of a second variable. For example, a nursing school faced with selecting students with the greatest chance of success could predict students' grade point averages based on their SAT scores. The predicted values would not be perfectly accurate unless the correlation between grade point averages and SAT scores was 1.00. However, if the correlation was fairly strong, the prediction would be reasonably good.

We will illustrate this point using the example in Table 9–3. Suppose that we only had the students' midterm test scores and wanted to predict how they would perform on the final exam. For the first subject, whose midterm score was 2, we would predict that the final exam score would be 3.3 [$Y' = 1.5 + .90 (2) = 3.3$]. If we applied the regression equation to each of the X values, we would obtain the predicted values of Y shown in column 8 of Table 9–3.

When we compare the *actual* values of Y (column 4) with the *predicted* values of Y (column 8), we see that the two are similar, but are identical for only one case (the third subject). The differences between Y and Y', shown in column 9, are known as the **errors of prediction** (*e*). In this example, the errors of prediction are rather small because the correlation between X and Y is high. When the correlation between the two variables is perfect, there are no errors of prediction; Y' would always be exactly equal to Y. Conversely, when the correlation is modest, the errors of prediction are more substantial.

The regression equation is the best linear representation of the relationship between X and Y because it is the line that minimizes the errors of prediction. More precisely, the regression equation minimizes the sums of squares of the prediction errors, and hence the origin of the term least squares. (Standard regression procedures are sometimes referred to as **OLS regression,** which stands for **ordinary least-squares regression**). In our example, the sum of the squared prediction errors, which are also called the **residuals,** is 5.28, shown at the bottom of column 10. *Any other value of* a *and* b—*i.e., any other line drawn through the data points—would have yielded a larger sum of the squared residuals.*

A graphic representation of this regression analysis is shown in Figure 9–6. The actual values of X and Y are shown as circles. The line running through the data points embodies the regression equation. The intercept a crosses the Y axis at 1.5. The regression coefficient (b) indicates the slope of the line. With $b = .90$, the line slopes such that for every five units on the X axis, we must go up 4.5 units ($.90 \times 5$) on the Y axis. Since the line embodies the equation, we can use it to determine Y' values. We would first find a value of X on the X axis, and then find the point directly vertical on the regression line. Next we would read the predicted value of Y by reading over horizontally to the Y axis. For example, if we wanted to predict a final exam score based on a midterm score of 5, we would find a Y' of 6 [i.e., $1.5 + .9(5) = 6$], indicated by a star on the regression line. We could use this line to make predictions about any value of X, just as the regression equation could be used for this purpose.

The Standard Error of Estimate

When the regression equation is used to make predictions, it is useful to have an index that indicates the accuracy of the predictions. The **standard error of estimate** is used

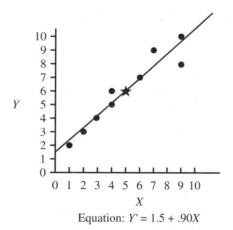

Equation: $Y' = 1.5 + .90X$

FIGURE 9–6.   GRAPHIC REPRESENTATION OF A REGRESSION EQUATION

for this purpose. This index indicates how "wrong," on average, a predicted value of Y might be expected to be. The formula for the standard error of estimate is:

$$S_{y \cdot x} = \sqrt{\frac{\Sigma(Y - Y')^2}{N - 2}}$$

where $s_{y \cdot x}$ = standard error of estimate for Y regressed on X
      $\Sigma(Y - Y')^2$ = sum of the squared errors of prediction for Y' (e^2)
      N = number of cases (sample size)

For our example of predicting final exam scores from midterm scores (Table 9–3), the standard error of estimate would be[9]:

$$s_{y \cdot x} = \sqrt{\frac{5.28}{8}} = .81$$

Thus, the average amount of error in predicting final exam scores would be less than one point. The smaller the standard error of estimate, the more accurate the predictions are likely to be.

Correlation and Regression

The formula we just presented for the standard error of estimate is a good definitional formula because it shows that the index represents the average of all the deviations about the predicted values of Y. In practice, an alternative formula is more convenient for computational purposes, and this formula is useful for a discussion of the link between correlation and regression. A good computational formula for the standard error of estimate is:

$$s_{y \cdot x} = \sqrt{\frac{\Sigma y^2 (1 - r^2)}{N - 2}}$$

where $s_{y \cdot x}$ = standard error of estimate for Y regressed on X
      Σy^2 = sum of the squared deviations for Y, i.e., $\Sigma(Y - \overline{Y})^2$
      r^2 = squared correlation coefficient between X and Y
      N = number of cases (sample size)

---

[9]The formula presented is for an index that allows us to draw inferences about the standard error of estimate in the population. If we wanted a purely descriptive index, the denominator of the formula would be N rather than $N - 2$. In our example, the value of the standard error of estimate would be .73 rather than .81.

From this formula, it can be seen that the larger the correlation coefficient, the smaller the numerator, and hence the smaller the standard error of estimate. In our example, using calculations shown in Table 9–3, the standard error of estimate would be:

$$s_{y \cdot x} = \sqrt{\frac{60\,(1 - .955^2)}{8}} = \sqrt{\frac{60\,(1 - .912)}{8}} = .81$$

We might note that if the correlation between midterm and final exam scores had been .80 rather than .955 with all else constant, the standard error of estimate would have been twice as large—1.64 rather than .81.

Another way to demonstrate the link between correlation and regression is to return to our discussion about the meaning of r^2. As noted previously, the square of the correlation coefficient tells us the proportion of variance in Y that can be explained or accounted for by X. In our example, 91% of the variability in final exam scores ($.955^2$) is accounted for by students' variability in midterm scores. The remaining 9% of Y's variability is from other sources. We can demonstrate that the residuals (errors of prediction) from Table 9–3 constitute 9% of Y's unexplained variability. Column 6 shows us that the sum of the squared deviations of the Y values from the mean of Y (i.e., the total amount of Y's variability) is 60. Thus, as a proportion of total variability the residuals are:

$$\frac{5.28}{60} = .09 = 1 - r^2$$

We can also calculate the degree to which each Y' deviates from the mean of all Y's ($y' = Y' - \bar{Y}'$).[10] If we squared these values and then summed them, we would find that $\Sigma y'^2$ is equal to 54.72. As a proportion of the variability in the *actual* Y scores, we find that:

$$\frac{54.72}{60} = .91 = r^2$$

Thus, the variability in the predicted final exam scores (the variation explained by X) represents 91% of the variability in the actual scores. These calculations reinforce the point that the stronger the correlation between the two variables, the better the power of regression-based predictions, and the smaller the errors of prediction. The closer the correlation coefficient is to zero, the more futile it is to use regression procedures to make accurate predictions. In fact, when the correlation is exactly zero, regression procedures predict the mean of Y for *all* values of X.

---

[10]Actual calculations are not shown.

THE COMPUTER AND SIMPLE LINEAR REGRESSION

Existing statistical software programs can readily be used to perform the calculations for correlation and regression. We illustrate a computer printout for a regression procedure, using the data from the example of students' midterm and final exam scores in statistics. We discuss only a portion of the printout here because Chapter 10 covers the computer output for regression analysis in greater detail.

As we will see in the next chapter, it is possible to have multiple predictor or independent variables in regression analysis, and the procedure is referred to as multiple regression—the term shown in the heading of Figure 9–7.[11] The multiple regression program in most software packages performs both simple and multiple regression. Panel A presents basic descriptive statistics (means and SDs) for the independent variable MIDTERM and the dependent variable FINAL.

Panel B of Figure 9–7 shows the correlation matrix. The correlation between MIDTERM and MIDTERM (the variable correlated with itself) is 1.000, while the correlation between MIDTERM and FINAL is .955, the same value we calculated manually. Beneath each correlation coefficient is the value of the relevant deviation scores, summed and squared. For example, the squared deviations of each midterm score from the mean of the midterm scores add up to 68.000, the same value shown as Σx^2 in column 3 of Table 9–3. The sum of the deviation cross products is 61.000, the same value shown as Σxy in column 7 of Table 9–3. Finally, the squared deviations of each final exam grade from the mean for FINAL add up to 60.000, the same value shown as Σy^2 in column 6.

Panel C indicates that the dependent variable in our example is FINAL and that the variable entered into the regression equation is MIDTERM. The value of r (shown here on the line labeled "Multiple R") is .95499, and the value of r^2 is .91201. The next line shows that the "Adjusted R Square" is somewhat lower, .90101. The SPSS regression program calculates an r^2 that is adjusted to reflect more closely the goodness-of-fit of the regression model in the population; the adjustment uses a formula that involves sample size and number of independent variables. The last line of panel C shows the standard error of estimate to be .81236, the value we obtained through manual calculations but to higher precision.

Panel D, labeled "Analysis of Variance," shows that the overall regression is statistically significant: the value of F is 82.91922, significant at the .000 level. The analysis of variance aspect of regression will be explained in greater detail in the next chapter. We can see here, though, that the total sums of squares for the dependent variable have been decomposed into (a) the sum of squares for regression (54.72059, the value we

---

[11]The SPSS/PC command that created the printout in Figure 9–7 is as follows:

```
REGRESSION VARIABLES = MIDTERM FINAL
    /DEPENDENT = FINAL /METHOD = ENTER
    /DESCRIPTIVES = DEFAULT XPROD.
```

```
* * * *   M U L T I P L E   R E G R E S S I O N   * * * *
```

Listwise Deletion of Missing Data

A   Mean   Std Dev   Label

MIDTERM   5.000   2.749
FINAL   6.000   2.582

N of Cases =   10

B   Correlation, Cross-Product:

                    MIDTERM   FINAL

MIDTERM   1.000   .955
                  68.000   61.000

FINAL   .955   1.000
                  61.000   60.000

C   Equation Number 1   Dependent Variable..   FINAL

Block Number 1. Method: Enter

Variable(s) Entered on Step Number
    1..   MIDTERM

Multiple R   .95499
R Square   .91201
Adjusted R Square   .90101
Standard Error   .81236

D   Analysis of Variance
                    DF   Sum of Squares   Mean Square
        Regression   1   54.72059   54.72059
        Residual   8   5.27941   .65993

        F =   82.91922   Signif F = .0000

E   ----------------- Variables in the Equation -----------------

Variable   B   SE B   Beta   T   Sig T

MIDTERM   .897059   .098513   .954992   9.106   .0000
(Constant)   1.514706   .555529   2.727   .0260

FIGURE 9–7.   COMPUTER PRINTOUT OF SIMPLE REGRESSION ANALYSIS

noted that represents $\Sigma y'^2$), and (b) the sum of squares of the residuals (5.27941, the value shown in column 10 of Table 9–3, to greater precision). Together, these two components total 60.000, which is the sum of the squared deviations for Y (column 6 of Table 9–3).

Finally, panel E shows the regression equation under the heading "Variables in the Equation." The regression coefficient for the X variable (MIDTERM) is .897059, which we rounded to .90 during our hand calculations. The intercept constant is shown here as 1.514706, which differs slightly from our calculated value of 1.50 because we used the rounded value of b (.90) in the formula to calculate a. We defer the discussion of the other elements of panel E until the next chapter.

RESEARCH APPLICATIONS OF CORRELATION AND REGRESSION

Bivariate correlation is a widely used inferential statistical procedure. Correlation coefficients are frequently displayed in research reports; they are efficient statistical indexes because they summarize concisely the magnitude, nature, and direction of a relationship between two variables. This section describes some of the applications of bivariate correlation and simple linear regression, and discusses methods of displaying the results of such analyses in reports.

The Uses of Bivariate Correlation and Simple Regression

Correlation and regression analysis are used by researchers in a variety of applications. Some of the descriptive applications of bivariate correlation analysis were discussed in Chapter 4. This section extends that discussion.

1. *Answering Research Questions.* The primary use of correlational procedures is for answering research questions and testing hypotheses. Many different types of research questions have been addressed through inferential correlation analysis. Table 9–4 illustrates some recent applications. It must be noted, however, that most researchers today go beyond bivariate correlation and extend their analyses to multiple correlation and regression, which we discuss in Chapter 10.
2. *Making Predictions.* Applied research is sometimes expressly performed to develop a regression equation for making predictions about some outcome. A graduate nursing program may, for example, undertake a regression analysis, using data from current and former students, that allows administrators to predict prospective students' graduate grade point averages based on their undergraduate grade point averages. As another example, a measure of depression at intake might be used to predict the length of hospitalization of psychiatric inpatients.
3. *Assessing an Instrument's Reliability.* Correlational procedures are used in a variety of ways to provide information about the adequacy of the measures used in nursing investigations. As one important example, correlations are often used to assess the

TABLE 9-4. EXAMPLES OF STUDIES USING INFERENTIAL CORRELATION ANALYSES

Research Question	Statistic	Result
What is the relationship between core pulmonary artery temperature and oral, axillary, FirstTemp Genius®, and IVAC Core-Check™? (Lattavo, Britt, & Dubal, 1995)	Pearson's r	$r = .75, .68, .74,$ and $.84$, respectively; all $p < .01$
What is the relationship between a patient's preoperative emotion and the use of (a) avoidance, (b) wishful thinking, and (c) problem-focused coping strategies? (Crumlish, 1994)	Pearson's r	(a) $r = .46, p < .001$ (b) $r = .57, p < .001$ (c) $r = .26, p < .05$
What is the correlation between cardiac patients' satisfaction with family function and the satisfaction of their spouses? (Hilbert, 1994)	Pearson's r	$r = .57, p < .001$
What is the relationship between the severity of erythema and severity of edema of nipple skin during the first week of breastfeeding? (Ziemer & Pigeon, 1993)	Spearman's r_S	$r_S = .41, p < .01$

reliability of research instruments—particularly scales that are designed to measure psychosocial traits (e.g., health beliefs, coping, social support, hopelessness).[12]

Reliability concerns the degree of dependability or accuracy with which an instrument measures the attribute it is designed to measure. The reliability of an instrument can be assessed in various ways, and several of them involve the calculation of Pearson's r.[13] In the context of a reliability assessment, the correlation coefficients are referred to as **reliability coefficients.** Like correlation coefficients, reliability coefficients can range between -1.00 and $+1.00$, but they are almost always positive. The higher the coefficient, the greater the reliability of the instrument. Reliability coefficients generally should be at least .70, and in some contexts may need to be even higher to be considered acceptable.

One approach to reliability assessment is known as the **test-retest approach.** If a researcher were interested in determining an instrument's stability over time, the instrument could be administered on two separate occasions. The correlation coefficient between individuals' scores at time 1 and scores at time 2 would provide evidence of the test-retest reliability of the instrument. For example, Martin (1994)

[12]For a more detailed discussion of methods of evaluating the reliability and validity of an instrument, a book on psychometric procedures sould be consulted (for example, Guilford, 1964, or Nunnally, 1978).

[13]The most widely used reliability coefficient is known as **Cronbach's alpha,** which is not a correlation coefficient in the usual sense, but has similar properties. Cronbach's alpha is an index of the degree to which all of the different items in a scale are measuring the same attribute. Although the formula for Cronbach's alpha looks different from the formula for a correlation coefficient, it is basically an index that summarizes the correlation between all items in a scale and the scale total, considered simultaneously.

assessed the test-retest reliability of the four subscales of the Chronic Respiratory Disease Questionnaire (CRQ). The reliability coefficients ranged from .20 to .90. The lowest coefficient, which was not significantly different from zero, was for the Fatigue subscale. The low reliability coefficient is consistent with the fact that fatigue is an attribute that does, indeed, change over time.

Another common situation is the assessment of the accuracy of observers' ratings. In a typical assessment of **interrater reliability,** two observers are asked to make observations and complete ratings independently. The correlation coefficient between the two sets of ratings provides an estimate of interrater reliability. As a research example, Hurley and her colleagues (1992) developed an objective observational scale for measuring discomfort in advanced Alzheimer patients. They evaluated the interrater reliability of the scale in two different sites on two separate occasions, and found that the correlations between the raters ranged between .86 and .98.

4. *Assessing an Instrument's Validity.* **Validity** concerns the degree to which an instrument is measuring what it is supposed to be measuring. Correlation procedures play an important role in estimating an instrument's validity.

For example, a researcher might want to assess the **criterion-related validity** of an instrument, an approach to validity assessment that involves examining the relationship between the instrument in question and some practical criterion. Thus, an observational scale designed to measure nursing effectiveness might be tested against supervisors' ratings of nurses' performance. The correlation between the two would provide information about the criterion-related validity of the scale. The higher the correlation, the stronger the evidence for criterion-related validity.

One of the most important aspects of validity is known as **construct validity,** which involves evidence that an instrument is really measuring the underlying construct of interest. Many approaches to establishing the construct validity of an instrument rely on the calculation of correlation coefficients. For example, Affonso and her colleagues (1994) developed and tested the Cognitive Adaptation to Stressful Events (CASE) scale to measure stress during and after pregnancy. They reasoned that if the CASE instrument were valid, scores on the scale should correlate with other measures of stress and adjustment—particularly with pregnancy-specific measures. In their validation sample, they found correlations in the vicinity of .50 between the CASE and the Stressful Events Related to Pregnancy (SERP) scale, both during the pregnancy and postpartum (all $p < .001$).

The Presentation of Correlation and Simple Regression in Research Reports

As noted in Chapter 4, correlational analyses are not usually displayed in scatterplots, but generally are reported either directly in the text, if there are only a handful of coefficients, or in a table. In the text, the write-up of an inferential correlational analysis normally should include the name of the test (especially if Pearson's r was not used), the value of the coefficient, the degrees of freedom, and the level of significance. As an example, the results for the fictitious study on grief resolution among widows might be reported as follows:

TABLE 9–5. EXAMPLE OF A CORRELATION MATRIX, SHOWING p LEVELS

Variable	1	2	3	4
1. Income				
2. Age	.04			
3. Functional Disability	−.24*	.29**		
4. Social Support	.06	−.18	−.09	
5. Perceived Purpose in Life	.13	−.03	−.33***	.20*

*$p < .05$ **$p < .01$ ***$p < .001$

Correlation Matrix of Key Study Variables (N = 102)

Among the 50 widows in the sample, the correlation between the deceased husbands' length of illness prior to death and the widows' grief resolution was positive but modest ($r = .26$). With 48 *df,* this correlation was nonsignificant at conventional levels for a two-tailed test ($p = .06$).

Tables for correlational analyses often involve a display of a correlation matrix, such as the one shown in Table 4–8 in Chapter 4. When a correlation matrix includes inferential information, as it usually does, asterisks are typically placed next to each coefficient that is statistically significant, with the number of asterisks corresponding to a level of significance specified in a key at the bottom of the table.[14] A fictitious example of such a tabular display for five variables is presented in Table 9–5. This table shows that one correlation (between functional disability and perceived purpose in life) was significant at the .001 level; two were significant at the .01 level; and one (between social support and perceived purpose in life) was significant at the .05 level. Six of the correlations—those without any asterisks beside them—were not statistically significant at conventional levels.

Note that in the example shown in Table 9–5, the diagonal was left blank. Computer printouts of correlation matrixes generally place 1.00 on the diagonal. When all of the variables in the correlation matrix are measured by psychosocial scales, researchers sometimes put the reliability coefficients on the diagonal, in parentheses, and then make a note to this effect at the bottom of the table.

Published research reports rarely present the results of a simple linear regression, in large part because multiple regression is far more common. However, when appropriate, the researcher could report the regression equation in the text (e.g., "The regression equation for predicting final exam scores from midterm scores was found to be $Y' = 1.5 + .90X$").

---

[14]In Neil's original table, reproduced in Table 4–3, individual asterisks were not used because *all* coefficients were significant at or beyond the .001 level, and this fact was noted in a footnote to the table.

RESEARCH EXAMPLE

Correlations are widely reported in the research literature, especially in studies that are nonexperimental. Here we describe a recent study that addressed its primary research questions through correlational procedures.

Sommers, Stevenson, Hamlin, and Ivey (1995) examined the relationship between, thermodilution cardiac output and cardiac index (CI) on the one hand and two noninvasive measures (skin temperature and limb blood flow) on the other hand. One of their goals was to determine whether the cardiac index could be reliably predicted by noninvasive devices so that iatrogenic complications associated with invasive devices could be prevented. The sample for their study was 21 patients undergoing coronary artery bypass grafting.

Measurements from the subjects were recorded after return from surgery and then every 2 hours for 8 hours in the immediate postoperative period (five time periods). The main study variables were CI, five measures of skin temperature (axilla, groin, knee, anterior ankle, and toe), and limb blood flow (LBF)—all either interval or ratio-level variables.

Correlations between CI and the five skin temperature measures were erratic over the five time periods. Of the 25 correlations (which were displayed in a table), only two were statistically significant. At time 1, CI was significantly correlated with axillary temperature ($r = .53$, $p = .01$), and at time 3, CI was significantly correlated with ankle temperature ($r = .44$, $p = .046$). All other correlations were small in magnitude and inconsistent in direction. For example, the correlations between CI and knee temperature ranged from $-.29$ to $.16$ in different time periods. And, at any given time period, some correlations with CI were negative and some were positive.

A similar pattern of inconsistency was observed with regard to the correlations between CI and LBF, as shown in a table that we have modified and present here as Table 9–6. This table shows the means for CI and LBF at all five time periods, the correlations between the two measures, and the significance levels. At time 1, LBF and CI were significantly correlated ($r = .43$, $p = .05$), but this relationship was not sustained for later measurements.

The investigators concluded that none of the noninvasive measures used in the study could be reliably used as a predictor of CI in the immediate postoperative period following coronary artery bypass grafting. It might be noted that the small sample size used in this study resulted in statistical tests that were very low in power. With only 21 subjects, the correlations between CI and the

TABLE 9–6. CORRELATIONS BETWEEN CARDIAC INDEX (CI) AND LIMB BLOOD FLOW (LBF) AT FIVE DATA POINTS ($N = 21$)

Time	Mean CI (L/min/m²)	Mean LBF (ml/100ml/min)	r	p
1	2.47	1.28	.43	.05
2	2.80	1.50	.18	.44
3	3.11	1.88	.02	.92
4	2.95	2.49	−.16	.49
5	3.08	2.37	−.02	.95

Adapted from Table 3 of Sommers et al.'s (1995) report.

predictor variables would need to be greater than .60 to achieve a power of .80. On the other hand, the modest and widely fluctuating values of the correlation coefficients do not suggest that increased power would have altered the researchers' conclusions.

SUMMARY

Pearson's r is both a descriptive and inferential statistic. As an inferential statistic, it is typically used to test the null hypothesis that the correlation between two variables in the population (symbolized as ρ, rho) is zero. To test that r is statistically different from zero, the obtained r is compared to critical values of r with $N - 2$ degrees of freedom. It is also possible to test the equivalence of two correlations by using the **r-to-z transformation.**

Pearson's r directly communicates the strength and nature of the relationship between two variables. However, the **coefficient of determination,** as r^2 is sometimes called, indicates the proportion of variance that is shared by the two variables and is generally preferred as the index of the magnitude of the relationship.

Several factors can reduce the magnitude of r, including the existence of a curvilinear relationship, restricting the range on one or both variables, and using unreliable measures. On the other hand, the use of extreme groups or the presence of an outlier can inflate the value of r.

There are several other statistics that can be used to describe and test relationships between two variables. Among these are **Spearman's rank order correlation** and **Kendall's tau** (τ), both of which are nonparametric tests.

Correlation is closely linked to **linear regression,** which is a technique used to analyze relationships between variables and to make predictions about the values of variables. Regression analysis can be used to identify the straight line that runs through data points with the best possible fit. The **regression equation** is $Y' = a + bX$, where Y' is **Y predicted,** a is the **intercept constant** (the point at which the line crosses the Y axis), and b is the **slope** (angle) of the line. The formulas for computing a and b are such that the **errors of prediction** (also called the **residuals**), when squared, are minimized. Thus, simple linear regression is said to use the **least-squares** criterion for determining the best-fitting line.

Regression is a useful tool for making predictions about variables that are linearly correlated. The **standard error of estimate** is the index used to indicate the accuracy of the predictions. The stronger the correlation between two variables, the more accurate the predictions.

EXERCISES

The following exercises cover concepts presented in this chapter. Exercises indicated with a dagger (†) can be checked against answers appearing in Appendix A. Additionally, Chapter 9 of the accompanying *Applications Manual* offers supplementary exercises, including ones that require computer analysis of a data set on diskette.

† 1. Given the following circumstances, determine whether the calculated values of r are statistically significant:

    a. $r = .29, N = 35, \alpha = .01$, two-tailed

    b. $r = .50, N = 15, \alpha = .05$, two-tailed

    c. $r = .12, N = 500, \alpha = .05$, two-tailed

    d. $r = .55, N = 12, \alpha = .05$, one-tailed

    e. $r = .44, N = 26, \alpha = .01$, one-tailed

† 2. For each correlation coefficient below, calculate what proportion of variance is shared by the two correlated variables:

    a. $r = .76$

    b. $r = .33$

    c. $r = .91$

    d. $r = .14$

† 3. For each coefficient of determination below, calculate the value of the correlation coefficient:

    a. $r^2 = .66$

    b. $r^2 = .13$

    c. $r^2 = .29$

    d. $r^2 = .07$

† 4. In a random sample of 100 people, the correlation between amount of daily exercise and weight was found to be $-.21$. What would be the likely effect on the *absolute value* of the correlation coefficient under the following circumstances:

    a. The sample is restricted to people who weighed under 180 pounds.

    b. The sample is restricted to people who get virtually no daily exercise versus those who exercise at least 30 minutes a day.

    c. The mean sample weight is 150 pounds, and one person is added to the sample who weighs 275 pounds.

† 5. Suppose that a researcher regressed surgical patients' lengths of stay in the hospital on a scale of functional ability measured 24 hours after surgery. Given the following, solve for the value of the intercept constant and write out the full regression equation:

Mean length of stay = 6.5 days; mean score on scale = 33; slope = $-.10$

† 6. Using the regression equation calculated in response to Question 5, compute the predicted value of Y (length of hospital stay) for patients with the following functional ability scores:

    a. $X = 52$

    b. $X = 68$

    c. $X = 23$

    d. $X = 10$

† 7. In a study that focused on the relationship between level of headache pain and number of pain relievers consumed, a researcher found that the correlation coeffi-

cient was .52 among the 200 women and .36 among the 200 men in the sample. Is there a significant difference between the two correlations at $\alpha = .05$?

† 8. A researcher studying the relationship between maternal age and length of breast-feeding in a sample of 75 primiparas found a correlation of .18, which was not statistically significant at the .05 level. What was the power of the statistical test? Conversely, what was the risk that a Type II error was committed?

† 9. Assuming in Question 8 that .18 is a good estimation of the population correlation, what sample size would be needed in a replication study to achieve power $= .80$ at $\alpha = .05$?

† 10. Compute Spearman's rank order correlation coefficient for the following pairs of ranks:

VAR1: 5 7 2 1 6 4 3
VAR2: 1 4 7 6 3 5 4

Is the correlation statistically significant at $\alpha = .05$?

Multiple Regression

This chapter focuses on multiple regression, a useful and versatile statistical procedure. First, however, we briefly discuss the general topic of multivariate statistics.

INTRODUCTION TO MULTIVARIATE STATISTICS

The inferential statistics we have examined thus far are bivariate. That is, they concern the relationship between two variables, typically one independent variable and one dependent variable. However, it has become increasingly clear that bivariate statistics are limited in their ability to unravel the complex phenomena in which researchers are interested. Phenomena such as infection, pain, coping, and blood pressure tend to have multiple determinants. Two-variable analyses cannot adequately capture the multiple influences on, or causes of, these phenomena. Thus, the trend toward the use of **multivariate statistics,** which involve three or more variables in a single analysis, is accelerating and is unlikely to be reversed. The widespread availability of computers has made it possible (and essential) for even novice researchers to learn complex statistical procedures.

This chapter and the four that follow describe the most widely used multivariate statistics. For the most part, these chapters have the same format as that adopted in preceding chapters. However, there are a few differences. First and foremost, formulas and actual calculations for multivariate procedures are minimized. Multivariate statistics are computationally formidable and are almost never done by hand, so no attempt is made to present fully worked-out examples. We use a few calculations heuristically to promote a better understanding of how multivariate statistics should be interpreted. At the same time, more attention is paid in these chapters to explaining how to read computer printouts. The chapters on multivariate statistics also devote less detailed coverage to the topic of power analysis.

BASIC CONCEPTS FOR MULTIPLE REGRESSION

The relationship between two variables is almost never perfect. When a researcher discovers that the correlation between two variables is .50, for example, it means that 25% ($.50^2$) of the variance in the dependent variable is explained by the independent variable, but a full 75% of the variance is *un*explained. Scientists generally strive to fully understand—and predict—the phenomena in which they are interested, and therefore they value research designs and statistical techniques that allow the complexity of the real world to be reflected in their investigations.

Multiple regression analysis, which is an extension of simple linear regression, allows researchers to improve their predictive power by using two or more independent variables to predict a dependent variable. For example, suppose we wanted to predict a person's weight. If we developed a regression equation using a person's gender as our sole predictor variable, the accuracy of our predictions would be modest. We would predict that men would be heavier than women, but we would sometimes be wrong. Moreover, the regression equation would always predict men to have the mean weight for males and women to have the mean weight for women, despite the fact that men's and women's weights can range over hundreds of pounds. If, however, we could use information on a person's height *and* gender, our ability to predict weight would be dramatically improved. Multiple regression produces an equation that provides the best prediction possible, given the correlations among all variables in the analysis.

The Basic Multiple Regression Equation

The multiple regression equation is, conceptually, a simple extension of the simple regression equation. The basic equation is:

$$Y' = a + b_1X_1 + b_2X_2 + \ldots + b_kX_k$$

where Y' = predicted value for variable Y
      a = intercept constant
      k = number of independent variables
      b_1 to b_k = regression coefficients for the k independent variables
      X_1 to X_k = values on the k independent variables

The multiple regression equation stipulates that the predicted value of Y is a linear combination of an intercept constant, plus predictor variables that are weighted by regression coefficients. Regression analysis yields best-fitting values of a and the bs, using the least squares criterion that the squared error terms (the differences between Y and Y') are at a minimum.

In the multiple regression equation, there is a regression coefficient (b weight) associated with each predictor variable. These coefficients are the optimal linear estimates of the dependent variable *when used in combination with the specified other independent variables.* The regression coefficients are thus the weights associated with a given independent variable when the other predictors are in the equation. If predictor variables were added to (or removed from) the regression equation, the bs would change.

As an example of an actual regression equation, suppose that a graduate nursing school program wanted to ensure the selection of the most worthy applicants. The school uses various pieces of information from its current graduate students to develop a regression equation to predict academic performance. Table 10–1 shows data for 20 students with regard to the dependent variable, graduate grade point average (GPA), and four independent variables—undergraduate GPA, scores on the Graduate Record Exam (GRE)-Verbal Test; scores on the GRE-Quantitative Test, and scores on an achievement motivation scale. Although we do not show the actual computations, the regression equation using these data is:

$$Y' = -1.636 + .793X_1 + .004X_2 - .0009X_3 + .009X_4$$

This equation specifies that graduate grade point average can be predicted by *subtracting* (because the value of the intercept constant is negative) 1.636 from the sum of the raw scores on the four predictors, multiplied by their respective regression coefficients. Note that in this equation, the b weight for GRE-Quantitative is negative, so this term also involves subtraction rather than addition.

To examine the equation's accuracy, suppose we used this equation to "predict" the graduate grade point average of the first student in Table 10–1:

$$Y' = -1.636 + .793(3.4) + .004(600) - .0009(540) + .009(75)$$
$$Y' = 3.649$$

The regression equation worked rather well in this instance. For this first subject, the error of prediction $(Y - Y')$ is only $-.049$ ($3.6 - 3.649$), and the squared error term is .0024. In the aggregate, the sum of the squared error terms is kept to a minimum through the regression analysis. Any values for the regression coefficients and intercept constant other than those in the regression equation would yield a larger sum of squared residuals.

The Standardized Multiple Regression Equation

In multiple regression, the independent variables are typically in different units of measure. In our example, GRE scores are on a scale that can range from 200 to 800, while undergraduate GPA can range from 0.0 to 4.0. The regression coefficients, then, neces-

TABLE 10–1. FICTITIOUS DATA FOR MULTIPLE REGRESSION EXAMPLE

	Independent Variables				Dependent Variable
Subject	Undergrad GPA X_1	GRE-Verbal X_2	GRE-Quant X_3	Motivation X_4	Graduate GPA Y
1	3.4	600	540	75	3.6
2	3.1	510	480	70	3.0
3	3.7	650	710	85	3.9
4	3.2	530	450	60	2.8
5	3.5	610	500	90	3.7
6	2.9	540	620	60	2.6
7	3.3	530	510	75	3.4
8	2.9	540	600	55	2.7
9	3.4	550	580	75	3.3
10	3.2	700	630	65	3.5
11	3.7	630	700	80	3.6
12	3.0	480	490	75	2.8
13	3.1	530	520	60	3.0
14	3.7	580	610	65	3.5
15	3.9	710	660	80	3.8
16	3.5	500	480	75	3.2
17	3.1	490	510	60	2.4
18	2.9	560	540	55	2.7
19	3.2	550	590	65	3.1
20	3.4	600	550	70	3.6
Mean	3.3	562.5	563.5	69.5	3.2
SD	0.3	57.2	74.9	10.7	0.4

sarily incorporate differences in the units of measure, and so the b weights in the basic regression equation cannot directly be compared.

To address this issue, the regression equation is sometimes presented in the following standardized form:

$$z_{Y'} = \beta_1 z_{x_1} + \beta_2 z_{x_2} + \ldots + \beta_k z_{x_k}$$

where $z_{Y'}$ = predicted value of the standard score for Y
    β_1 to β_k = standardized regression weights for k independent variables
    z_{x_1} to z_{x_k} = standard scores for k independent variables

In standardized form, the raw values of the predictor variables are converted to z scores, each of which has a mean of 0.0 and an SD of 1.0. The z scores are weighted by standardized regression coefficients that are usually referred to as **beta weights** (βs).[1] In the standardized regression equation, there is no intercept constant because the intercept is always 0.0. In our example, the standardized regression equation is:

$$z_{Y'} = .53z_{x_1} + .48z_{x_2} - .14z_{x_3} + .21z_{x_4}$$

This equation indicates that the predicted standard score for graduate GPA equals the sum of the standard scores for the four predictors multiplied by their respective beta weights. Note that, as in the original regression equation, the regression coefficient for GRE-Quantitative is negative and so the third term is subtracted from, rather than added to, the others.

Multiple Correlation

Multiple regression analysis allows researchers to address a number of important questions about the relationships among variables. One of the questions that most researchers are interested in is how well a group of independent variables, taken together, predicts a dependent variable. In our example, this question becomes, how well do undergraduate GPA, GRE-Verbal and GRE-Quantitative scores, and motivation scores predict graduate GPA?

This question is addressed by considering the **multiple correlation** between the dependent variable on the one hand and the predictor variables on the other. Just as simple linear regression is closely linked to bivariate correlation, so multiple regression is closely related to multiple correlation.

The **multiple correlation coefficient,** symbolized as *R,* is an index that summarizes the magnitude of the relationship between a dependent variable and several independent variables, considered simultaneously. *R* represents the highest possible correlation between a least-squares linear composite of the predictor variables and the dependent variable.

Unlike Pearson's *r, R* cannot take on negative values. *R* ranges from a low of 0.0 to a high of 1.00, with higher values indicating a greater magnitude of relationship between several independent variables and a dependent variable. *R* conveys no information about the *direction* of relationship, which is sensible when you consider that some independent variables could be negatively correlated with the dependent variable, while others could be positively correlated.

Like *r,* the square of *R* indicates the proportion of variance in the dependent variable accounted for by the predictors. R^2 thus provides a direct means of evaluating the accuracy of the multiple regression equation. When R^2 is 1.0, perfect prediction can be achieved. When R^2 is, say, 0.10, prediction errors will be large.

---

[1]Beta weights in regression analysis should not be confused with β as the risk of a Type II error in power analysis.

The calculation of R^2 also allows researchers to determine how much the accuracy of their predictions is *improved* by the addition of independent variables. In our example of predicting graduate GPA, the multiple correlation coefficient is quite high—.95. Therefore, the total proportion of explained variance in graduate GPA is .90 ($.95^2$). Table 10–2 presents the full correlation matrix for the four predictors and the dependent variable. This matrix shows that the bivariate correlation (sometimes referred to as the **zero-order correlation**) between undergraduate GPA and graduate GPA is .85, so that r^2 for this relationship is .72 ($.85^2$). Thus, the inclusion of three additional predictors in the regression equation increased the proportion of variance explained by .18 (i.e., from .72 to .90).

Several features of the multiple correlation coefficient should be noted. First, R cannot be less than the highest bivariate correlation between Y and the Xs. By inspecting Table 10–2, we can see that the independent variable that is correlated most strongly with graduate GPA is X_1 (undergraduate GPA), $r = .85$. Thus, R could not have been less than .85.

A second important point is that as predictors are added to the equation, R tends to increase most notably when the predictor variables are not themselves highly correlated with each other. If all the independent variables were perfectly correlated, the value of R would be the same as the r between any X and Y—all rs would be identical, and additional independent variables beyond the first one would contribute no new information. By contrast, if two independent variables (X_1 and X_2) are totally *un*correlated (i.e., $r_{12} = .00$), the rs between Y and the Xs could be added together to determine the value of R (i.e., $R = r_{y1} + r_{y2}$). When the bivariate correlations among the independent variables are between zero and 1.00, as they almost always are, the increment to R as variables are added to the equation tends to be relatively small. Thus, R in our example is not substantially higher than the r between Y and X_1 alone (.95 versus .85). This phenomenon is the result of the fact that there is redundancy of information among correlated predictors. When the correlations among the independent variables are high, each predictor has little new information to add. When correlations among predictors are low, each variable has the potential to explain a unique portion of the variability in the dependent variable.

TABLE 10–2. CORRELATION MATRIX FOR MULTIPLE REGRESSION EXAMPLE

	Undergrad GPA X_1	GRE-Verbal X_2	GRE-Quant X_3	Motivation X_4	Graduate GPA Y
X_1	1.00				
X_2	.49	1.00			
X_3	.45	.67	1.00		
X_4	.71	.38	.21	1.00	
Y	.85	.73	.47	.74	1.00

A third and related point is that increments to R tend to decrease as additional predictors are included in the regression equation. Redundancy among predictors is the rule, not the exception, and redundancy increases as the number of predictors increases. In our example, Table 10–2 shows that the correlations among the independent variables are moderate to strong. We can see the decline in the increment to R as successive predictors are added:

$$
\begin{aligned}
r_{y1} &= .85 \\
R_{y12} &= .92 \\
R_{y123} &= .94 \\
R_{y1234} &= .95
\end{aligned}
$$

The correlation coefficient increases from .85 for X_1 and Y alone to .92 (an increment of .07) when X_2 is added to X_1 for the prediction of Y. However, the increment is smaller at each subsequent addition of predictors. Typically, the inclusion of independent variables beyond the first four or five does little to improve the value of R.

Adjustments to R^2

In bivariate correlation, coefficients from samples are expected to fluctuate above and below the population value. In multiple correlation, however, the value of R cannot be negative, so that all chance fluctuations are in a direction that inflates the magnitude of R. Since sampling fluctuation tends to be more severe in small samples, overestimation of R is usually greatest in small samples. For this reason, R^2 is often adjusted to yield a better estimate of the population value, and sample size is taken into account in the adjustment. In some textbooks, the result is called **adjusted R^2,** while in others it is referred to as **shrunken R^2.**

The formula for the adjusted value (which we label $\tilde{R}^2$) is straightforward:

$$
\tilde{R}^2 = 1 - (1 - R^2)\left[\frac{N - 1}{N - k - 1}\right]
$$

In our example of predicting graduate GPA with all four independent variables, the R^2 was .90. Applying the adjustment formula, we would get the following:

$$
\tilde{R}^2 = 1 - (1 - .90)\left[\frac{20 - 1}{20 - 4 - 1}\right] = .87
$$

Most computer programs routinely print both R^2 and $\tilde{R}^2$.

Statistical Control: Partial and Semipartial Correlation

Regression coefficients in multiple regression must be interpreted somewhat differently than regression coefficients in bivariate regression. In simple regression, the value of b

indicates the amount of change in the predicted value of Y for a specified rate of change in X. In multiple regression, the coefficients represent the number of units the dependent variable is predicted to change for each unit change in a given predictor *when the effects of the other predictors are held constant.* In the example we have been using, the partial regression coefficient of .793 associated with undergraduate GPA in our equation means that, holding constant GRE and motivation scores, graduate GPA is predicted to increase by .793 units for every unit change (i.e., change of 1.0) in undergraduate GPA.

The concept of "holding constant" other predictor variables is an important one that relates to a central topic of research design and analysis: control. In a research context, **control** usually means the control of variance in the dependent variable. Control can be achieved in a number of ways,[2] but here our concern is with statistical control. **Statistical control** uses statistical methods to isolate or nullify variance in a dependent variable that is associated with variables that are extraneous to the relationship under study. For example, in studying the relationship between a teenager's self-esteem and use of drugs, the researcher would want to control other factors that are known to be related to drug usage (e.g., family income, prior academic performance, presence of one versus two parents in the household). Multiple regression and other multivariate analyses provide a mechanism for achieving such control. The process can best be explained through visual representations of partial and semipartial correlation.

Partial correlation provides a measure of the relationship between a dependent variable (Y) and an independent variable (X_1) while controlling for the effect of a third variable (X_2). Figure 10–1 presents a Venn diagram that portrays relationships among variables. As explained in Chapter 4, the circles represent total variability in the variables, and the degree to which circles overlap indicates the magnitude of the correlation between them, i.e., how much of their variance is shared. Figure 10–1 illustrates a situation in which Y is correlated with both X_1 and X_2, which in turn are correlated with each other. Y's variability in this diagram has four components—variability that is uniquely shared with X_1 (labeled a), variability that is uniquely shared with X_2 (labeled c), variability that is common to all three variables (labeled b), and variability that Y does not share with the other two variables (d). With partial correlation, the influence of X_2 on Y (areas b and c) is removed statistically. Then the partial correlation between X_1 and Y (symbolized as $r_{y1\cdot2}$) indicates the degree to which these two variables are correlated after the influence of X_2 is partialled out. Thus, the squared partial correlation reflects a as a proportion of $a + d$, not as a proportion of the entire circle.[3]

---

[2]For a discussion of alternatives to statistical control, a research text such as that by Polit and Hungler (1995) should be consulted.

[3]When one variable is partialled out, the correlation is sometimes referred to as a **first-order partial correlation.** It is possible to hold constant, or partial out, more than one variable. A **second-order partial correlation** ($r_{y1\cdot23}$), for example, is the correlation between Y and X_1 with the effects of X_2 and X_3 removed.

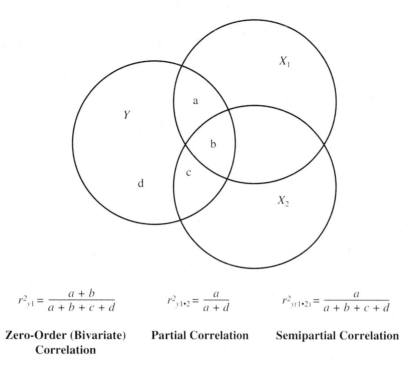

$$r^2_{y1} = \frac{a + b}{a + b + c + d} \qquad r^2_{y1\cdot2} = \frac{a}{a + d} \qquad r^2_{y(1\cdot2)} = \frac{a}{a + b + c + d}$$

Zero-Order (Bivariate)   **Partial Correlation**   **Semipartial Correlation**
Correlation

FIGURE 10–1.   VENN DIAGRAM ILLUSTRATING PARTIAL AND SEMIPARTIAL CORRELATION

In partial correlation, the effect of the extraneous variable is removed from the independent and dependent variables. **Semipartial correlation** is the correlation between *all* of Y and X_1, from which X_2 has been partialled out. It is called *semi*partial because the effect of the extraneous variable is removed from X_1 but not from Y. In the diagram, the area *a* corresponds to the squared semipartial correlation coefficient between Y and X_1 (symbolized as $r_{y(1\cdot2)}$); this squared semipartial coefficient represents *a* as a proportion of the entire circle. The area *c* corresponds to the squared semipartial correlation coefficient between Y and X_2 ($r_{y(2\cdot1)}$). These two squared coefficients represent the unique areas of overlap between Y and each of the two X variables.

Multiple correlation may be viewed as a combination of correlations and semipartial correlations. A formula for R^2 that demonstrates this concept is:

$$R^2_{y12} = r^2_{y1} + r^2_{y(2\cdot1)}$$

That is, the squared correlation between Y and the two X variables is equivalent to the squared correlation between Y and X_1, plus the squared semipartial correlation between

Y and X_2 with X_1 partialled. This equation can be extended indefinitely. The term for a third predictor variable, for example, would be $r^2_{y(3\cdot12)}$—the squared semipartial correlation of Y with X_3, with X_1 and X_2 partialled out.

In regression analysis, the regression coefficients—the b weights—are sometimes referred to as **partial regression coefficients.** This signifies that the coefficients are the weights associated with a given predictor when partialling out or controlling for the effects of the other predictors in the equation.

TESTS OF SIGNIFICANCE FOR MULTIPLE REGRESSION

Thus far we have considered multiple regression in a purely descriptive sense; the regression equation and R are specific to the sample being used. However, researchers are almost always interested in generalizing their results to the population, and therefore tests of significance are needed to facilitate the required inferences. There are several relevant tests of significance, each used to address a different research question.[4]

Tests of the Overall Equation and R

The most basic statistical test in multiple regression is a test of the null hypothesis that the population value of R is zero. This is equivalent to testing the null hypothesis that all the regression coefficients in the multiple regression equation are zero.

The test for the significance of R is based on principles analogous to those discussed in connection with analysis of variance in Chapter 7. The total amount of variability in the dependent variable is partitioned into contributing components, and an F ratio is constructed. The computed F statistic is then compared to tabled values for the F distribution.

In ANOVA, the F ratio involves two sums of squared deviations for the dependent variable—the sum of squares between (in the numerator) and the sum of squares within (in the denominator). For multiple regression, the general form of the F ratio is similar:

$$F = \frac{SS_{\text{regression}}/df_{\text{regression}}}{SS_{\text{residuals}}/df_{\text{residuals}}}$$

The underlying principle for the overall test in multiple regression is the same as in ANOVA; variability in the dependent variable that is attributable to the independent variables ($SS_{\text{regression}}$) is contrasted with variability attributable to other factors or error ($SS_{\text{residuals}}$).

---

[4]Several assumptions underlie statistical tests associated with multiple regression. These are discussed in a subsequent section.

There are several formulas for computing the multiple regression F statistic, but the most convenient is:

$$F = \frac{R^2/k}{(1 - R^2)/(N - k - 1)}$$

where k = number of predictor (independent) variables
N = total number of cases (sample size)

We can use this formula to test the significance of the regression for predicting graduate GPA, for which the value of R^2 with four predictor variables is .90. Therefore, the value of the F statistic would be:

$$F = \frac{.90/4}{.10/15} = \frac{.225}{.0067} = 33.58$$

In regression, $df_{regression}$ is equal to k, the number of predictors, and $df_{residuals}$ is equal to $N - k - 1$. In this example, then, there are 4 and 15 degrees of freedom. In Table B–3 of Appendix B we find that the critical value of F with 4 and 15 df for $\alpha =$ .05 is 3.06. Since our calculated value of F is considerably larger than the critical value, we can reject the null hypothesis that the population value of R is zero.

Tests of the Regression Coefficients

In addition to an overall test, researchers are often interested in the significance of individual predictors in the regression equation. Most computer programs compute a t statistic for each regression coefficient. These t statistics test the unique contribution of each independent variable. A significant t value indicates that the regression coefficient is significantly different from zero. This means that the variable associated with the regression coefficient contributes significantly to the regression, once the other independent variables are taken into account.

In our example of predicting graduate GPA, the t statistic associated with the regression coefficient for undergraduate GPA ($b = .793$ for X_1) is 4.03. (The calculations are not shown, but a subsequent section of this chapter presents computer output for this analysis.) For individual regression coefficients, the appropriate degrees of freedom are $df_{residual}$, which in this case is 15. For $df = 15$ and $\alpha = .05$, the critical value of t (Table B–2) is 2.13. Thus the regression coefficient associated with undergraduate GPA is statistically significant. Each coefficient in the equation would be evaluated in a similar fashion.

Tests for Added Predictors

A question that is frequently of interest to researchers is whether adding predictors significantly improves the predictive power of the regression equation. That is, does adding

X_{k+1} to the regression equation significantly increase R over that which was achieved with X_k predictors?

In the context of the graduate GPA example, we might ask a question such as the following: Does adding the two GRE scores and the motivation scores to the regression equation as a set increase our ability to predict graduate GPA over what we could achieve using undergraduate GPA alone? As noted earlier, the bivariate correlation between undergraduate and graduate GPA (r_{y1}) is .85, and thus $r_{y1}^2 = .72$. The multiple correlation between Y and all four predictors (R_{y1234}) is .95, so $R_{y1234}^2 = .90$. We can readily determine that the inclusion of three predictors improved R^2 by .18—but is this increase statistically significant? In other words, does the added predictive power reflect chance fluctuations for this sample only, or is the increase likely to be observed in the population?

An F statistic is computed for answering this question. The general formula for testing the significance of variables added to the regression equation is:

$$F = \frac{(R^2_{yk_1} - R^2_{yk_2})/(k_1 - k_2)}{(1 - R^2_{yk_1})/(N - k_1 - 1)}$$

where $R^2_{yk_1}$ = R^2 for Y correlated with k_1 predictors
$\quad k_1 \quad$ = the larger of the two sets of predictors
$\quad R^2_{yk_2}$ = R^2 for Y correlated with k_2 predictors
$\quad k_2 \quad$ = the smaller of the two sets of predictors

In our current example, the calculated F statistic for testing whether the addition of GRE and motivation scores as a set results in a significant improvement in predicting graduate GPA over predictions using undergraduate GPA alone would be:

$$F = \frac{(.90 - .72)/(4 - 1)}{(1 - .90)/(20 - 4 - 1)} = \frac{.06}{.0067} = 8.96$$

The appropriate degrees of freedom for this F test are ($k_1 - k_2$) for the numerator and ($N - k_1 - 1$) for the denominator, which in this case are 3 and 15. Consulting Table B–3, we find that the critical value of F for $\alpha = .05$ with 3 and 15 degrees of freedom is 3.29. Since our calculated value of F is larger, we can conclude that the addition of X_2, X_3, and X_4 as a set to the regression equation significantly improved the accuracy of predictions of Y over what could be achieved using X_1 alone.

STRATEGIES FOR ENTERING PREDICTORS IN MULTIPLE REGRESSION

There are several analytic strategies for selecting and entering independent variables in regression equations. Differences among the alternative strategies involve what happens to overlapping variability among correlated independent variables, and how the order of entry of predictors into the equation is determined.

Venn diagrams help to illustrate how three prominent strategies allocate overlapping variability differently. Figure 10–2 shows a schematic diagram of the relationship between four variables—a dependent variable, Y, and three independent variables, X_1, X_2, and X_3. In this example, all three predictor variables are correlated with the dependent variable. Based on the extent of overlap between the X and Y variables, it can be seen that Y is most strongly correlated with X_1, and least strongly correlated with X_3. The diagram also indicates that X_2 is correlated with both X_1 and X_3. However, X_1 and X_3 do not overlap at all—they are totally uncorrelated. What is at issue is how to allocate the variability that the three predictor variables have in common with Y—the areas designated as m and o in Figure 10–2(A).

The Simultaneous Multiple Regression Model

The standard multiple regression strategy enters all independent variables into the regression equation simultaneously, and hence the name **simultaneous multiple regression.** A single regression equation is developed, and the regression coefficients indicate the relationship between each predictor when all other predictors have been taken into

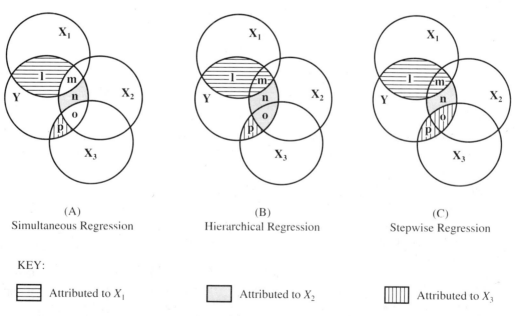

(A)   (B)   (C)
Simultaneous Regression   Hierarchical Regression   Stepwise Regression

KEY:

▤ Attributed to X_1 ▢ Attributed to X_2 ▥ Attributed to X_3

FIGURE 10–2. VENN DIAGRAMS ILLUSTRATING ALTERNATIVE REGRESSION STRATEGIES

account. The regression equation presented earlier for the prediction of graduate GPA used the simultaneous multiple regression model.

Figure 10–2 (A) illustrates this analytic strategy. The shaded areas of the circles (labeled *l, n,* and *p*) indicate the variability allocated to X_1, X_2, and X_3, respectively, with this procedure. As this figure shows, each independent variable is assigned only the portion of Y's variability that it contributes uniquely—the portions we described earlier as corresponding to the squared semipartial correlations. The areas of overlap—areas *m* and *o*—contribute to the prediction of Y and to the magnitude of R. However, these areas are not attributed to any particular independent variable.

Thus, in the standard multiple regression model, all independent variables are dealt with on an equal footing. This strategy is most appropriate when there is no theoretical basis for considering that any particular independent variable is causally prior to another, and when all independent variables are of equal importance to the research problem.

The Hierarchical Multiple Regression Model

In **hierarchical multiple regression,** independent variables are entered into the model in a series of steps, and the order of entry is controlled by the researcher. Hierarchical regression allows the researcher to observe what an independent variable (or set of independent variables) adds to the equation at the point that it is entered.

The order of entry of predictors should be based on logical or theoretical considerations. For example, some independent variables may be conceptualized as being causally or temporally prior to other independent variables, and these could be entered early in the analysis. Suppose, for instance, that we wanted to predict breast self-examination practices on the basis of health beliefs and age. It could be argued that age should be entered into the equation first, since age (or, to think of it another way, year of birth) is temporally and perhaps even causally prior to health beliefs.

Another common reason for using hierarchical regression is to examine the effect of certain independent variables after the effect of other variables has been controlled. For example, suppose our main research interest was in examining the relationship between a woman's alcohol consumption during pregnancy and infant birth weight. Hierarchical regression could be used to first control (remove the effect of) extraneous variables that also influence infant birth weight (e.g., length of gestation, maternal weight prior to pregnancy, and so on). With these variables entered in an early step, it would be possible to determine what alcohol consumption *adds* to the equation.

Figure 10–2(B) illustrates hierarchical regression. In this example, the researcher has decided to enter X_1, X_2, and X_3 in three successive steps. The *process* of variable entry is shown in Figure 10–3. Panel A shows that in the first step, all of the variability that is shared between X_1 and the dependent variable is attributed to X_1, and this variability is removed from further consideration. Thus, referring back to Figure 10–2, the over-

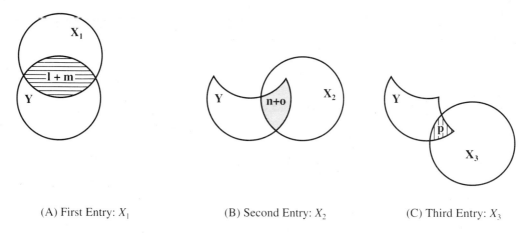

(A) First Entry: X_1 (B) Second Entry: X_2 (C) Third Entry: X_3

FIGURE 10–3.   ILLUSTRATION OF HIERARCHICAL REGRESSION

lapping area between X_1 and X_2 (the area labeled m) is assigned to X_1. In the next step of the analysis (panel B of Figure 10–3), only a portion of Y's variability remains to be explained; the variability associated with X_1 has been "controlled" or held constant. When X_2 is entered into the equation, the variability that remains between Y and X_2 is assigned to X_2, and this includes the area labeled o in Figure 10–2. In the third phase, only the variability that is unique to X_3 is attributed to this predictor because all overlapping variability has already been accounted for.

In hierarchical regression, the number of steps and the number of variables included at each step are determined by the researcher. When several variables are added as a block, the analysis is a simultaneous regression for those variables at that stage. Thus, hierarchical regression can be viewed as a series of simultaneous regressions.

Stepwise Multiple Regression

A third alternative strategy, **stepwise multiple regression,** is a somewhat controversial procedure because variables are entered into the regression equation based solely on statistical, rather than theoretical or logical, criteria. The basic stepwise model involves successive steps in which predictors are entered, one at a time, in the order in which the increment to R is greatest. The computer, rather than the researcher, determines the order of entry of predictor variables.

The first independent variable entered in stepwise regression is the variable that has the highest bivariate correlation with the dependent variable. In the example illustrated in Figure 10–2, X_1 has the highest correlation, and so X_1 is the first variable included in the equation. As shown in panel C of this figure, all of the shared variability between X_1 and Y (areas l and m) is attributed to this first predictor, as was true in hierarchical regression.

The predictor variable selected to enter in the second step is not necessarily the one with the second highest correlation with Y. The selected variable is the independent variable that accounts for the largest portion of what *remains* of Y's variability after the first variable entered has been taken into account. In our example, X_2 is more strongly correlated with Y than is X_3. However, much of the predictive power of X_2 has already been accounted for by X_1 because these two predictors are correlated. By contrast, X_3 is not correlated with X_1, and thus X_3 can account for a greater proportion of what remains of Y's variability—and thus contribute more to R. Thus, X_3 is entered in step 2 of the stepwise regression. Panel C of Figure 10–2 shows that all of the variability shared between X_3 and Y is attributed to X_3, including the area labeled o that represents overlap between X_2 and X_3. In the third step, X_2 is finally entered, but X_2 now accounts for only a small portion of Y's variability (area n).

When stepwise regression is used, there are typically more than three variables. At each step, the predictor entered into the equation is the one that accounts for the greatest proportion of variability in Y *after removing the effect of previous variables.* Typically, the analysis proceeds as long as there are predictors that can contribute significantly to R; when there are no more independent variables that can yield a significant increment to R, the analysis stops.

Within stepwise regression, there are a variety of options. The one we have just described is called **forward selection.** The equation starts from scratch and is built forward, a step at a time, with the addition of variables that meet statistical criteria. A second option is **backward deletion,** which starts out with *all* independent variables entered into the equation—as in simultaneous regression. Then, in successive steps, variables that fail to contribute to the regression are deleted. A third alternative is a **true stepwise solution,** which proceeds in a similar fashion to forward selection, except that variables already in the equation are reevaluated and dropped in later steps if they fail to contribute significantly to the regression once later-added variables are in the equation.

Stepwise regression procedures are controversial because there is no underlying theoretical or logical rationale to the entry or inclusion of variables in the equation. Decisions about which variable to enter next may be based on relatively minor differences between remaining variables, and the differences could reflect sampling error. Thus, the regression equation from any single sample may not be the best reflection of population values. Stepwise regression is perhaps best suited to exploratory work. Even then, caution should be exercised in using stepwise regression, and replication with a second sample is strongly advised. As an alternative, if a single sample is sufficiently large, **crossvalidation** can be accomplished by dividing the sample in half (preferably at random) to determine if a similar regression equation results from both subsets of data.

NATURE OF THE INDEPENDENT VARIABLES

Multiple regression is used to predict a dependent variable that is measured on an interval or ratio-level scale. There is, however, considerable flexibility with regard to the form of the independent variables. This section reviews the major options for the properties of independent variables used in regression analysis.

Interval- and Ratio-Level Independent Variables

Independent variables used in multiple regression are often variables that have been measured on an interval- or ratio-level scale, or on a scale that approximates interval characteristics. In our example of predicting graduate GPA, the four predictors were measured on scales that are reasonably close approximations to interval-level measurement.[5]

The use of variables measured on interval and ratio scales is straightforward. The values typically do not have to be transformed or manipulated—the raw data values are used directly in the analysis.

Nominal-Level Independent Variables

Nominal-level variables can also be included in regression analysis, but care must be taken with regard to how they are represented. Nominal-level variables must be **coded** in a manner that allows for appropriate interpretation of the regression coefficients. Let us take as an example the variable of race/ethnicity. Suppose that in our original data set we have assigned four codes to this variable: 1 = white, 2 = African American, 3 = Hispanic, and 4 = other. The raw data for this variable could not meaningfully be used in the regression analysis because the analysis assumes that 4 means "more of" the variable than 3, and so on. The original coding scheme has no inherent quantitative meaning, so the regression coefficients for this variable could not be sensibly interpreted. Thus, nominal-level variables almost always have to be recoded before using them in regression analysis.

Several alternative systems can be used to code nominal variables. Whichever option is chosen, the value of R remains the same, but the values of the regression coefficients and the intercept constant are affected. The coding options share one feature in common: the coding involves creating $c - 1$ newly coded variables to represent the original variable, where c is the number of categories of the original variable. Thus, for gender (male/female), there would only need to be one newly coded variable ($2 - 1 = 1$), but for our four-category race/ethnicity variable, there would need to be three created variables ($4 - 1 = 3$).

---

[5]Ordinal-level variables can also be used in regression analyses, if there are a sufficiently large number of categories and the distribution is reasonably close to being normal, so long as the ordinal variable has a linear relationship with other variables. If an ordinal-level variable has only a few categories (e.g., assistant professor, associate professor, and full professor), it should be treated like a nominal-level variable.

TABLE 10–3. DUMMY CODING OF RACE/ETHNICITY VARIABLE

Race/Ethnicity	Original Code	WHITE X_1	AFROAMER X_2	HISPANIC X_3
White	1	1	0	0
African American	2	0	1	0
Hispanic	3	0	0	1
Other	4	0	0	0

Dummy Coding. The most widely used coding scheme for regression analysis is referred to as **dummy coding.** Dummy coding involves the creation of a series of dichotomous **dummy variables** that contrast members in one category with everyone else. The code of 1 is used to designate membership in the specified category, and 0 is used to designate nonmembership. For example, if we were coding gender, the code of 1 could be assigned to all females, and the code of 0 could be assigned to all males (or vice versa).

When there are more than two categories, there need to be $c - 1$ variables, all of which are coded either 1 or 0. Table 10–3 shows how our race/ethnicity variable would be handled. The original codes for the four-category variable are shown in the second column. In the next three columns are three new variables, which are labeled as they might be for a computer analysis: WHITE, AFROAMER, and HISPANIC. Any subject whose code on the original variable was 1 would be coded 1 for the variable WHITE, and any subject whose original code was 2, 3, or 4 (i.e., those who were nonwhite) would be coded 0. In effect, the new variable represents "whiteness" and the codes indicate yes or no for each subject's status on this variable. For the variable AFROAMER, only subjects with an original code of 2 would be coded 1 and all others would be coded 0, while for HISPANIC, those originally coded 3 would be coded 1 and all others would be 0.

Since there need to be $c - 1$ new variables, there is always a category that is omitted and serves as a **reference group.** In this case, the reference group is "other." For example, Native American subjects in the sample, who would be coded 4 on the original race/ethnicity variable, would be coded 0 on WHITE, AFROAMER, and HISPANIC. A fourth variable is not necessary because the information would be redundant; a person who is nonwhite, non-African American, and non-Hispanic can be designated by having all 0s for these three variables.[6] It does not really matter which group is omitted, but the omitted category is often the one that has the smallest membership.

The new coded variables can then be used as predictors in a multiple regression analysis. Suppose we wanted to predict infant birth weight based on mothers' race/ethnicity. The multiple regression equation would be:

---

[6]If a variable for OTHER were created and used in the multiple regression analysis with the other three race/ethnicity variables, the computer analysis would print an error message. No predictor variable that is perfectly correlated with other independent variables (which is what happens when there is total redundancy) can be included in the regression equation.

$$\text{BWEIGHT}' = a + b_1\text{WHITE} + b_2\text{AFROAMER} + b_3\text{HISPANIC}$$

In this analysis, the intercept term reflects the mean on the dependent variable (BWEIGHT) for the reference group; for this group all the dummy variables are equal to zero, and therefore all other expressions after a in the equation would also equal zero. The regression coefficient on each dummy variable is the estimate of the difference in the dependent variable between the designated group and the reference group. Thus, the coefficient for WHITE estimates the difference in infant birth weight between white mothers and mothers of other racial/ethnic backgrounds. In significance tests, the t-test associated with the coefficient on a particular dummy variable tests whether that group differs significantly from the reference group.

Effect Coding. **Effect coding** is similar to dummy coding, except that the reference group is assigned -1 rather than 0 for each newly created variable. Thus, if effect coding were used rather than dummy coding for the race/ethnicity variable, subjects who were originally coded 4 (Other) would be assigned -1 on the WHITE, AFROAMER, and HISPANIC variables. All other subjects would be coded with 1s and 0s as for dummy coding, as shown in Table 10–4.

With effect coding, the a in the equation is the grand mean—the mean of the entire sample—on the dependent variable rather than the mean of the reference group. The regression coefficient associated with each predictor now indicates the group's mean on the dependent variable relative to the grand mean, and the t-test associated with each coefficient tests the significance of the group's difference from the grand mean.

Using effect coding in our example, we could compare the mean birth weights for white, African American, and Hispanic mothers against the overall grand mean. To find the mean for mothers of other races/ethnicities, we would have to perform a calculation. All bs—including that for the omitted group—must total zero, since the b weights reflect deviations from the mean. Thus, if the regression coefficients for white, African American, and Hispanic mothers were $+4$, -3, and $+1$, respectively, the coefficient for the "other" category would be -2 $(4 - 3 + 1 - 2 = 0)$.

TABLE 10–4. EFFECT CODING OF RACE/ETHNICITY VARIABLE

Race/Ethnicity	Original Code	WHITE X_1	AFROAMER X_2	HISPANIC X_3
White	1	1	0	0
African American	2	0	1	0
Hispanic	3	0	0	1
Other	4	−1	−1	−1

Orthogonal Coding. If dummy or effect coding is used, the researcher cannot draw conclusions about differences between all pairs of group means. In our above example, the regression analysis would not enable us to conclude that the birth weights of African American and white babies differed significantly.[7] When researchers have specific hypotheses about group differences, they sometimes use **orthogonal coding** to test these differences. Orthogonal coding provides a means of performing planned (a priori) comparisons that yield a more powerful statistical test than post hoc comparisons.

The term **orthogonal** refers to a perfect *non*relationship between variables. If variable X and variable Y are orthogonal ($r = .00$), knowledge of the value of X tells us nothing about the value of Y. Orthogonal coding sets up contrasts among groups that are independent.

In our example of four racial/ethnic groups, suppose that 40% of the population of interest was white, 40% was African American, 10% was Hispanic, and 10% was in the "other" group. We might, therefore, want to contrast the two "majority" groups (whites and African Americans) with the two "minority" groups (Hispanics and Others). We can do this by assigning codes of ½ and −½, as we show for the first contrast in Table 10–5. This contrast compares the mean for whites and African Americans *combined* with the mean for Hispanics and Others *combined*. Next, suppose that we wanted to test the hypothesis that whites and African Americans were different. This contrast is represented with a code of 1 for whites and a code of −1 for African Americans; the other two groups that are not being compared are coded 0 (contrast 2 in the table). Our final hypothesis (contrast 3 in the table) concerns differences between Hispanics and others.

To set up orthogonal codes, there are three requirements. First, there must be $c - 1$ contrasts. Second, the codes established *within* a contrast must add up to 0. In Table 10–5, the sum of codes for contrast 1 is zero (½ + ½ − ½ − ½ = 0), as is the sum of codes for contrast 2 (1 − 1 + 0 + 0 = 0) and contrast 3 (0 + 0 + 1 − 1 = 0). Finally, the sum of crossproducts must also equal zero. For example, the summed crossproducts for the first two contrasts equal zero [(½)(1) + (½)(−1) + (−½)(0) + (−½)(0) = 0]. The summed crossproducts for contrasts 1 with 3 and contrasts 2 with 3 must also equal zero, as they do in this example.

TABLE 10–5. ORTHOGONAL CODING OF RACE/ETHNICITY VARIABLE

Race/Ethnicity	Original Code	Contrast 1 X_1	Contrast 2 X_2	Contrast 3 X_3
White	1	½	1	0
African American	2	½	−1	0
Hispanic	3	−½	0	1
Other	4	−½	0	−1

---

[7]Post hoc multiple comparisons in a multiple regression context are described in Pedhazur (1982), chapter 9.

When orthogonal coding is used, a is the grand mean of the dependent variable. Each regression coefficient (b) represents one of the hypothesized contrasts.

Interaction Terms

In addition to using continuous variables and coded nominal-level variables as predictors in multiple regression, interactions between variables can be represented in the equation. As explained in Chapter 7, an interaction refers to the combined effect of two variables—e.g., the effect of a specific "cell" when two independent variables are crossed, as in a randomized block or factorial design. In multiple regression, interaction terms can be constructed between nominal-level and continuous variables and used as variables in the equation.

It is beyond the scope of this book to explain interaction within multiple regression in detail and to fully discuss how interaction terms should be interpreted.[8] However, we briefly illustrate the use of interaction terms here with a simple example that involves two nominal-level variables that have been dummy coded. Suppose that we designed an experiment to test the effectiveness of an intervention to alleviate pain in male versus female cancer patients using a randomized block design. As shown in Table 10–6, the first independent variable (X_1) is GROUP; those in the experimental group are coded 1, while controls are coded 0 on this variable. For GENDER (X_2), females are coded 1 and males are coded 0. The interaction term for the interaction between GROUP and GENDER (X_3) is constructed by multiplying the two codes for X_1 and X_2 together, as shown in the right-hand column of Table 10–6. In this example, females in the experimental group are coded 1 as a result of the multiplication of codes, while all others are coded 0. Conceptually, it makes sense to multiply; the interaction term represents the *joint effect of two variables over and above any additive combination of their separate effects.* The

TABLE 10–6. CODING OF INTERACTIONS FOR TWO DUMMY VARIABLES

Cell	GROUP X_1	GENDER X_2	INTERACT X_3
Experimental, Female	1	1	1
Experimental, Male	1	0	0
Control, Female	0	1	0
Control, Male	0	0	0

[8]For further information on interaction in multiple regression, the reader can consult Pedhazur (1982) or Cohen and Cohen (1975).

regression coefficient for the interaction term (b_3) equals the *difference* between the regression coefficient of X_1 for males and females. If the regression coefficient for the interaction is significant, we can conclude that the regression of the pain measure on experimental group status is conditional—that is, it depends on whether the patients are male or female.

A Note on the Link Between Regression and ANOVA

Since categorical variables and interaction terms can be represented as independent variables in multiple regression, you may have wondered if there is a connection between multiple regression and ANOVA. In fact, ANOVA and multiple regression are virtually identical. All of the examples used in the chapter on ANOVA could have been analyzed through multiple regression analysis, and the conclusions would have been identical. Both ANOVA and regression require a continuous dependent variable, and both involve partitioning variance into a component associated with the independent variables and a component for unexplained or error variance. Both techniques involve the computation of an F ratio to test for significant effects. And both provide information about the total amount of variation explained by the independent variable: through R^2 for multiple regression and through eta^2 for ANOVA.

By convention, researchers whose research design is experimental (i.e., those who manipulate and control the independent variable) usually use ANOVA, while those whose research is nonexperimental are more likely to use regression. However, any data for which ANOVA is appropriate could, through the use of coded nominal variables and interaction terms, be analyzed through multiple regression. When one or more independent variables are continuous, however, ANOVA cannot be used; the data must be analyzed by multiple regression.

SPECIAL ISSUES IN MULTIPLE REGRESSION

Multiple regression analysis is a complex statistical procedure to which entire textbooks have been devoted. This book provides primarily an overview of the major features of regression, but a few additional topics merit brief discussion.

Relative Importance of Predictors

If the main purpose of the regression analysis is for prediction—as in our example of a nursing school predicting graduate GPA for admissions purposes—the goal is to achieve the most accurate prediction possible by maximizing R^2. However, multiple regression analysis is also used by scientists to help them better understand phenomena of interest, and for this reason they often seek to determine which of the independent variables in their regression equation are most important in explaining the dependent variable. With regard to graduate GPA, a researcher might be interested in learning how important achievement motivation is in graduate school performance, relative to cognitive skills and earlier school performance.

When the predictor variables in a regression analysis are correlated—which is almost always the case—the assessment of the relative importance of the predictors is difficult. There is no totally satisfactory way of untangling the effects of correlated independent variables.

It should be clear that the solution is *not* to compare the b weights in the regression equation. Because the regression coefficients are in the original units of measurement, their values cannot be compared. In the regression equation for predicting graduate GPA, the b for undergraduate GPA was .793, while that for GRE-Verbal scores was .004. Undergraduate GPA is not 200 times more important than the verbal GRE scores, but the weight is 200 times larger because of differences in the units of measurement.

Perhaps, then, the solution is to compare standardized regression coefficients, which are all in the same unit of measurement. In the standardized regression equation for predicting graduate GPA, the beta weight for undergraduate GPA (.53) was about 10% larger than that for verbal GRE scores (.48). Does that mean that undergraduate GPA has 10% more explanatory power than verbal GRE scores? Unfortunately, although some researchers compare beta weights in this fashion, it is not really judicious to do so. Beta weights tend to be unstable, fluctuating in value from sample to sample. Moreover, beta weights change as variables are added to or subtracted from the regression equation. For example, if we were to omit GRE-Verbal scores (X_2) from the regression analysis, the standardized regression equation would be:

$$z_{Y'} = .57z_{x_1} + .14z_{x_3} + .31z_{x_4}$$

In this new equation, the beta weights for all three variables are higher than before. The biggest change is the beta weight for GRE-Quantitative, which was previously negative and is now positive. Because beta weights are not fixed relative to other beta weights in the analysis, it is difficult to attach much theoretical importance to them.

Another approach is to consider the proportion of Y's variability that is explained by different predictors, but this is problematic, too. Returning to our graduate GPA example, the most highly correlated predictor was undergraduate GPA, which accounts for .72 of Y's variance ($r^2 = .85^2 = .72$). When GRE-Verbal is added to the equation, R^2 increases by .13 to .85. Should we conclude, then, that undergraduate grades are about 5.5 times as important as GRE-Verbal scores ($.72 \div .13 = 5.5$) in explaining graduate school grades? Unfortunately, this would be inappropriate because the relative contribution of the two variables is completely determined by which one is entered into the regression first. If GRE-Verbal were the first variable used to predict graduate GPA, the proportion of variance it would account for would be $r^2 = .73^2 = .53$. If undergraduate GPA were *then* added, the R^2 for the two predictors would stay the same at .85, so that the apparent contribution of undergraduate GPA is only .32 ($.85 - .53 = .32$); this is

60% *less than* verbal GRE scores, rather than 5.5 times greater. This situation results from the fact that any overlapping variability in the predictor variables (the area labeled *b* in Figure 10–1) is attributed to the first variable into the equation.

One of the better solutions is to compare the squared semipartial correlations of the predictors. This would mean comparing the area labeled *a* with that labeled *c* in Figure 10–1. The semipartial correlations are useful because they indicate a predictor's unique contribution to Y', i.e., the contribution after the effect of other predictors is taken into account. Semipartial correlations can be produced by the regression programs of all the major software packages. In the present example, the semipartial correlation of graduate GPA and undergraduate GPA while partialling GRE-Verbal scores is .57, while that of graduate GPA and verbal GRE with undergraduate grades partialled is .35. Thus, when these two independent variables are used to predict graduate grades, the unique contribution of undergraduate grades is about 60% greater than that for GRE-Verbal scores.

Suppression in Multiple Regression

There are instances in which a predictor variable has an effect on the regression equation that appears inconsistent with that variable's relationship with the dependent variable. This can occur through a phenomenon known as **suppression.**

For example, it is sometimes possible for an independent variable to contribute significantly to R^2 even though it is totally uncorrelated with the dependent variable. This situation, which is sometimes called **classical suppression,** is illustrated in Figure 10–4(A). Here, X_1 is correlated with Y, but X_2 is not. However, because of the correla-

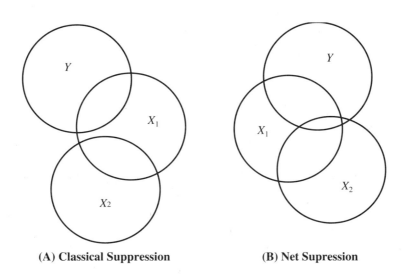

(A) Classical Suppression   (B) Net Supression

FIGURE 10–4.   VENN DIAGRAM ILLUSTRATING SUPPRESSION

tion between the two predictors, the inclusion of X_2 in the regression equation increases the variance accounted for in the dependent variable by suppressing some of the variability in X_1 that is irrelevant to Y.

An illustration may clarify how this works. Suppose we wanted to predict new nurses' clinical performance as rated by their supervisors (Y) on the basis of the nurses' score on a global nursing achievement test (X_1). Test scores are influenced not only by actual nursing knowledge, but also by test anxiety (X_2). Test anxiety does not affect the nurses' day-to-day performance in clinical settings, and so these two variables are uncorrelated. However, part of the reason that test scores and clinical performance do not correlate more highly than they do is because the test scores of some are depressed by their anxiety—their real nursing knowledge is artificially masked. By removing the portion of test score variability that reflects the influence of test anxiety, the prediction of clinical performance based on test scores improves.

There are several other types of suppression, one of which is illustrated in Figure 10–4(B). In **net suppression,** there are correlations among all the variables. That is, r^2_{y1} > 0, r^2_{y2} > 0, and r^2_{12} > 0. However, the correlation between Y and X_2 is relatively small, and yet the contribution of X_2 in the regression equation is not insubstantial. This results from the fact that the contribution of X_2 occurs mainly through suppressing a portion of the variance of X_1 that is uncorrelated with Y.

The presence of suppressors can be detected by comparing the bivariate correlations of Y and each X with the corresponding beta weights for each X. If the regression coefficients are significant, suppression is present when the bivariate correlation and the beta weight have opposite signs,[9] or when the value of the correlation coefficient is substantially smaller than the value of the beta weight.

Problems Relating to Multiple Regression

Multiple regression is a powerful statistical procedure, but the researcher needs to pay attention to a few potential problems in using this analytic technique. This section discusses a few issues of concern.

Multicollinearity. A problem known as **multicollinearity** can occur in multiple regression analysis when the independent variables are too highly intercorrelated.[10] In general, researchers should avoid the use of a set of independent variables when there are intercorrelations that are .85 or higher.

[9]There is some suppression in our graduate GPA example, as evidenced by the fact that the bivariate correlation between graduate grades and the CRE-Quantitative scores is positive, while the regression coefficient is negative. However, this coefficient is not statistically significant, so that a suppression effect in the population cannot be assumed.

[10]Another problem, called **singularity,** occurs if independent variables are *perfectly* correlated. The calculation of regression coefficients is done through **matrix algebra,** and singularity prohibits some of the necessary operations. Singularity would occur, for example, if four (rather than three) dummy variables were included in a regression analysis to represent a four-category nominal variable.

Multicollinearity should be avoided for several reasons. First, from a logical point of view, it is unnecessary; if the independent variables are highly correlated, they add little new information to the regression equation when used in combination. Moreover, the inclusion of two highly intercorrelated variables raises the critical value of F required to reject the null hypothesis, because each additional predictor lowers the degrees of freedom for residuals. Second, the results of a regression analysis when multicollinearity is present tend to be unstable; when independent variables are highly correlated, the computations required for the regression coefficients are seriously jeopardized. And third, as a result of the second problem, the regression coefficients can be very misleading and render interpretation of the results problematic.

The easiest way to prevent multicollinearity is to avoid including highly intercorrelated independent variables in the regression equation. However, it is not always possible to detect multicollinearity by simply inspecting bivariate correlation coefficients, because *combinations* of variables sometimes create multicollinearity.

Computer programs that perform multiple regression can be instructed to avoid multicollinearity by establishing a **tolerance.** The tolerance of a predictor is computed by treating each one as the dependent variable in a multiple regression analysis, and determining the R^2 when the other independent variables are used as predictors; tolerance is 1 minus this R^2 value. Thus, if a predictor variable were totally uncorrelated with other independent variables, the tolerance would be 1.00; the tolerance would be 0.00 if the variables were perfectly intercorrelated. In almost all instances, tolerance is between .00 and 1.00, with higher values being more desirable. The computer can be instructed to automatically exclude any predictor whose tolerance falls below a level specified by the researcher (e.g., .01). However, it might be preferable to make your own choice about variables to be excluded, rather than letting the computer mechanically rule out predictors. This can be accomplished by inspecting the tolerances for all variables and then rerunning the analysis after deciding which, if any, should be omitted.

Violation of Assumptions. Like all statistical techniques, the use of multiple regression as an inferential tool is based on certain assumptions. First, **multivariate normality** is the assumption that each variable and all linear combinations of the variables are normally distributed. Second, linearity is assumed—i.e., it is assumed that there is a straight line relationship between all pairs of variables. Third, there is an assumption of homoscedasticity, i.e., that the variability in scores for one variable is approximately the same at all values of another variable.[11]

In bivariate statistics, frequency distributions of individual variables and scatterplots of the two variables in the analysis are used to assess the violation of underlying

---

[11]There is also an assumption that the errors of prediction are independent of one another. This might not be the case if, for example, systematic changes occurred over the course of collecting data (e.g., systematic improvements over time when implementing an intervention). If there is a reason to suspect nonindependence of errors that is related to the order of cases, there are tests in all major computer programs (e.g., the **Durbin-Watson statistic**) to detect this problem.

assumptions. In multiple regression, researchers examine **residual scatterplots** that plot errors of prediction on one axis and predicted values of the dependent variable on the other. Residual scatterplots can be produced by all major software packages.

When the assumptions for multiple regression are met, the residuals are distributed approximately in a rectangular form, with a concentration of values along a straight line in the center. Figure 10–5 (A) presents an example of a residual scatterplot in which all assumptions are met. When multivariate normality is achieved, the errors of prediction are normally distributed around each value of Y′, and so there should be a clustering of residuals along the center line, with residuals trailing off on either side. Figure 10–5 (B) illustrates a residual scatterplot in which the distribution of residuals is skewed (i.e., there are more values above the center line than below it). If nonlinearity is present, the overall shape of the scatterplot would be curved rather than rectangular, as illustrated in Figure 10–5 (C). Finally, Figure 10–5 (D) illustrates a violation of the assumption of homoscedasticity, showing that the errors of prediction are not equal for all predicted values of Y′.

If there is evidence that assumptions have been violated, it may be possible to address the problem through transformations of the original data. Transformations such as computing the square root, taking logs, or computing the reciprocal of variables can help to stabilize the variance and achieve linearity and normality. A fuller discussion of transformations and their effects may be found in Cohen and Cohen (1975), Ferketich and Verran (1993), or Norušis (1992).

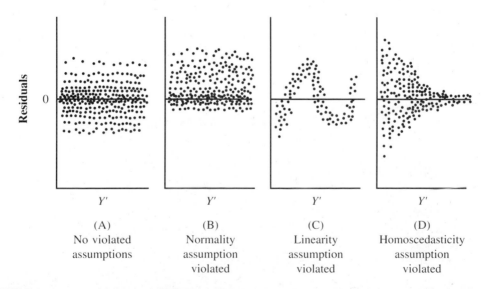

FIGURE 10–5.   RESIDUAL SCATTERPLOTS ILLUSTRATING VIOLATIONS OF ASSUMPTIONS

Outliers. Extreme cases that are legitimate outliers can have a strong impact on the regression solution and therefore need to be diagnosed and addressed. Outliers for individual variables can be detected by examining frequency distributions for the variables in the analysis. Even when there are no univariate outliers, however, there can be multivariate outliers that represent extreme combinations of independent variables in the context of the dependent variable.

Multivariate outliers can also be detected through an analysis of the residuals. Standardized residual values that are greater than 3 or less than -3 are considered multivariate outliers. (In our example of predicting graduate GPA, the standardized residuals ranged from -2.11 to 1.74, indicating the absence of outliers.) Most computer programs for multiple regression also provide other residual analyses that help the researcher evaluate extreme cases. When extreme cases are found, they should usually be eliminated from the analysis or rescored.

Sample Size Considerations

One of the practical matters that needs to be considered in using multiple regression is whether the sample size is sufficiently large to support the analysis. Inadequate sample size can increases the risk of Type II errors. It also can yield unstable and meaningless regression coefficients. There are two ways of approaching the sample size issue, as discussed below.

Ratio of Predictors to Cases. If the number of subjects for the regression analysis is too small, the regression equation may well yield a good solution for the sample data, but yet be of little predictive value when applied to a new sample. This is particularly likely to occur if there are many independent variables, and if a stepwise solution to variable selection has been used. Since most research studies involve the collection of a considerable amount of data, and since multiple regression can readily be performed on a computer, it is sometimes tempting to include many independent variables in the analysis. However, potential predictor variables should be chosen with care because having too many predictors can actually reduce the utility of the regression equation and can raise the risk of Type I and Type II errors.

Various statistical experts have offered sample size guidelines that concern the appropriate ratio of cases to predictors. Tabachnick and Fidell (1989) suggest that the *barest minimum* requirement is 5 times more cases than predictors. However, they recommend a ratio of 20 to 1 for standard and hierarchical regression, and a ratio of 40 to 1 for stepwise regression. A larger sample size is required for stepwise regression because this procedure tends to capitalize on idiosyncrasies of the specific data set. Also, by having a larger sample, crossvalidation may become a viable option.

These general guidelines may result in too small a sample under certain conditions. One of these conditions is a small effect size, an issue we discuss in the next section.

Other situations that require a larger case-to-predictor ratio include having a dependent variable that is skewed rather than normally distributed, and having variables that have substantial measurement error.

Power Analysis. A more precise and reliable way to determine sample size requirements for multiple regression is to perform a power analysis. As we have seen, power analysis takes estimated effect size—the estimated magnitude of the relationship between independent and dependent variables—into account in determining the sample size needed to reduce the risk of a Type II error.

The number of subjects needed to reject the null hypothesis that R^2 is zero is a function of effect size, number of predictors, desired power, and the significance criterion to be used. For multiple regression, the estimated population effect size is:

$$\gamma = \frac{R^2}{1 - R^2}$$

As with other power analyses used to determine sample size, the researcher must estimate the effect size during the planning phase of the study on the basis of prior research or pilot work. An alternative (which should be used only if there is no information about the likely value of R^2) is to use Cohen's (1987) convention of estimating that the effect will be either small ($R^2 = .02$), moderate ($R^2 = .13$), or large ($R^2 = .30$).

The next step is to apply the following formula:

$$N = \left[\frac{L}{\gamma} \right] + k + 1$$

where N = estimated number of cases needed
   L = tabled value for a specified α and power
   γ = estimated effect size
   k = number of predictor variables

Values of L for various power levels when $\alpha = .05$, for up to 20 predictors (k), are presented in Table 10–7.[12]

Suppose we were planning a study to predict preoperative anxiety on the basis of five predictor variables and had reason to believe that R^2 would be approximately .10. The estimated population effect size would be .111 (.10 ÷ .90). For $\alpha = .05$ and a power of .80 with five predictors, the value of L is 12.83. Substituting the appropriate values into the formula, we find:

---

[12]For $\alpha = .01$, or for a larger number of predictors than 20, the tables in Cohen and Cohen (1975) can be consulted.

TABLE 10–7. POWER TABLE FOR MULTIPLE REGRESSION: VALUES OF L FOR $\alpha = .05$

k^*	Power								
	.10	.30	.50	.70	.80	.85	.90	.95	.99
1	.43	2.06	3.84	6.17	7.85	8.98	10.51	13.00	18.37
2	.62	2.78	4.96	7.70	9.64	10.92	12.65	15.44	21.40
3	.78	3.30	5.76	8.79	10.90	12.30	14.17	17.17	23.52
4	.91	3.74	6.42	9.68	11.94	13.42	15.41	18.57	25.24
5	1.03	4.12	6.99	10.45	12.83	14.39	16.47	19.78	26.73
6	1.13	4.46	7.50	11.14	13.62	15.26	17.42	20.86	28.05
7	1.23	4.77	7.97	11.77	14.35	16.04	18.28	21.84	29.25
8	1.32	5.06	8.41	12.35	15.02	16.77	19.08	22.74	30.36
9	1.40	5.33	8.81	12.89	15.65	17.45	19.83	23.59	31.39
10	1.49	5.59	9.19	13.40	16.24	18.09	20.53	24.39	32.37
15	1.84	6.71	10.86	15.63	18.81	20.87	23.58	27.84	36.58
20	2.14	7.65	12.26	17.50	20.96	23.20	26.13	30.72	40.10

$^*k$ = number of predictor variables.

$$N = \left[\frac{12.83}{0.111} \right] + 5 + 1 = 121.6$$

Thus, a sample of about 122 patients is needed to detect a population R^2 of .10 using five predictors, with a 20% risk of a Type II error and a 5% risk of a Type I error.

Table 10–7 can also be used to estimate the power of a completed multiple regression analysis. Suppose we had a sample of 50 subjects and calculated R^2 to be .07 on the basis of three predictors; the null hypothesis is retained. In this example, the effect size is .075 (.07 ÷ .93). Thus:

$$50 = \left[\frac{L}{.075} \right] + 3 + 1$$

$$50 - 4 = \frac{L}{.075}$$

$$L = 46 \, (.075) = 3.46$$

Looking in Table 10–7 in the row for $k = 3$, we find that when $L = 3.30$, power is .30, and so in this example where L is slightly greater than 3.30, the estimated power would be about .31. Thus, in this hypothetical example, the probability of committing a Type II error was about .69 (1 − .31).

Power analysis can also be used to determine the sample size requirements to test null hypotheses about individual regression coefficients. The procedures are described in Cohen and Cohen (1975).

COMPUTER ANALYSIS AND MULTIPLE REGRESSION

Multiple regression analyses are almost always performed by computer, and therefore it is important to know how to read output from a regression analysis. This section discusses printouts for the analysis of the graduate GPA data presented in Table 10–1.

Computer Example of Simultaneous Regression

Figure 10–6 presents the printout for the standard (simultaneous) regression of graduate GPA regressed on the four predictor variables.[13] Panel A begins by identifying the dependent variable, GPA@G. All of the independent variables (MOTIV, GRE@Q, GRE@V, AND GPA@U) are entered as a block (listed under the heading "Variable(s) Entered . . ."). The values of the multiple R (.94611) and R^2 (.89513) are shown next, followed by the value of the adjusted (shrunken) R^2 (.86716) and the standard error (.16123). The standard error could be used to build confidence intervals around predicted values of graduate grades.

The overall test for the significance of the regression is presented in Panel B (labeled "Analysis of Variance"). The printout shows the degrees of freedom, sum of squares, and mean square due to regression and due to residuals. The overall F ratio for this analysis is 32.00815; the probability is .0000, i.e., less than 1 in 10,000 that an F this large occurred by chance alone. This means that the independent variables, as a group, are significantly correlated with the dependent variable.

The next two panels provide information about individual predictors. In Panel C, the first column lists all of the independent variables, and the column labeled B lists the regression coefficients (b weights) associated with each. It is these values, together with the value of the intercept constant (shown as Constant), that are represented in the regression equation we presented earlier in this chapter. (In our presentation of the equation, we rounded values to two decimal places.) The next column indicates the standard errors associated with each b weight. Coefficients with large standard errors are unreliable and their values may vary from sample to sample. Next, the standardized regression coefficients (β weights) are presented in the column headed Beta. The next three columns show the zero-order (Correl), semipartial (Part Cor), and partial correlation coefficients, respectively, for each independent variable with GPA@G. Note that the semipartial correlation coefficients for the full equation indicate that the unique contribution of GRE@V and GPA@U is about equal when the other two predictors are in the equation (i.e., about .33).

---

[13] The SPSS/PC command that generated the printout in Figure 10–6 is as follows:
    REGRESSION VARIABLES=GPA@U GRE@V GRE@Q MOTIV GPA@G
        /STATISTICS=DEFAULT ZPP TOL
        /DEPENDENT = GPA@G
        /METHOD=ENTER.

```
* * * *   M U L T I P L E   R E G R E S S I O N   * * * *
```

Listwise Deletion of Missing Data

A Equation Number 1   Dependent Variable..   GPA@G   GRADUATE GRADE PT AVERAGE

Block Number 1. Method: Enter

Variable(s) Entered on Step Number
```
  1..    MOTIV    MOTIVATION SCALE SCORE
  2..    GRE@Q    QUANTITATIVE GRE SCORE
  3..    GRE@V    VERBAL GRE SCORE
  4..    GPA@U    UNDERGRAD GRADE PT AVERAGE
```

```
Multiple R            .94611
R Square              .89513
Adjusted R Square     .86716
Standard Error        .16123
```

B Analysis of Variance

	DF	Sum of Squares	Mean Square
Regression	4	3.32809	.83202
Residual	15	.38991	.02599

F =   32.00815   Signif F = .0000

C ---------------------- Variables in the Equation ----------------------

Variable	B	SE B	Beta	Correl	Part Cor	Partial
MOTIV	.008849	.005074	.213474	.743091	.145817	.410575
GRE@Q	-8.52152E-04	7.02197E-04	-.144329	.465765	-.101471	-.299003
GRE@V	.003716	9.30824E-04	.480598	.726917	.333844	.717782
GPA@U	.793487	.196990	.531715	.854531	.336804	.720846
(Constant)	-1.635591	.461711				

D ----------- Variables in the Equation -----------

Variable	Tolerance	VIF	T	Sig T
MOTIV	.466580	2.143	1.744	.1016
GRE@Q	.494282	2.023	-1.214	.2437
GRE@V	.482529	2.072	3.993	.0012
GPA@U	.401234	2.492	4.028	.0011
(Constant)			-3.542	.0030

FIGURE 10–6.   COMPUTER PRINTOUT OF SIMULTANEOUS REGRESSION

Panel D is a continuation of the previous panel, presenting various statistics for each predictor. The Tolerance column provides information on possible multicollinearity. All of these values are well above the standard default for excluding a multicollinear variable, which is normally .01 or lower.[14] The next column shows the variance inflation factor, labeled VIF, which is the reciprocal of tolerance (i.e., 1 divided by tolerance).

The last two columns of panel D show information on the statistical tests associated with individual regression coefficients. The t statistic is computed by dividing a b-weight by its standard error (i.e., B ÷ SE B), and the value of t is shown in the column headed T. The final column (labeled Sig T) indicates the actual probability that the regression coefficients reflect sampling fluctuation. In this example, the coefficients for GRE@V and GPA@U are both significant well beyond the .05 level. However, the other two variables (MOTIV and GRE@Q) are not statistically significant. Their inclusion in the regression analysis does not significantly improve our prediction of graduate grades over that which is achieved through GRE@V and GPA@U.

Computer Example of Stepwise Regression

Figure 10–7 shows the output for a stepwise regression of the same data set, i.e., the data in Table 10–1.[15] The top of the first panel shows that the dependent variable is GPA@G, that the method is stepwise, and that PIN = .0500 and POUT = .1000. In stepwise regression, statistical criteria must be indicated for variables to enter and exit the equation. PIN indicates the *probability* level that must be achieved by a regression coefficient for a variable to go *in* the equation. POUT is the *probability* used to determine variables going *out*. Both of these are set to the default values in this example and could be modified by the analyst. The remainder of panel A shows information analogous to that in panel A for the simultaneous regression (Figure 10–6), with one important exception: all of the information on R, R^2, analysis of variance, and so on relates to the regression of GPA@G on a single independent variable. That variable is the predictor entered in the first step, GPA@U, which is the variable with the highest bivariate correlation with graduate grades. With only GPA@U used to predict GPA@G, the adjusted R^2 is .71524. The overall regression is highly significant ($F = 48.72178$, $p = .0000$).

Panel B of Figure 10-7 shows information about individual predictors and is divided into two parts: variables *in* the equation (at this point only GPA@U) and variables *not in* the equation (at this point, the remaining three predictors). For the variables in the equation, the printout lists the regression coefficient (B), standard error of the coeffi-

---

[14]In the version of SPSS/PC used to run this analysis, the tolerance default was .0001.

[15]The SPSS/PC command that created the printout in Figure 10–7 is as follows:
    REGRESSION VARIABLES=GPA@U GRE@V GRE@Q MOTIV GPA@G
        /STATISTICS=DEFAULT CHA
        /DEPENDENT=GPA@G
        /METHOD=STEPWISE.

```
* * * *   M U L T I P L E   R E G R E S S I O N   * * * *

Listwise Deletion of Missing Data

Equation Number 1     Dependent Variable..   GPA@G   GRADUATE GRADE PT AVERAGE
```

A `Block Number  1.  Method:  Stepwise     Criteria   PIN  .0500   POUT  .1000`

```
Variable(s) Entered on Step Number
   1..    GPA@U     UNDERGRAD GRADE PT AVERAGE


Multiple R              .85453
R Square                .73022        R Square Change    .73022
Adjusted R Square       .71524        F Change          48.72178
Standard Error          .23606        Signif F Change    .0000

Analysis of Variance
                        DF     Sum of Squares      Mean Square
Regression               1         2.71497            2.71497
Residual                18         1.00303             .05572

F =       48.72178      Signif F =   .0000
```

B `------------------ Variables in the Equation ------------------`

```
Variable              B          SE B         Beta          T   Sig T

GPA@U          1.275232      .182695      .854531       6.980  .0000
(Constant)    -1.004642      .606111                   -1.658  .1147


------------ Variables not in the Equation -------------

Variable    Beta In  Partial  Min Toler        T   Sig T

GRE@V       .403929  .676724   .757213      3.790  .0015
GRE@Q       .100119  .171963   .795870       .720  .4815
MOTIV       .276526  .375788   .498217      1.672  .1128
```

FIGURE 10–7. COMPUTER PRINTOUT OF STEPWISE REGRESSION

cient (SE B), Beta weight, t statistic for the regression coefficient, and significance of t. The b weight for GPA@U is highly significant ($t = 6.980$, p = .0000).

For variables *not* yet entered in the regression, the statistical information indicates *what would happen if the variables were entered in the next step.* For example, the value under Beta In is the standardized regression coefficient for each predictor *if* the variable were to enter the regression equation in step 2. The partial correlation for the predictor, holding GPA@U constant, is shown in the next column, followed by information on the minimum tolerance (Min Toler). This represents the smallest tolerance any variable *already in* the equation would have if the specified predictor were included. In this example, all of the Min Toler values exceed .01, indicating no problem with multicollinearity

C Variable(s) Entered on Step Number
      2..   GRE@V   VERBAL GRE SCORE


```
Multiple R            .92400
R Square              .85377         R Square Change       .12355
Adjusted R Square     .83656         F Change          14.36270
Standard Error        .17883         Signif F Change       .0015

Analysis of Variance
                    DF      Sum of Squares       Mean Square
Regression           2             3.17431           1.58716
Residual            17              .54369            .03198

F =      49.62708       Signif F =    .0000
```

D ------------------ Variables in the Equation ------------------

```
Variable                 B          SE B         Beta         T   Sig T

GPA@U                 .978217     .159055     .655501      6.150  .0000
GRE@V                 .003124  8.24202E-04    .403929      3.790  .0015
(Constant)          -1.780016     .502697                -3.541  .0025
```

------------- Variables not in the Equation -------------

```
Variable     Beta In   Partial  Min Toler        T   Sig T

GRE@Q       -.195428  -.370724    .500663    -1.597  .1299
MOTIV        .250073   .460901    .440626     2.077  .0542
```


End Block Number   1   PIN =   .050 Limits reached.

FIGURE 10–7.   (CONTINUED)

for any variables that might enter. Finally, the value of the t statistic for each regression coefficient, if entered next, is shown with its associated probability level. In this case, we see that only one variable, GRE@V, has a t value that reaches a significance level at or below .05 (i.e., .0015).

It is this variable, GRE@V, that is entered in the next step, as shown in Panel C. The predictor that is entered is always the one with the lowest p value of those not yet in the equation, assuming it meets the PIN criterion. Panel C is comparable to Panel A, showing information on the overall regression when GPA@G is regressed on both GPA@U and GRE@V. In panel A, the R^2 was .73022, and here R^2 is .85377. Thus, the inclusion of GRE@V added .12355 to R^2. This information is shown in the row labeled R Square Change, and below that is the F statistic that tests the significance of *adding* GRE@V to the regression equation (F Change). In this case, $F = 14.36270, p = .0015$. The analysis of variance summarizes the test of the overall regression with both predictors. The overall test ($F = 49.62708$) remains highly significant.

Panel D presents information on individual variables that are in or not in the equation. For the two variables in the equation, we learn from the coefficients in the column headed B that the regression equation now is:

$$GPA@G' = -1.780016 + .978217(GPA@U) + .003124(GRE@V)$$

Note that the information for GRE@V in this panel corresponds exactly to the information that was shown in panel B when GRE@V was not yet entered. For example, the beta weight of .403929 is identical, as is the value of t.

As was true for panel B, the bottom portion of panel D shows statistics for variables not yet in the equation as they would be if the variable were to enter in the next step. This time, however, we can see that neither of the two remaining variables, GRE@Q and MOTIV, has a regression coefficient that would be statistically significant at the .05 level. For MOTIV, the t value of 2.077 has a probability value of .0542, which just misses achieving statistical significance. Thus, as indicated at the bottom of this printout, the regression stops at this point because "PIN = .050 Limits reached."

In a stepwise regression, remaining predictors can be forced to enter the regression equation as a block. If we had done this, the regression coefficients and R^2 would be identical to that shown in the simultaneous regression analysis. However, we would also find that the R^2 change from .83656 to .89513 would not be statistically significant.

RESEARCH APPLICATIONS OF MULTIPLE REGRESSION

Multiple regression is a widely used statistical procedure in nursing research. It is used primarily to analyze nonexperimental data, but it can also be applied in experimental studies. This section describes the major research applications of multiple regression and discusses the presentation of multiple regression results in research reports.

The Uses of Multiple Regression

Nurse researchers use multiple regression extensively to address a variety of research questions regarding the relationships among variables. Multiple regression is also used for prediction and for other purposes as well.

1. Answering Research Questions. Multiple regression is a complex and versatile analytic technique. As we have seen in describing some of its features, multiple regression can help to answer a number of different types of questions. These questions include those listed in Box 10-1.

   As discussed earlier, the last question in Box 10-1 is difficult to answer unequivocally when the predictor variables are correlated. But multiple regression is also the basis for a sophisticated technique known as path analysis, which is an approach to **causal modeling.** Although correlations cannot in general be used to

10-1

RESEARCH QUESTIONS FOR MULTIPLE REGRESSION ANALYSIS

• How well does a particular group of independent variables explain or predict a dependent variable? (For example, how well do undergraduate grades, GRE scores, and achievement motivation explain graduate grades?)

• How much does any single independent variable add to the prediction of a dependent variable, over that accomplished by other independent variables? (For example, how much do motivation scores add to the prediction of graduate GPA over that which undergraduate GPA and GRE scores contribute?)

• What is the relationship between any given independent variable and the dependent variable, once the other predictor variables are taken into account? (For example, what is the relationship between undergraduate GPA and graduate GPA, once the relationship between graduate GPA and the other three predictors is controlled?)

• What is the relative importance of one predictor in explaining a dependent variable in comparison with other predictors? (For example, what is the relative importance of verbal versus quantitative GRE scores in predicting graduate GPA?)

establish causality, path analytic procedures can provide some evidence regarding the nature and direction of causal influence among variables. An overview of path analysis is presented in Chapter 14.

2. *Prediction.* Multiple regression provides an excellent vehicle for making predictions about a dependent variable when only information on the independent variables is available. Such predictions are typically undertaken for utilitarian purposes. As an example, Beckstrand and her colleagues (1990) used multiple regression analysis to predict insertion distance for orogastric and nasogastric feeding tubes on the basis of children's height and esophagal lengths.

3. *Missing Values Replacement.* As noted in earlier chapters, researchers are often confronted with the problem of missing data for some subjects on one or more variable. There are a number of different solutions to the missing values problem. For example, as discussed in Chapter 3, the missing value sometimes is replaced with

the mean value for the variable in question. One of the better approaches is to use multiple regression to predict what the missing value would have been, had it not been missing, and to substitute that predicted value for the missing data. Let us suppose that the first subject in Table 10–1 did not have a score on the motivation scale. We could predict this person's MOTIV score by regressing MOTIV on the other three variables, using data from the other 19 subjects. The regression equation in this example would be:

$$MOTIV' = 16.90 + 6.31(GPA@U) \quad .04(GRE@V) \quad .01(GRE@Q) + 19.35(GPA@G)$$

Using this equation to predict MOTIV for the first subject, we would obtain:

$$MOTIV' = 16.90 + 6.31(3.4) - .04(600) - .01(540) + 19.35(3.6)$$
$$MOTIV' = 78.6$$

The predicted value of the motivation score for the first subject is 78.6, which is reasonably close to the actual score of 75. Had we used mean substitution to replace the missing value, we would have used 68.9, which is considerably less accurate. Ideally, the variables used as predictors for the missing values equation should not be variables that would also be used in the substantive analyses (i.e., variables used in the analyses for which prediction of missing values is necessary). In our present example, we used GRE scores and grades to predict MOTIV purely to illustrate the process; other variables available in the data set would be preferable for predicting missing values.

Nurse researchers have used multiple regression for many purposes. Examples of some studies that involved multiple regression analysis are presented in Table 10–8.

TABLE 10–8. EXAMPLES OF STUDIES USING MULTIPLE REGRESSION

Research Question	Type of Regression
What are the factors that contribute to the prediction of stress experienced during treatment for childhood cancer? (Hockenberry-Eaton, Kemp, & Dilorio, 1994)	Stepwise
What are the effects of maternal employment, maternal employment attitude/behavior consistency, and mothers' satisfaction with the employment decision on family functioning and preterm infant development? (Youngblut, Loveland-Cherry, & Horan, 1994)	Hierarchical
Which demographic characteristics, social influences, environmental resources, and previous health care experiences predict the number of health services used by elders with heart disease? (Wallace, Lockhart, & Boyle, 1995)	Simultaneous
What is the effect of perceived control over pain on distress and disability among patients with chronic nonmalignant pain, after controlling for pain intensity? (Wells, 1994)	Hierarchical

TABLE 10–9 EXAMPLE OF A TABLE FOR SIMULTANEOUS REGRESSION

Predictor Variable	Graduate GPA		Comprehensive Exam	
	r	Beta	r	Beta
Undergraduate GPA	.85***	.53**	.39	.17
GRE-Verbal Scores	.73***	.48**	.57**	.12
GRE-Quantitative Scores	.46*	−.14	.77***	.65
Motivation Scores	.74***	.21	.11	−.19
R^2		.90		.62
Adjusted R^2		.87		.52
$F(4,15)$		32.01***		6.05**

$^*p < .05$ $^{**}p < .01$ $^{***}p < .001$

Multiple Regression of Graduate Grade Point Average and Scores on Comprehensive Examination on Four Predictors ($N = 20$)

The Presentation of Multiple Regression in Research Reports

Multiple regression analyses are typically so complex that they cannot adequately be summarized in the text of a report without tables. The exception is when the main focus of the analysis is to determine the value of R^2, information that can readily be reported in one or two sentences. However, this is rarely the only information sought in a multiple regression analysis, so tables are almost always needed.

Unfortunately, there is no standard format for the tabular presentation of regression results. This stems in part from the fact that regression is used to address many different questions, but it also is due to the absence of widely accepted guidelines.[16] In this section we discuss the elements that we believe should be included in regression tables, along with some options. The overall guiding principle in laying out a regression table is to be parsimonious while conveying critical pieces of information about the analysis.

Tables for Simultaneous Regression Results. Tables for presenting regression results are most straightforward when the regression analysis has used the simultaneous (standard) model of entering predictors. Table 10–9 presents a table summarizing the standard regression of the graduate GPA data (i.e., for the computer printout shown in Figure 10–6). Because researchers often use tables to present results for more than one regression analysis, we have added a second dependent variable (students' scores on their comprehensive examination) to illustrate how this can be accomplished.

At a bare minimum, a table for standard regression should include the following: the sample size, the names of the dependent variables, the names of all predictor vari-

[16]Suggestions have been offered by Knapp (1994), but relatively few published tables conform to these suggestions.

ables, the regression coefficients for the predictors, the value of R^2, the significance of the overall regression, and the significance of individual predictors. Table 10–9 has all of these elements, as well as some additional information.

The sample size is sometimes specified in the title of the table, as it is in this example, or sometimes in a footnote to the table. The names of the dependent variables should appear in the title, as well as in headings that indicate which analysis is being described, if there is more than one analysis. (These headings could also indicate the Ns if they differed from one analysis to another.)

Predictor variables are typically reported in the left column of the table, in sufficient detail that a person can understand the nature of the variable without having to refer to the text. In standard regression, the order of the variables in the list is not important. The vast majority of researchers present standardized regression coefficients (βs) rather than b weights with each predictor, as we have done in this example in the Beta column. If an aim of the report is to communicate a regression equation for prediction purposes, however, unstandardized b weights (and the intercept constant) should be used instead of, or in addition to, beta weights.

The value of R^2 for each analysis must be reported and, unless the sample size is large, it is also wise to report the adjusted R^2, as in this example. Although some researchers report the value of R in addition to R^2, it is unnecessary to do so because it is easy to compute R from R^2.

The results of statistical tests can be presented in various ways. In this example, we did not present the actual values of the t statistics associated with each regression coefficient (e.g., 4.028 for undergraduate GPA as a predictor of graduate GPA). It would have been possible to do so by adding a third column for each dependent variable, to the right of the column labeled Beta. However, the value of the t statistic in itself is not normally of great interest, and so it was omitted to conserve space. The level of significance could also be presented in a separate column labeled either Sig or p, and this column could present *actual* probabilities (e.g., .0011 for undergraduate GPA). However, in most cases it is adequate to use asterisks to indicate the level of significance of individual predictors.

Most regression tables show the value of F for the overall regression, as we do in Table 10–9. Here again, asterisks are used to indicate level of significance, but the actual probability could have been presented in a separate row. The table also shows the degrees of freedom for the F test in parentheses (4,15).

There are some optional elements that can be included in a regression table for simultaneous regression. One is the value of the bivariate correlation coefficients between the dependent variable and each predictor, which we have included in Table 10–9 under the column labeled r. This is extremely useful information, but is unnecessary if a full correlation matrix is presented in a separate table. Another option is to include a column for squared semipartial correlations, showing the unique proportion of variance associated with each predictor.

Tables for Hierarchical Regression. All of the basic elements for a simultaneous regression table should also be included in a hierarchical regression table—i.e., sample size, names of dependent and predictor variables, regression coefficients, the value of R^2, and the results of significance tests. In addition, information on the changes to R^2 at each step of the analysis and the significance of the changes should be presented.

Table 10–10 presents the results of three hierarchical regression analyses for a large sample of teenage mothers, in which Depression Scale scores, Parenting Stress Scale scores, and a measure of alcohol abuse are regressed on three blocks of predictors. Block 1 consists of variables on the young mother's household composition—whether her mother (the maternal grandmother) is living in the household, whether her partner is living in the household, and number of her own children. Block 2 involves variables on the young mother's economic situation—whether she is receiving welfare, whether she is employed, and whether she has received a high school diploma. The third block involves psychosocial variables—scores on the Difficult Life Circumstances Scale (items include whether someone close to the teen is in jail and whether she has been mugged or assaulted in the past year), scores on a self-esteem scale, and scores on a social support scale. These predictors are shown in the left column, grouped in blocks in the order of entry into the regression.

The standardized regression coefficients (beta weights) for each independent variable are shown under the columns labeled Beta, for each dependent variable. Asterisks adjacent to the beta weights indicate whether the t-tests for the predictors are statistically significant. For the Depression Scale outcome variable, for example, all three of

TABLE 10–10. EXAMPLE OF A TABLE FOR HIERARCHICAL REGRESSION

Step Predictor	Depression Beta[a]	Depression R^2 Change	Parenting Stress Beta[a]	Parenting Stress R^2 Change	Alcohol Abuse Beta[a]	Alcohol Abuse R^2 Change
1 *Household Composition*		.01**		.01***		.02***
Mother present	−.03		−.01		−.08***	
Partner present	−.03		−.07**		−.09***	
No. of children	.00		.07*		−.09***	
2 *Economic Variables*		.02**		.01**		.00
Receiving welfare	.00		.07**		.00	
Employed	−.03		.01		.00	
Has HS diploma	−.11***		−.04*		.06**	
3 *Psychosocial Variables*		.24***		.07*		.04***
Diff. Life Circs.	.39***		.18***		.19***	
Self-Esteem scale	−.24***		−.18***		.02	
Social Support scale	−.07***		.04		−.02	
Cumulative R^2	.27***		.09***		.06***	

[a]Betas shown are for the last step.
*$p < .05$ **$p < .01$ ***$p < .001$

Hierarchical Multiple Regression of Depression, Parenting Stress, and Alcohol Abuse in Low-Income Teenage Mothers (N = 1892)

the psychosocial predictor variables, plus the young mother's educational attainment, are statistically significant. For each dependent variable there is also a column labeled R^2 Change[17] that shows the increment to R^2 as each of the three blocks is stepped into the equation. The asterisks next to this value indicate whether the F test for the increment to R^2 is statistically significant. In this example, even though the increments to R^2 are often quite small, each change is statistically significant; this is because there are nearly 2000 cases in the sample ($N = 1892$). The final row of the table shows the cumulative R^2—the amount of variance explained when all predictors are in the equation—which equals all of the R^2 changes added together. Asterisks are used again here to indicate the level of significance for the overall equation. In this example, the cumulative R^2s range from .06 (alcohol abuse) to .27 (depression), and all are statistically significant. Note that adjusted R^2s are not included in this table; because of the large sample size, original and adjusted R^2 values are virtually identical.

One of the dilemmas in creating tables for hierarchical regression is how to present the regression coefficients. The betas change at each step, and yet the format shown in Table 10–10 presents only one beta for each predictor. A footnote to the table indicates that the betas are for the final step, when all predictors are in the equation.[18]

If it is theoretically important to show how the betas change as successive blocks of predictors are stepped into the equation—or if the addition of blocks dramatically changes the betas and these changes are of interest—all beta values should be shown in the table. Usually, however, changes to betas can only be presented for one or two dependent variables in one table, especially if there are more than three blocks of predictors. An example of this type of table, for the regression of the Depression Scale and Parenting Stress Scale scores only, is shown in Table 10–11. There are three sets of beta weights for the variables entered in step 1, two sets for the variables entered in step 2, and one set for those entered in the final step. The R^2 changes and cumulative R^2 values are shown in the bottom two rows of the table, corresponding to the values of these statistics at each of the three steps. In this example, the beta changes for predictors entered in the equation early tend to be relatively small (e.g., for the presence of the mother in the household, the betas are $-.01$, $-.01$, and $-.03$ at steps 1 through 3, respectively), and so in this example the expanded format is not especially informative. Variants of the format used in Table 10–10 are far more common in research journals than the format used in Table 10–11.

These tables illustrate how dummy-coded predictor variables can be handled in tables. When effect coding or orthogonal coding is used, the coding *must* be explicitly specified, either as part of the label for the predictor or in a footnote. However, this is not necessary for dummy variables. Five of the variables in Tables 10–10 and 10–11 are

---

[17]To economize on space, some researchers label this column $R^2 \Delta$ (delta); Δ is the standard scientific symbol for change.

[18]An alternative would have been to use the heading Beta for Last Step. Regrettably, most tables for hierarchical regression in research reports neglect to specify whether the betas shown are the values when the predictor first enters the equation or at the final step.

TABLE 10–11. EXAMPLE OF A TABLE FOR HIERARCHICAL REGRESSION WITH BETAS SHOWN AT EACH STEP

Step Predictor	Depression			Parenting Stress		
	Step 1	Step 2 Beta Weights	Step 3	Step 1	Step 2 Beta Weights	Step 3
1 *Household Composition*						
Mother present	−.01	−.01	−.03	−.01	−.01	−.01
Partner present	−.04	−.03	−.03	−.09***	−.07**	−.07**
No. of children	.04	.02	.00	.09***	.08***	.07*
2 *Economic Variables*						
Receiving welfare		.01	.00		.08**	.07**
Employed		−.04	−.03		.00	.01
Has HS diploma		−.14***	−.11***		−.06**	−.04*
3 *Psychosocial Variables*						
Diff. Life Circs.			.39***			.18***
Self-Esteem scale			−.24***			−.18***
Social Support scale			−.07***			.04
R^2 Change	.01**	.02*	.24***	.01***	.01**	.07*
Cumulative R^2	.01**	.03***	.27***	.01***	.02***	.09***

*$p < .05$ **$p < .01$ ***$p < .001$

Hierarchical Multiple Regression of Depression and Parenting Stress in Low-Income Teenage Mothers ($N = 1892$)

dummy coded: mother present, partner present, receiving welfare, employed, and has high school diploma. The labels for these variables indicate the condition that is coded 1. For example, the variable labeled Employed is, by convention, understood to represent the employed condition, which is coded 1, while the unemployed condition is coded 0. Of course, the coding scheme *can* be explicitly indicated. For example, the employment variable could have had the following label: Employment status (1 = employed, 0 = not employed).

Tables for Stepwise Regression. The basic information for stepwise regression is similar to that for simultaneous regression. In stepwise regression, however, the listing of the independent variables is critical, because the list indicates the order of entry of predictors. Since stepwise regression normally ends when predictors cease to be statistically significant, it is often unnecessary to show the amount of change and significance of R^2 changes. Thus, the headings for each dependent variable in the table might simply be Beta and Cum R^2. (The reader can compute the R^2 change at each step simply by subtracting the value of R^2 in one row from the value of R^2 in the preceding row.) If it is not too cumbersome to do so, the names of the predictors that did *not* get stepped into the equation at statistically significant levels should be specified in a footnote.

Narrative Presentation of Regression Results. The features of a regression table that a researcher chooses to highlight in the text depend to a great extent on the nature of the research questions posed. We present one example of the narrative that might be used to describe Table 10–10, and urge you to consult journal articles (e.g., for studies listed in Table 10–8) for other examples.

As shown in Table 10–10, the predictor variables as a group did a modest job of explaining variation in the three dependent variables. The overall R^2 for alcohol abuse was especially low ($R^2 = .06$) and was only slightly better for the Parenting Stress Scale ($R^2 = .09$). The regression was substantially more successful in explaining Depression Scale scores ($R^2 = .27$). In all three cases, the overall regression was statistically significant beyond the .001 level.

Despite differing degrees of success in predicting the dependent variables, there were several common features across the regression analyses. First, the variables in the household composition block, entered in the first step, accounted for only a very small (albeit significant) proportion of the explained variance in all three analyses. None of the three household variables were, taken individually, significantly related to Depression Scale scores, once other factors were taken into consideration. However, the presence of a husband or boyfriend in the teen mothers' household was associated with significantly less parenting stress and lower abuse of alcohol. The mothers' presence in the household also had a beneficial effect on alcohol abuse. The larger the number of children in the household, the higher was the amount of parenting stress, but the lower was the amount of alcohol abuse.

The block of economic variables also made only a modest contribution to explained variance for all three outcome variables, with R^2 increments ranging from .00 to .02. Interestingly, the young mothers' employment status was unrelated to depression, parenting stress, and alcohol abuse. Welfare receipt was associated with increased parenting stress but was unrelated to depression and alcohol abuse, once other independent variables were controlled. The educational attainment variable was significantly related to all three dependent variables; women who had a high school diploma were less depressed and reported less parenting stress, but were *more* likely to abuse alcohol.

The inclusion of the three psychosocial variables greatly improved the explanatory power of all three regressions. The increments to R^2 ranged from .04 for alcohol abuse to .25 for Depression Scale scores; all increments were statistically significant. The single most powerful predictor appears to be scores on the Difficult Life Circumstances Scale, a measure of ongoing, daily stress. Young women with a lot of daily stress were significantly more likely to be depressed, to feel stressed as parents, and to abuse alcohol. High self-esteem was associated with a lower risk of depression and parenting stress, but was unrelated to alcohol abuse. Women with greater amounts of social support tended to be less depressed, but social support was not related to parenting stress or alcohol abuse.

RESEARCH EXAMPLE

Examples of multiple regression analyses abound in the nursing and health care literature. The study described below is a good example of a practical application of multiple regression.

Hays (1995) conducted a study to determine the amount of variance in nursing resource consumption among public health nursing clients that could be explained by an instrument called the Community Health Intensity Rating Scale (CHIRS). The CHIRS is an instrument that uses client need as the basis for classifying community health nursing clients. Hays noted that prediction of resource consumption is an essential element in controlling health care costs, and that such pre-

TABLE 10–12. VARIANCE IN NURSING EFFORT EXPLAINED BY CHIRS TOTAL SCORE AFTER CONTROLLING FOR LENGTH OF STAY

Variables, by Program	n	Cum R^2	R^2 Change	Beta	t	p	Bivariate r
Frail Older Adult	47						
Length of Stay		.486	.486	.702	6.452	<.001	.697
CHIRS Total Score		.487[a]	.001	.038	.350	.728	−.055
High-Risk Prenatal	44						
Length of Stay		.075	.075	.236	1.713	.094	.273
CHIRS Total Score		.227[b]	.152	.392	2.838	.007	.414
High-Risk Infant	42						
Length of Stay		.513	.513	.662	7.125	<.001	.716
CHIRS Total Score		.670[c]	.157	.399	4.296	<.001	.489

[a]Adj. R^2 = .464;   [b]Adj. R^2 = .189;   [c]Adj. R^2 = .653
Adapted from Table 2 of Hays' (1995) report.

dictions could also be used for planning and implementing quality improvement efforts.

Hays' analysis focused on the intensity of need of three client groups served by a city-county health department: frail older adults, high-risk prenatal clients, and high-risk infants. The clients' intensity rating (client need at the beginning of service) was determined by application of CHIRS to the clinical records of 133 discharged clients.

Multiple regression analysis was used to predict two measures of resource consumption: number of public health nursing visits and nursing effort. The nursing effort variable was a composite measure of various indicators of resource consumption (e.g., number of nursing attempted visits, number of telephone calls, etc.). Hierarchical multiple regression was used to predict these two outcomes on the basis of CHIRS scores, after first controlling for length of stay. Length of stay (number of days between admission for care and discharge from the caseload) was entered on the first step of the analysis to control the confounding effect of the amount of time the client was available to receive services.

After controlling length of stay, the CHIRS total score was found to contribute significantly to the prediction of the number of public health nursing visits for only one of the three client groups, the high-risk infants (R^2 change = .073, p = .013). However, as shown in Table 10–12, the CHIRS total score made a significant contribution to explaining variance in the composite nursing effort measure for two groups: high-risk prenatal clients (R^2 change = .152, p = .007) and high-risk infants (R^2 change = .157, i.e., p < .001). Resource consumption for frail older adults could not be reliably predicted on the basis of the CHIRS scores. Hays concluded that ". . . the cost implications of this finding reside in the use of CHIRS as a basis for distinguishing which high-risk prenatal clients and infants require the most public health nursing resources" (p. 109).

SUMMARY

Multiple regression is a statistical procedure for understanding and predicting a dependent variable on the basis of two or more independent variables. The basic multiple regression equation for predicting Y (Y') involves an intercept constant, plus the values of the predictor variables weighted by corresponding regression coefficients (**b weights**). When the equation is specified in standardized form, the regression coefficients are called **beta weights** (β).

The **multiple correlation coefficient (R)** represents the magnitude (but not direction) of the relationship between the dependent variable and the predictor variables, taken together. The square of R (R^2) indicates the proportion of variance in Y accounted for by the predictors. R^2 is often presented after an adjustment for sample size is made, and the new value is referred to as **adjusted R^2** or **shrunken R^2.**

Multiple regression offers the potential for **statistical control;** the regression coefficients indicate the number of units Y' is expected to change for each unit change in a given predictor, when the effects of the other predictors are held constant. Control is achieved through partialling out overlapping variability in the predictors. The **partial correlation** between X_1 and Y ($r_{y1.2}$) is the degree to which X_1 and Y are correlated after the influence of a third variable, X_2, is removed. **Semipartial correlation** ($r_{y(1.2)}$) is the correlation between all of Y and X_1, from which X_2 has been partialled out. Squared semipartial correlation coefficients are sometimes used to compare the relative contribution that predictors uniquely make to the prediction of Y.

An F ratio statistic that contrasts the sum of squares due to regression against the sum of squares due to residuals is used to test the overall significance of the regression. An F statistic can also be used to test the significance of variables added to the regression equation—i.e., the significance of the increment to R^2. The significance of individual regression coefficients is determined through t statistics.

Predictor variables are entered into the regression equation either through a **simultaneous regression model** (all predictors entered at the same time), through a **hierarchical regression model** (variables entered in a sequence determined by the researcher), or through a **stepwise regression model** (variables entered in the order that contributes most to the increment of R^2). The main difference between these methods concerns what happens to overlapping variability among intercorrelated independent variables.

In multiple regression, the dependent variable should be a continuous variable measured on an interval or ratio scale. The independent variables can be continuous, but they can also be coded nominal-level variables. Alternative coding schemes for nominal-level variables include **dummy coding, effect coding,** and **orthogonal coding.** Interaction terms can also be included in the analysis, and thus data that are amenable to ANOVA can also be analyzed through multiple regression.

Researchers using multiple regression need to attend to potential problems, such as **multicollinearity**—the inclusion of independent variables that are too highly correlated. Multicollinearity can be detected by examining the **tolerance** of predictors. Researchers should also check to determine that the assumptions for multiple regression have not been violated, and this is usually done through inspection of **residual scatterplots.** In interpreting regression results, researchers should also be alert to the possibility of **suppression,** a phenomenon that makes a predictor with little or no correlation with the dependent variable look important, because the predictor suppresses irrelevant variability in other predictors. Finally, care should be taken to ensure an adequate number of cases for multiple regression, preferably through a power analysis.

EXERCISES

The following exercises cover concepts presented in this chapter. Exercises indicated with a dagger (†) can be checked against answers appearing in Appendix A. Additionally, Chapter 10 of the accompanying *Applications Manual* offers supplementary exercises, including ones that require computer analysis of a data set on diskette.

† 1. Using the regression equation for predicting graduate GPA presented in this chapter, find the predicted value of Y for the last three cases in Table 10–1 (subjects 18 through 20).

† 2. Using the following information for R^2, k, and N, calculate the value of the F statistic for testing the overall regression equation and determine whether F is statistically significant at the .05 level:
   a. $R^2 = .53, k = 5, N = 120$
   b. $R^2 = .53, k = 5, N = 30$
   c. $R^2 = .28, k = 4, N = 64$
   d. $R^2 = .14, k = 4, N = 64$

† 3. Which, if any, of the tests described in Exercise 3 would be statistically significant with $\alpha = .001$?

† 4. Below is a correlation matrix:

	VARA	VARB	VARC	DEPVAR
VARA	1.00			
VARB	.62	1.00		
VARC	.77	.68	1.00	
DEPVAR	.54	.36	.48	1.00

   a. If DEPVAR were regressed on VARA, VARB, and VARC, what is the *lowest* possible value of R^2?
   b. In a stepwise regression, what would the first predictor variable into the equation be?
   c. In a stepwise regression, what would the second predictor variable into the equation be?

5. How does a semipartial correlation coefficient differ from a partial correlation coefficient? If $r_{y1.2} = .31$, would the value of $r_{y(1.2)}$ likely be smaller or larger?

† 6. Suppose that, using dummy codes, smokers were coded 1 and nonsmokers were coded 0 on SMOKSTAT, and that males were coded 1 and females were coded 0 on GENDER. What would the four codes for the interaction term be?

† 7. Using the following information for R^2, k, and N, calculate the *adjusted* R^2:

      a. $R^2 = .53, k = 5, N = 120$
      b. $R^2 = .28, k = 4, N = 64$
      c. $R^2 = .28, k = 10, N = 64$
      b. $R^2 = .28, k = 4, N = 564$

† 8. Suppose that $R^2_{y123} = .41$ and $R^2_{y12} = .38$ and that there are 50 subjects in the sample.

      a. What is the increment to R^2 of adding a new predictor to the equation?
      b. What is another name for the increment? How would this be symbolized?
      c. What is the value of the F statistic for testing the increment to R^2? Is the increment statistically significant at the .05 level?

† 9. Use dummy coding to create new variables (use 8-character variable names) for the following nominal-level variables:

      a. Employment status: 1 = employed full time; 2 = employed part time; 3 = not employed
      b. Menopausal status: 1 = premenopausal; 2 = perimenopausal; 3 = menopausal; 4 = postmenopausal
      c. Hospitalization: 1 = hospitalized past 12 months; 2 = not hospitalized past 12 months

10. Compare the beta weights for GPA@U and GRE@V in panel D of Figure 10–7 with the beta weights for the same two variables in panel C of Figure 10–6. How does the relative importance of the two variables differ from one analysis to the other? Why does this difference occur? What does this say about the interpretation of beta weights?

† 11. Using power analysis, determine the sample size needed to achieve power = .80 for $\alpha = .05$:

      a. estimated $R^2 = .15, k = 5$
      b. estimated $R^2 = .04, k = 2$
      c. estimated $R^2 = .21, k = 8$
      d. estimated $R^2 = .33, k = 6$

12. Write a narrative description of the regression results presented in Table 10–9.

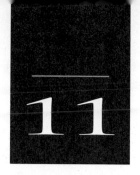

Analysis of Covariance, Multivariate ANOVA, and Canonical Analysis

This chapter focuses primarily on multivariate extensions of analysis of variance. As we have seen in the previous chapter, there is a close link between ANOVA and multiple regression. That link will become more apparent as we discuss ANOVA's extensions.

ANALYSIS OF COVARIANCE

A statistical procedure known as **analysis of covariance (ANCOVA)** is used to make comparisons between two or more groups, after statistically removing the effect of one or more extraneous variables on the dependent variable. The central question for AN-COVA is the same as for ANOVA: Are mean differences between groups "real," or are observed mean differences in a sample likely to have occurred by chance?

Basic Concepts for ANCOVA

Conceptually, it is useful to think of ANCOVA as a combination of multiple regression and ANOVA. In the first (regression) stage of the analysis, the effects of extraneous variables (referred to as **covariates** in the context of ANCOVA) are removed from further consideration. This first stage is analogous to the first step of a hierarchical regression analysis. In the next stage, variability in the dependent variable *that remains to be explained* is analyzed in an ANOVA-type format. That is, the group means are compared after they have been statistically adjusted for the effect of the covariates. Because extraneous (error) variance is reduced, ANCOVA permits a more sensitive test of group differences than is achieved with ANOVA.

Figure 11–1, which shows a visual representation of the ANCOVA procedure, is quite similar to the depiction of hierarchical regression in Figure 10–3. The shaded area

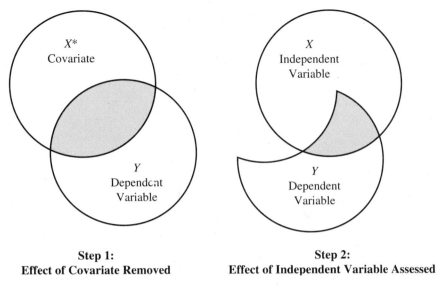

Step 1:
Effect of Covariate Removed

Step 2:
Effect of Independent Variable Assessed

FIGURE 11–1.   VENN DIAGRAM DEPICTING ANALYSIS OF COVARIANCE

of the circle in step 1 shows the extent to which the dependent variable Y is correlated with the covariate X^*. The dependent variable is regressed on X^*, and the portion of Y's variability that is accounted for by X^* is removed from further consideration. Then, in step 2, the analysis focuses on the ability of the independent variable X to explain any *remaining* variability in Y. The independent variable in ANCOVA is always a nominal-level variable, such as experimental versus control, male versus female, and so on.

An example might help to clarify the ANCOVA process. Suppose we were interested in testing the effectiveness of an intervention to improve motor function in nursing home residents. The dependent variable (Y) is a measure of motor performance administered after the intervention, and the independent variable (X) is group status (i.e., membership in the experimental group that received the intervention versus in a control group that did not). The covariate (X^*) is the motor performance score prior to the intervention. Preintervention motor performance scores would presumably be highly correlated with postintervention scores; regardless of the intervention, some people would have better motor performance than others. In this example, we have controlled individual differences in motor function by using preintervention motor performance scores as the covariate. Thus, the analysis would examine the effect of the intervention on what remains of the variability in postintervention motor performance scores after individual differences in motor function are statistically controlled.

Partitioning Variance in ANCOVA

As with ANOVA and multiple regression, ANCOVA involves the partitioning of variance into different components. It may be recalled from Chapter 7 on ANOVA that the total sum of squares for the dependent variable (SS_T) can be partitioned into variance attributable to the independent variable (sum of squares between groups or SS_B) and to variance associated with other factors such as individual differences (sum of squares within or SS_W). The F ratio involves contrasting these two sources of variation.

In ANCOVA, the F ratio contrasts sums of squares that have been adjusted for the covariate's relationship with the dependent variable. That is, the adjusted sum of squares between (SS'_B) is contrasted to the adjusted sum of squares within (SS'_W). The adjustments involve subtracting terms relating to the correlation of the covariate and the dependent variables from the unadjusted SS_B and SS_W.

A concrete example should help to clarify the process. Suppose that we randomly assigned 30 people with lower back pain to three treatment groups: a bedrest group, an exercise group, and a control group. Pain is measured both before the treatment (the covariate) and after the treatment (the dependent variable) on a visual analog scale that can range from 0 to 100. Some hypothetical data for this example are shown in Table 11–1. As the means at the bottom of this table show, the pretest pain scores (the $\overline{X}$*s) for the bedrest, exercise, and control groups were 67.5, 69.5, and 62.5, respectively. An analysis of variance comparing these three pretest means indicates that the groups were not significantly different at the outset of the study ($F = 0.35, p = .71$); the initial group dif-

TABLE 11–1. FICTITIOUS DATA FOR ANCOVA EXAMPLE

Bedrest Group (A)		Exercise Group (B)		Control Group (C)	
Pretest Pain X^*_A	Posttest Pain Y_A	Pretest Pain X^*_B	Posttest Pain Y_B	Pretest Pain X^*_C	Posttest Pain Y_C
95	85	75	60	35	30
80	70	80	45	50	40
60	50	50	30	45	45
45	30	85	70	30	20
55	45	70	55	85	85
50	40	85	65	60	50
75	65	60	35	90	85
80	70	65	40	90	75
40	35	80	60	80	65
95	85	45	10	60	60
$\overline{X}^*_A = 67.5$	$\overline{Y}_A = 57.5$	$\overline{X}^*_B = 69.5$	$\overline{Y}_B = 47.0$	$\overline{X}^*_C = 62.5$	$\overline{Y}_C = 55.5$

ferences likely reflect chance sampling fluctuations. The posttest means (the $\bar{Y}$s) show greater variability, ranging from a low of 47.0 for the exercise group to a high of 57.5 for the bedrest group. The research question is whether the three groups differ significantly in terms of posttest pain scores.

Table 11–2 summarizes, in the top panel, the results of the simple ANOVA for posttest pain scores. The table indicates how total variance was partitioned for the ANOVA:

$$SS_T = SS_B + SS_W$$
$$11,916.67 = 621.67 + 11,295.00$$

As the table indicates, the ANOVA yielded a nonsignificant F statistic ($F = 0.74$, $p = .49$). On the basis of ANOVA, we would conclude that neither a bedrest nor an exercise treatment had an effect on lower back pain.

Panel B of Table 11–2 demonstrates that ANCOVA can dramatically alter the conclusions. We see that in the first step of the analysis, which involves the regression of the dependent variable on the covariate, variation in pretest pain scores accounts for a considerable portion of the total variance in posttest pain scores. We can use the information in the table to determine that about 81% of the variance in posttest scores is accounted for by the covariate. The r^2 between pretest and posttest pain is determined by dividing the total sum of squares by the sum of squares attributable to the covariate:

$$r^2_{yx*} = \frac{9,703.17}{11,916.67} = .81$$

This strong relationship merely indicates that people who started out in especially severe pain tended to end up with high levels of pain, regardless of which group they were in, while people with less pain initially also tended to have less pain later. The F

TABLE 11–2. COMPARISON OF ANOVA AND ANCOVA RESULTS

Source of Variation	Sum of Squares	df	Mean Square	F	p
A. *ANOVA*					
Between Groups	621.67	2	310.83	0.74	.49
Within Groups	11,295.00	27	418.33		
Total	11,916.67	29			
B. *ANCOVA*					
Step 1 Covariate	9,703.17	1	9,703.17	290.02	.000
Step 2 Between Groups	1,343.61	2	671.80	20.08	.000
Within Groups	869.89	26	33.46		
Total	11,916.67	29			

test for the covariate, which contrasts the sum of squares for the covariate against the adjusted sum of squares within, after dividing by the appropriate degrees of freedom, is a highly significant 290.02 ($p < .0005$).

The second step of the ANCOVA involves partitioning what remains in Y's variability after the covariate is accounted for; the residual sum of squares is:

$$SS_T - SS_{covar} = SS_{residual}$$
$$11,916.67 - 9,703.17 = 2,213.50$$

The residual sum of squares, in turn, can be partitioned into two components: the adjusted sum of squares between and the adjusted sum of squares within—which are SS'_B and SS'_W:

$$SS_{residual} = SS'_B + SS'_W$$
$$2,213.50 = 1,343.61 + 869.89$$

Total variability in posttest pain scores can now be partitioned as follows:

$$SS_T = SS_{covar} + SS'_B + SS'_W$$
$$11,916.67 = 9,703.17 + 1,343.61 + 869.89$$

The critical F ratio for testing group differences contrasts the adjusted sum of squares between (which is *larger* than the original SS_B) against the adjusted sum of squares within (which is *smaller* than the original SS_W), after dividing by the appropriate degrees of freedom:

$$F = \frac{1,343.61 / 2}{869.89 / 26} = \frac{671.80}{33.46} = 20.08$$

As Table 11-2 shows, the resulting F ratio of 20.08 is highly significant. The conclusion now is that, after controlling for initial pain levels, there is a statistically significant difference in posttest pain levels resulting from exposure to different treatments.

This example was deliberately contrived to have the ANCOVA results differ from the ANOVA results, and in most actual studies the effects of ANCOVA are less dramatic. Nevertheless, it is true that if you can select important covariates, then ANCOVA will result in a more sensitive test than ordinary ANOVA. The increased sensitivity results from the fact that the error term, against which treatment effects are compared, is usually smaller in ANCOVA. In our example, the error term in panel A of Table 11–2 is extremely large, thereby masking the effect of the treatment variable.

Adjusted Means

The posttest pain scores for the three groups in our example reflect not only the effects of the different conditions, but also individual differences in pretreatment pain levels. It is possible, and often desirable when reporting the results of ANCOVA, to adjust the group means, through a process that is sometimes referred to as **multiple classification analysis.** Adjusted means allow researchers to observe **net effects**—i.e., group differences on the dependent variable *net* of the effect of the covariate.

With one covariate, the formula for adjusting the mean—here, for group A—is:

$$\bar{Y}_{A(adj)} = \bar{Y}_A - b(\bar{X}^*_A - \bar{X}^*)$$

where $\bar{Y}_{A(adj)}$ = adjusted mean on the dependent variable for Group A
$\bar{Y}_A$ = unadjusted mean on the dependent variable for Group A
b = regression coefficient for the covariate
$\bar{X}^*_A$ = mean of the covariate for Group A
$\bar{X}^*$ = grand mean of the covariate for all groups

From this formula, it can be seen that when all the treatment groups have identical means on the covariate (here, when $\bar{X}^*_A = \bar{X}^*$), the unadjusted and adjusted means for the dependent variable are identical. The larger the group differences on the covariate, the larger the adjustments will be.

In our example, the grand mean for X^* is 66.5, and b is 1.02 (calculations not shown). Thus, we can compute the three adjusted means by using the above formula and replacing values for group A with those for groups B and C, as appropriate:

$$\bar{Y}_{A(adj)} = 57.5 - 1.02(67.5 - 66.5) = 56.48$$
$$\bar{Y}_{B(adj)} = 47.0 - 1.02(69.5 - 66.5) = 43.94$$
$$\bar{Y}_{C(adj)} = 55.5 - 1.02(62.5 - 66.5) = 59.58$$

ANCOVA tests the null hypothesis that the adjusted means for the groups being compared are equal. In this example, an inspection of the adjusted means clarifies why the ANCOVA resulted in statistically significant group differences, while the ANOVA did not. The ANOVA compared the posttest means for the three groups, and these scores ranged from 47.0 to 57.5, a spread of 10.5 points. However, the range for the adjusted means is from 43.94 to 59.58, a spread of 15.64 points. In essence, the ANCOVA takes into consideration how much the groups *changed* from pretest to posttest. We can see from Table 11–1 that the mean pretest-posttest *changes* in pain scores ranged from a low of 7.0 points for the control group, to a high of 22.5 points for the exercise group.

Multiple Comparisons among Adjusted Means

When ANCOVA results in a significant F test, as in the example we have been using, the researcher is in a position to reject the null hypothesis that the adjusted group means are equal. However, as in ANOVA, further analysis is needed to determine which pairs of adjusted group means are significantly different from one another.

The following formula can be used to compute an F statistic for comparing adjusted group means, illustrated here for groups A and B:

$$F = \frac{(\bar{Y}_{A(adj)} - \bar{Y}_{B(adj)})^2}{MS_W \left[\dfrac{1}{n_A} + \dfrac{1}{n_B}\right]\left[1 + \dfrac{SS_{between(X*)}}{df_B (SS_{within\ (X*)})}\right]}$$

where $\bar{Y}_{A(adj)}$ = adjusted mean of dependent variable for Group A
$\bar{Y}_{B(adj)}$ = adjusted mean of dependent variable for Group B
MS'_W = adjusted mean square within from ANCOVA
n_A = number of subjects in Group A
n_B = number of subjects in Group B
$SS_{between(X*)}$ = sum of squares between in an ANOVA with $X*$ as the dependent variable and X as the independent variable
df_B = degrees of freedom between groups
$SS_{within(X*)}$ = sum of squares within in an ANOVA with $X*$ as the dependent variable and X as the independent variable

As this formula indicates, to calculate the F for the pairwise comparisons, we must first perform an ANOVA in which the covariate (in our example, the pretest pain scores) is the dependent variable and group is the independent variable. For the example we have been using in this chapter, the sum of squares between for this ANOVA ($SS_{between(X*)}$) equals 260.0 and the sum of squares within ($SS_{within(X*)}$) is 10097.5 (calculations not shown). Thus, the F statistic for comparing the adjusted group means for groups A and B is:

$$F = \frac{(56.48 - 43.94)^2}{33.46 \left[\dfrac{1}{10} + \dfrac{1}{10}\right]\left[1 + \dfrac{260.0}{2(10097.5)}\right]} = 23.20$$

For this F test, the degrees of freedom are 1 and $N - df_B - 2$. In our example, then, the df are 1 and 26; the F value of 23.20 is highly significant ($p < .001$), indicating that the adjusted posttest pain scores for groups A and B are significantly different. Similar calculations comparing other pairs of adjusted group means results in an F of 1.42 for the group A/group C comparison (not significant) and an F of 36.09 for the group B/group C comparison ($p < .001$). Thus, the multiple comparison of adjusted group means indicates that the exercise treatment resulted in significantly lower pain scores, after removing the effect of pretreatment pain, than the bedrest and the control conditions, and that the latter two conditions were not significantly different from each other.

Selection of Covariates

Covariates can be either continuous interval-or ratio-level variables, but they can also be dummy-coded nominal variables. In our example, the covariate was measured on an interval scale, but we could have used, say, gender as the covariate.

Although we have used examples with a single covariate, ANCOVA can be used to make adjustments for multiple covariates simultaneously.[1] However, it is not usually wise to use more than five or six covariates, and with small samples even fewer are recommended. When a lot of covariates are used in the analysis, it is inevitable that they will be intercorrelated, and this in turn could introduce problems of multicollinearity. Moreover, if the covariates are intercorrelated, they are redundant in terms of reducing error variance, and they actually *lower* the power of the analysis. This is because degrees of freedom are subtracted from the denominator of the error term, while error variance is not subtracted from the numerator.

A pretest measure of the dependent variable is almost always a very powerful covariate. Important demographic characteristics—e.g., age, gender, marital status, race/ethnicity, socioeconomic status, and educational attainment—are typically correlated with a broad array of human attributes and may therefore be attractive as covariates. The stronger the correlation between a covariate and the dependent variable, the better is the covariate. It is usually prudent to consult the research literature for factors that have been found to influence the dependent variable, and to use these as covariates. Ideally, such a literature search would have occurred prior to initiating the research so that measures of the most relevant characteristics could be included in the design of the study.

In selecting covariates, care should be taken to choose ones that can be measured reliably. Measurement errors can lead to either overadjustments or underadjustments of the mean, and can contribute to either Type I or Type II errors. For physiological and demographic variables (age, gender, ethnicity), measurement error is not typically a problem, but the same cannot be said for psychosocial variables. Tabachnick and Fidell (1989) recommend limiting covariates to those whose reliability is .80 or greater.

Applications of ANCOVA

ANCOVA is an extremely powerful and effective procedure that is used in several different contexts. Its general purposes are to maximize the equivalence of groups prior to assessing the effect of the independent variable of interest on the dependent variable, and to reduce error variance. ANCOVA can be used with a single independent variable,

---

[1] When more than one covariate is used, all covariates enter the first step simultaneously and are treated as a set, as in simultaneous regression. Within that set, the significance of each covariate is assessed as if it were the last to enter the equation. Thus, an individual covariate is significant in the ANCOVA only if its unique contribution to explaining variance in the dependent variable is significant.

as in the examples we have been using, and can also be used in multifactor and repeated measures designs.

Strictly speaking, ANCOVA is appropriate primarily in experimental situations in which subjects have been randomly assigned to groups. In a true experimental design, groups are in theory already equivalent across an infinite number of traits because of random assignment. However, in reality, groups are never perfectly equal, and thus AN-COVA can enhance the groups' comparability with respect to the chosen covariates. Moreover, ANCOVA increases the sensitivity of the F test for the effect of the independent variable by removing the variability attributable to the covariates from the error term (the sum of squares within groups). Unless the covariates are totally uncorrelated with the dependent variable, ANCOVA increases the power of the analysis and can reduce the risk of a Type II error.

Although the use of ANCOVA in nonexperimental and quasiexperimental studies has been the subject of some controversy, it is precisely in these situations where AN-COVA has been used most extensively. When subjects cannot be randomly assigned to groups, the researcher is always confronted with the possibility that groups being compared are not equivalent, thereby potentially obscuring the relationship between the independent and dependent variables. For example, suppose we implemented the pain management strategy to patients in clinic A and then compared them to patients in clinic B, who did not receive the intervention. If we compared mean pain scores for the two groups after the intervention, we could not really be sure that any differences were the result of the interventions, rather than due to preexisting differences in pain levels, because the subjects were not randomly assigned to the treatments. By using preintervention pain scores as a covariate, however, the two groups would essentially be equated on initial levels of pain. Differences between the two groups with regard to the covariate (initial pain levels) are removed so that, presumably, remaining differences can be attributed to the effect of the independent variable (intervention versus no intervention).

ANCOVA is also used as a statistical matching procedure to enhance the comparability of groups that are being compared in a totally nonexperimental fashion. For example, if the stress levels of recently widowed and recently divorced persons were being compared, we would want to ensure that the two groups were comparable with respect to characteristics that might influence stress (e.g., age, financial circumstances, length of marriage, and so on). These characteristics could be statistically controlled through ANCOVA.

While ANCOVA can be productively applied in studies that do not involve random assignment, its use is sometimes criticized because of possible misinterpretations of the results. At issue is the concept of causality. When subjects are randomly assigned to treatment groups, statistically significant group differences usually justify an inference of causality; the treatment variable (X) is presumed to have *caused* differences in the dependent variable (Y). ANCOVA allows a more sensitive test of real group differences than ANOVA. When subjects are not randomly assigned to groups, however, even the use of ANCOVA does not usually justify causal inferences. The researcher is usually only in a position to conclude that the groups continued to be different *even after* differences in the covariates were taken into account. But since not all possible human characteristics could ever be statistically controlled, there remains the possibility that group differences in the dependent variable are due to attributes that were not used as covariates, rather than being "caused by" the independent variable.

When ANCOVA is used in studies that are not experimental, there is one more difficulty. ANCOVA adjusts the group means on the dependent variable such that they reflect the means that would have occurred *if* all subjects had the same values on the covariates. But this "if" might be a totally unrealistic condition. For example, in comparing stress levels in divorced and widowed persons, suppose we had a measure of marital satisfaction 1 year prior to the divorce or death of spouse. We could control marital satisfaction statistically, but in some sense this is not a meaningful thing to do; differences in marital satisfaction may be fundamental to the process by which the divorced people are no longer married. Great care must be taken, then, in the interpretation of ANCOVA results in nonexperimental studies.

Assumptions for ANCOVA

As with all other inferential statistics, ANCOVA is based on a number of assumptions, including all of those that were discussed with regard to ANOVA in Chapter 7—random selection of subjects, a normally distributed dependent variable, and homogeneity of variance among the groups. With a reasonably large sample size—and if the number of subjects in the groups is equal or approximately so—ANCOVA, like ANOVA, is robust to the violation of the last two assumptions.

ANCOVA also assumes that the relationship between the dependent variable and each covariate is linear, and that there is a linear relationship between all pairs of covariates. When this assumption is not true, the power of the statistical test is reduced, and the risk of a Type II error increases. Scatterplots can be used to evaluate for possible curvilinearity. When a covariate is found to have a curvilinear relationship with the dependent variable, it is probably best to eliminate it from the analysis, although transformations of the covariate may be another alternative.

Another assumption is referred to as **homogeneity of regression across groups**—the covariate should have the same relationship with the dependent variable in every group being compared. Homogeneity of regression is illustrated in Figure 11–2 (A). Here we see that the slopes of the three groups are equal—that is, the regression lines are parallel. When there is heterogeneity of regression—illustrated in Figure 11–2 (B)—there is an interaction between the covariate and the independent variable. The regression lines are no longer parallel. Some computer software programs for ANCOVA automatically test for homogeneity of regression, but most do not. However, all major software programs can perform tests for the null hypothesis that the slopes for the co-

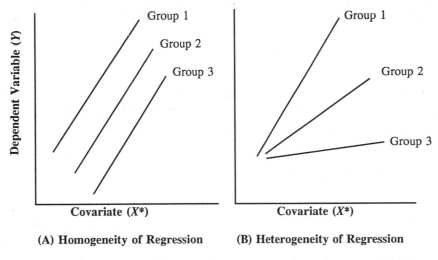

(A) Homogeneity of Regression   **(B) Heterogeneity of Regression**

FIGURE 11–2.   HOMOGENEITY AND HETEROGENEITY OF REGRESSION

variate are equal, and these tests should be performed if there is any reason to suspect heterogeneity of regression.[2] If the slopes are significantly different, ANCOVA should not be used.

Special Issues in ANCOVA

The major features of ANCOVA have been described. This section briefly covers a few additional issues relating to ANCOVA that deserve mention.

The Magnitude of the Relationship. Once a researcher determines that the independent variable is significantly related to the dependent variable, after adjustments for the covariates are made, it may be of interest to determine the *magnitude* of the relationship. Eta^2, which we discussed in connection with ANOVA, is the appropriate index. Here, eta^2 is a measure of the *adjusted* relationship between the independent and dependent variable. The formula for eta$'^2$ *is:*

$$\text{eta}'^2 = \frac{SS'_B}{SS'_B + SS'_W}$$

where eta$'^2$ = eta^2 for the adjusted means

---

[2]In SPSS, the MANOVA program can be used to test homogeneity of regression.

In the example we have used to illustrate ANCOVA (Table 11–2), the value of eta^2 for adjusted means is:

$$\text{eta}'^2 = \frac{1343.61}{1343.61 + 869.89} = .61$$

We can thus conclude that 61% of the variance in the adjusted posttest pain scores is associated with the independent (treatment) variable. Said another way, 61% of the variance *remaining* in posttest pain scores, after removing variance accounted for by pretest pain scores, is attributable to the treatment variable.

Power and ANCOVA. In general, when ANCOVA is used appropriately with carefully selected covariates, the analysis of group differences is more powerful with ANCOVA than with ANOVA because error variance is reduced. The degree of increased power is a function of *how much* error variance is removed—i.e., how correlated the covariates are with the dependent variable.

As described for other statistical analyses, power analysis for ANCOVA can be used to estimate required sample size before the study begins, or to estimate the power of a completed analysis. The estimated effect size for ANCOVA is the adjusted eta^2, the index described in the previous section as representing the proportion of variance explained by the independent variable after removing variance explained by the covariates (Cohen, 1977). The procedures and tables described in the power analysis section of Chapter 7 for ANOVA are appropriate for ANCOVA, substituting the adjusted eta^2 for eta^2.

In the example used in this chapter, the value of eta$'^2$ was .61. Referring back to Table 7–6, we see that with eta^2 = .60 and number of subjects per group = 8, the power is .99 for α = .05. Thus, since there were 10 subjects per group in our example, the power exceeds .99. We can conclude that there was less than a 1% risk of committing a Type II error in this fictitious study.

Multicollinearity. As with multiple regression, the researcher must be careful not to include in the ANCOVA analyses independent variables and covariates that are too highly intercorrelated. The possibility of multicollinearity is most likely to occur when there are multiple covariates. Certain software packages that perform ANCOVA automatically protect against multicollinearity by computing the tolerance, as we described for multiple regression. However, other packages (such as SPSS) do not. If there is a potential risk of multicollinearity, one option is to use a multiple regression program to examine tolerance levels prior to running the ANCOVA.

Alternatives to ANCOVA. Researchers may in some cases want to, or may need to, consider alternatives to ANCOVA. Alternatives are most readily available if the covariate and the dependent variable are measures of the same attribute measured at 2 points in time, as in the example we have used in this chapter. When this is the case, one option is to use a repeated measures ANOVA with a within-subjects and a between-subjects factor. This option is often less attractive than ANCOVA, however, because the effect of the independent variable is evaluated as the interaction between the independent variable and the pretest versus posttest scores, rather than as a main effect.

Another alternative is to compute difference scores between the pretest and posttest measures, and to then treat these differences—often referred to as **change scores**—as the dependent variable in ANOVA. For example, using the data in Table 11–1, the change score for the first subject in group A would be 10 (95 − 85). One of the main problems with change scores is that there are often **ceiling effects** or **floor effects** than constrain the magnitude of change. That is, the amount of change may be artificially small simply because pretest scores are at the upper or lower end of the scale, leaving little room for changes resulting from the treatment. To illustrate, the pretest pain score of the first subject in group A in our example could not have increased by more than 5 points, no matter how much more pain was felt at posttest. ANCOVA is generally preferable to ANOVA with change scores.

Another option that does not require the covariate to be measured on the same scale as the dependent variable is **blocking.** This essentially involves using the covariate as another independent variable in a multifactor design, with ANOVA used to perform the statistical tests. If the covariate is a continuous variable, it must first be converted to a categorical variable (e.g., continuous pretest pain scores could be categorized as low, medium, and high based on some cutoff points). An advantage of this approach is that it can be used when the covariate's relationship with the dependent variable is curvilinear. Moreover, if there would have been heterogeneity of regression between the original covariate and the dependent variable in ANCOVA, this can be detected in multifactor ANOVA as an interaction between the blocked covariate and the independent variable. However, when ANCOVA's assumptions are met, ANCOVA is usually preferable to blocking the covariate because converting the covariate to several levels of a blocked variable results in lost information and a smaller reduction of the error term.

MULTIVARIATE ANALYSIS OF VARIANCE AND COVARIANCE

Multivariate analysis of variance (often abbreviated **MANOVA**) is an extension of ANOVA that is designed to test differences between two or more groups on two or more dependent variables simultaneously. For example, suppose an intervention with cancer patients is designed to both reduce stress and increase hopefulness. Or suppose a treatment for insomniacs is evaluated in terms of its effect on several measures of sleep (e.g., minutes of sleep, intrasleep awakenings, sleep efficiency, etc.). In such situations, MANOVA is the appropriate statistical technique. It is beyond the scope of this book to describe MANOVA in detail because of its extreme complexity, but its major features are described.

Basic Concepts for MANOVA

The F statistic in ANOVA tests whether any group differences on the mean of a single dependent variable are likely to have occurred by chance alone. In MANOVA, statistical tests evaluate whether mean group differences on a *combination* of dependent variables are likely to have resulted by chance. MANOVA involves the creation of a new dependent variable that is a linear combination of the original dependent variables, combined in such a way that groups are as different as possible. Analysis of variance is then performed on the newly created composite dependent variable.

Like ANOVA, MANOVA involves the partitioning of variance into various components. For the most basic MANOVA situation—a one-way MANOVA—variance in the composite dependent variable is partitioned into two components—variance attributable to differences between groups, and error variance, that is, differences within groups. In ANOVA, the partitioned components are computed by summing the squared differences between individual scores and various means. By contrast, MANOVA involves a matrix of scores on the dependent variables, and complex matrix operations are required to partition variance in the composite dependent variable. These matrix operations are described in such texts as Tabachnick and Fidell (1989), Finn (1974), or Timm (1975).

Typically, MANOVA is used in the context of experimental designs in which the investigator has randomly assigned subjects to different treatment groups. Although MANOVA *can* also be used to analyze nonexperimental data, the interpretations of results are necessarily different. In practice, researchers analyzing nonexperimental data are more likely to use multiple regression or canonical analysis than MANOVA.

Advantages and Disadvantages of MANOVA

When faced with an ANOVA-type situation with several dependent variables, the majority of researchers perform multiple ANOVAs rather than MANOVA. Strictly speaking, it is incorrect to perform a series of ANOVAs with the same subjects. The main problem with multiple ANOVAs is that the risk of a Type I error becomes inflated when the dependent variables are correlated, as they almost always are.[3] This is a similar problem to using multiple t-tests rather than ANOVA when there are more than two groups. MANOVA takes the correlations among dependent variables into account when it creates the composite dependent variable, and therefore the risk of a Type I error is maintained at the desired level (i.e., at .05 or lower).

---

[3]A statistical test known as **Bartlett's test of sphericity** can be used to test whether dependent variables are correlated. It is used to test the hypothesis that the population correlation matrix is an **identity matrix**—i.e., a matrix that has all 1s on the diagonal and 0s for all off-diagonal entries.

Another reason for using MANOVA is that it may reveal group differences that were undetected with individual ANOVAs. Figure 11–3 illustrates how this might occur. In this figure, the axes of the coordinates represent two dependent variables, Y_1 and Y_2. Frequency distributions for three groups being compared (A, B, and C) are portrayed directly on the axes. These distributions indicate considerable overlap among the three groups on the two dependent variables when they are considered separately; the group means for Y_1 and Y_2 are fairly similar. However, the ellipses in this figure, which represent the composite of the two dependent variables, make group differences stand out more clearly. Sometimes, then, MANOVA can be more powerful than a series of ANOVAs.

More often, however, MANOVA is actually *less* powerful than ANOVA. For example, it usually requires more subjects to reject the null hypothesis for MANOVA than for ANOVA, given the same effect size, significance criterion, and desired power. Moreover, MANOVA involves even more assumptions than ANOVA and may lead to ambiguities when interpreting the effects of the independent variable on any individual dependent variable. However, if the research inherently involves more than one dependent variable, MANOVA may be the required statistical procedure.

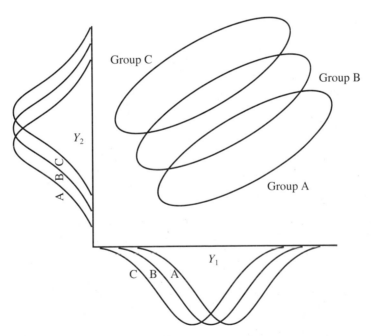

FIGURE 11–3.   COMPOSITE OF TWO DEPENDENT VARIABLES FOR THREE GROUPS

Statistical Tests for MANOVA

To illustrate the information obtained from MANOVA, suppose that in our fictitious experiment to evaluate the effectiveness of bedrest versus exercise versus no intervention in reducing lower back pain we had two dependent variables: posttreatment pain scores and number of pain medications taken within 5 days of treatment. For the moment, we omit from the analysis the pretreatment pain scores. Data for this example are presented in Table 11–3.

The most basic research question in MANOVA is whether the group differences on the dependent variables are true population differences or whether sample differences likely occurred by chance. In ANOVA, the F statistic is the appropriate statistic to consider, but in MANOVA there are four alternative statistics that can be examined and that are available in most software programs: **Wilks' lambda (λ), Hotelling's trace criterion, Pillai's trace criterion,** and **Roy's gcr** (greatest characteristic root) **criterion.** An F test in ANOVA is the ratio of the mean squares for the treatment to the mean squares for error. In MANOVA, there is no longer a single number to represent the two sums of squares, but rather there are several matrices with sums of squares and crossproducts. The matrices must be combined into a test statistic, and the four statistics just described use different criteria for creating the test statistic. When there are only two groups being compared in a one-way MANOVA, all four statistics are identical. When there are three or more groups, the values of these statistics may differ, but the conclusions (i.e., whether to reject or accept the null hypothesis) are usually—though not always—the same.

TABLE 11–3. FICTITIOUS DATA FOR MANOVA EXAMPLE

Bedrest Group (A)		Exercise Group (B)		Control Group (C)	
Posttest Pain Y_{1A}	Medication Y_{2A}	Posttest Pain Y_{1B}	Medication Y_{2B}	Posttest Pain Y_{1C}	Medication Y_{2C}
85	12	60	9	30	2
70	7	45	4	40	5
50	4	30	0	45	4
30	2	70	6	20	1
45	8	55	4	85	10
40	5	65	8	50	6
65	7	35	5	85	14
70	9	40	3	75	8
35	2	60	8	65	6
85	11	10	1	60	4
$\bar{Y}_{1A}=57.5$	$\bar{Y}_{2A}=6.7$	$\bar{Y}_{1B}=47.0$	$\bar{Y}_{2B}=4.8$	$\bar{Y}_{1C}=55.5$	$\bar{Y}_{2C}=6.0$

For the data shown in Table 11–3, the MANOVA statistics for testing group differences are as follows:

Statistic	Value
Pillai's trace criterion	.06
Hotelling's trace criterion	.07
Wilks' lambda	.94
Roy's gcr	.06

The most widely used of the test statistics is Wilks' lambda. This statistic represents the pooled ratio of error variance in the composite dependent variable to error variance plus treatment variance. This may sound vaguely similar to the R^2 statistic—in fact, Wilks' lambda may be defined as:

$$\lambda = 1 - R^2$$

In other words, Wilks' lambda is a direct measure of the proportion of variance in the composite dependent variable that is *un*accounted for by the independent variable. Thus, one of the reasons that Wilks' lambda is popular as the test statistic in MANOVA is that it provides a direct measure of the strength of the relationship between the independent variable and the dependent variables, taken together. In our example, the proportion of variance accounted for by the treatment variable is .06, i.e., $1 - .94$.

However, Pillai's criterion is the most robust of the four statistical tests, meaning that it yields results that are most likely to be correct even when the assumptions for MANOVA are violated. Thus, when the sample is relatively small, when there are unequal ns in the groups, or when basic assumptions (described below) are known to be violated, Pillai's criterion may be the most appropriate test statistic.

The exact distributions for the four MANOVA test statistics differ somewhat. While tables of the exact distributions can be found in some advanced textbooks, the more usual procedure is to transform the statistics such that they have approximately an F distribution.[4] For the Wilks' lambda statistic in our example (.94), the F statistic is .44, $p = .78$. Based on this MANOVA analysis, we must conclude that the three groups do not differ significantly in terms of posttreatment pain scores and number of pain medications consumed. We would have come to the same conclusion regardless of which of the four test statistics had been used.

If we *had* found statistically different group means for the overall MANOVA test, we would naturally want to identify which dependent variable was influenced by the independent variable. This is, unfortunately, not a straightforward task if the dependent

---

[4]There is, however, no convenient way of transforming Roy's gcr into a statistic with a known distribution, so programs typically display the gcr statistic without transformation or significance level.

variables are correlated. The situation is similar to that encountered in trying to determine the relative importance of the independent variables in multiple regression.

Perhaps the most common approach is to examine the univariate ANOVA results for each dependent variable separately. The dependent variables can be rank-ordered, in terms of their contribution to a significant MANOVA statistic, by the magnitude of *significant* univariate F statistics. However, when this procedure is adopted, more stringent alpha levels should be used in determining which dependent variables are significant, using a Bonferroni-type adjustment. The formula for determining the risk of a Type I error when evaluating multiple dependent variables is:

$$\alpha = 1 - (1 - \alpha_1)(1 - \alpha_2). \ . \ .(1 - \alpha_j)$$

where
$$\alpha = \text{overall risk of Type I error}$$
$$\alpha_1. \ . \ .\alpha_j = \text{risk of Type I error for } Y_1 \text{ to } Y_j$$
$$j = \text{number of dependent variables}$$

Thus, if our significance criterion for the univariate F tests was set at .05, the overall risk of committing a Type I error for our example of two dependent variables actually would be:

$$\alpha = 1 - (1 - .05)(1 - .05) = .098$$

With two dependent variables, there would be about a 1 in 10 chance of committing a Type I error if we used .05 as the significance criterion for individual ANOVA tests. If we wanted our overall risk of a Type I error to be kept at the 5% level, we would have to conclude that a dependent variable was nonsignificant if the p value for the univariate ANOVA F test exceeded .025.[5]

Another alternative for evaluating dependent variables in the context of significant overall MANOVA results is referred to as **stepdown analysis.** This procedure is comparable to using hierarchical regression in multiple regression to test the importance of independent variables. In the first step, the highest priority dependent variable (as specified by the researcher) is tested by means of ordinary ANOVA. Remaining dependent variables are "stepped in" in a series of ANCOVAs that use previously entered dependent variables as covariates to see whether the new dependent variable adds anything to the combination of dependent variables already tested. Stepdown analysis is available in several computer programs for MANOVA.

---

[5]For a significance criterion of .05, the p value for individual ANOVA F tests would have to be .017 (or lower) with three dependent variables, .013 with four dependent variables, .010 with five dependent variables, and .005 with ten dependent variables.

MANCOVA and Other Procedures Related to MANOVA

Like ANOVA, MANOVA can be extended in various ways to accommodate different research designs.[6] For example, although we have been describing one-way MANOVAs, **multifactor MANOVAs** can also be performed. A two-way MANOVA would be used to test hypotheses about multiple dependent variables when there are two independent variables (e.g., the effect of the three treatment conditions on posttreatment pain scores and pain medication usage, separately for those who have or have not had back surgery). In this case, the analysis provides tests of two main effects (treatment and surgery history) and an interaction effect on the composite dependent variable.

Another variant includes having a within-subjects factor. For example, the same subjects could be exposed to two or more treatment conditions, and then the effects of the treatment could be examined for more than one outcome. This analysis would be a **repeated measures MANOVA,** sometimes abbreviated R-MANOVA.

Another important extension of MANOVA is **multivariate analysis of covariance (MANCOVA).** MANCOVA involves adjustments to the composite dependent variable prior to assessment of the effects of the independent variable. Just as ANCOVA generally adds considerable power to the statistical test in comparison with ANOVA, so too does MANCOVA generally make it less likely that a Type II error will be committed in comparison with MANOVA. The power increases as the correlation between the covariates and the dependent variables increases.

In the example we used to illustrate MANOVA, we could use MANCOVA to first statistically remove the effect of pretreatment pain scores, and then examine the effect of the treatment variable on both posttreatment pain scores and medications. In fact, when we do this, the conclusions are different than when MANOVA is used. It may be recalled that without pretreatment pain scores controlled, the value of Wilks' lambda for the effect of the treatment variable on the composite dependent variable was .94—only 6% of the variance explained. After removing the effect of initial pain scores, the treatment variable accounts for a full 62% of the variance in the composite dependent variable (i.e., $\lambda = .38$). This effect is significant beyond the .001 level.

Assumptions and Requirements for MANOVA and MANCOVA

The dependent variables for MANOVA and MANCOVA should be measured on a scale that is ratio-level or interval-level. Covariates for MANCOVA can be either continuous variables or dummy-coded dichotomous variables.

Significance tests for MANOVA and MANCOVA assume random sampling from the population of interest. These tests also assume a multivariate normal distribution.

---

[6]A variant not discussed here at length is **Hotelling's T^2** statistic, which is the multivariate analog of the t-test with multiple dependent variables. That is, Hotelling's T^2 is used to test differences on multiple dependent variables in a two-group between-subjects design, or in a one-sample design.

MANOVA is fairly robust to the normality assumption when there are at least 20 cases in each cell of the design, but if any dependent variable is known to be severely skewed, a transformation should be used.

The multivariate analog of the assumption of homogeneous variances for individual dependent variables is **homogeneity of the variance-covariance matrices.**[7] If sample sizes are equal in the groups being compared, MANOVA is robust to violations of this assumption. With unequal sample sizes, the **Box M test,** available in several MANOVA computer programs, should be used to assess homogeneity. Since this test tends to be overly sensitive, Tabachnick and Fidell (1989) recommend that an alpha of .001 be used as the criterion for concluding that the MANOVA may not be adequately robust, and they also recommend using Pillai's criterion as the statistical test when the significance of the Box M test exceeds .001.

Linearity is also assumed—linearity between all pairs of dependent variables, all pairs of covariates in MANCOVA, and all covariate-dependent variable combinations. If there is reason to assume a curvilinear relationship, scatterplots of pairs of variables should be examined. Departures from linearity can reduce the power of the statistical tests.

In both stepdown analysis and MANCOVA, homogeneity of regression is assumed. If an interaction between a covariate and an independent variable exists, MANCOVA is not the appropriate procedure. An interaction implies that a different covariate adjustment on the dependent variable is needed in different groups.

When using MANOVA, there should always be more cases than dependent variables in every cell of the design. If a cell has more dependent variables than subjects, the cell becomes singular and the assumption of homogeneity becomes untestable.

CANONICAL ANALYSIS

Canonical analysis is a statistical procedure that is appropriate whenever a researcher wants to analyze the relationship between two variable *sets,* each of which has two or more variables. For example, a researcher might want to understand the relationship between a woman's demographic characteristics on the one hand (e.g., age, gender, race/ethnicity, educational attainment, employment), and various health-promoting behaviors engaged in during pregnancy (e.g., higher vitamin intake, reduced alcohol consumption, number of prenatal visits) on the other. Canonical analysis is often used when the researcher has one set of independent variables (sometimes called the **variables on the left**) and a second set of dependent variables (the **variables on the right**).

---

[7]A **variance-covariance matrix** is a square matrix with the variances of the variables on the diagonal and the covariances of pairs of variables off the diagonal. (The **covariance** of two variables is the sum of the crossproducts of each variable's deviation scores, divided by degrees of freedom. When each covariance is divided by the standard deviations of the two variables, the result is the correlation between the two.)

Canonical analysis can also be used, however, even when the sets of variables are not conceptualized as independent or dependent—that is, when the researcher is simply exploring relationships between two separate sets of variables.

Canonical analysis has not been widely used, in part because of its complexity and in part because it is problematic as a hypothesis-testing technique. We present an overview of canonical analysis, and urge interested readers to consult Tabachnick and Fidell (1989) or Pedhazur (1982) for a more detailed description.

Basic Concepts for Canonical Analysis

Canonical analysis can be thought of as an extension of—or a generalization of—multiple regression analysis. In multiple regression, the independent variables are weighted by regression coefficients and then combined to form a linear composite that yields the highest possible correlation with the dependent variable. In canonical analysis, the underlying principle of forming linear combinations is the same, except that there are now several variables on both sides of the equation. As a result, two linear composites, called **canonical variates,** must be formed—one combination on the independent variable side *(X)* and the other on the dependent variable side *(Y)*.

The canonical variates can be correlated in more than one way. Canonical analysis yields several *pairs* of canonical variates, sometimes called **roots.** Each root yields a separate **canonical correlation coefficient,** symbolized as R_c. Canonical analysis differentially weights both the X and Y variables in such a way that the maximum possible correlation between the two sets is obtained. After yielding the highest possible R_c, additional canonical correlations are computed, but subsequent R_cs are subject to a restriction: successive pairs of canonical variates of the Xs and Ys cannot be correlated with previously created roots. Thus, the second R_c is based on a linear composite of the X and Y variables that is not correlated with the first root, *and* that yields the second largest R_c possible within the data set.

The canonical correlation coefficient, R_c, can be interpreted like a multiple correlation coefficient, with values ranging from 0.0 to 1.00. The square of a canonical correlation, R^2_c, represents the variance shared by the specific linear combination of the two sets of variables. The maximum number of R_cs in any canonical analysis is the number of variables in the smaller of the two sets. For example, if there were five X variables and three Y variables, there would be a maximum of three R_cs.

The concept of more than one correlation coefficients stemming from the same analysis is best explained with an illustration. In the example cited earlier, we had a set of demographic variables as independent variables and a set of variables measuring healthcare behaviors during pregnancy as dependent variables. Canonical analysis might reveal that there are at least two reliable ways in which the sets of canonical variates are related. The first way might concern the financial circumstances of the women (e.g., measures of the consumption of vitamins and number of prenatal visits might be correlated with income and employment). A second way might concern a person's knowledge of health-promoting behaviors (e.g., measures of smoking and alcohol consumption might be correlated with the women's educational attainment). Thus, each R_c essentially captures a *dimension* of the relationship between the two sets of variables. Each dimension needs to be interpreted by considering the pattern of coefficients associated with the variables in the two sets.

Indexes Associated with Canonical Analysis

In addition to canonical correlation coefficients, canonical analysis yields other indexes that can be used to better understand the relationships among the variables in the two sets. As in multiple regression, canonical analysis provides information on how variables in the analysis should be weighted to form the canonical variate. **Canonical weights** are standardized weights (like beta weights) associated with each X and Y variable. The canonical weights can be used in connection with each subject's standard *(z)* scores on all the X and Y variables to yield a **canonical variate score.**[8] A canonical variate score can be created for each root—that is, for each dimension identified in the analysis. Sometimes the magnitudes of the canonical weights are interpreted in terms of the relative importance of individual X and Y variables in forming the canonical variate. However, canonical weights, like beta weights, tend to be somewhat unstable and generally suffer from the same interpretive limitations as beta weights in regression analysis.

Structure coefficients are often used for interpreting canonical analysis results. Structure coefficients (or **loadings** as they are sometimes called) represent the correlation between the original X and Y variables and the canonical variate scores. Thus, there are structure coefficients for each variable with each canonical variate pair. The higher the absolute value of the structure coefficient for a variable, the more important that variable is in defining the underlying dimension of that canonical variate pair.[9] In our example, for instance, income, prenatal visits, and vitamin use would have high loadings on the first pair of canonical variates, while education, smoking, and alcohol use would have high loadings on the second pair. Generally, structure coefficients that have an absolute value of .30 or higher are considered high enough to be meaningful for interpretation purposes.

Another index in canonical analysis is referred to as the **redundancy index.** Redundancy is a measure of how much variance the canonical variates from the independent variables extract from the dependent variables, and vice versa. For example, the

---

[8]Canonical variate scores are not often computed in practice. However, if canonical variates are readily interpretable and conceptually interesting, canonical variate scores can be used as new independent or dependent variables in subsequent analyses.

[9]Structure coefficients can be negative or positive, as with correlation coefficients. The square of the structure coefficient indicates the proportion of variance of the variable that is accounted for by the canonical variate pair.

independent variable redundancy in a canonical variate pair is the percentage of variance it extracts from the independent variable set times R^2_c for that canonical variate pair. Thus, there is a redundancy index for each of the two sets of variables, for each R_c. When the redundancy indexes for a variable set are added together, the value indicates the total percentage of variance extracted in the other variable set. For example, suppose in our example of demographic variables and health-promoting behaviors in pregnant women, the redundancy index for the demographic variables was .294 for the first canonical variate pair and .167 for the second. This means that 46.1% (29.4 + 16.7 = 46.1) of the variance in health-promoting behaviors is extracted by the demographic characteristics in the analysis.

Statistical Tests in Canonical Analysis

Several approaches have been used regarding significance testing in canonical analysis, but the most widely used test is **Bartlett's test** of Wilks' lambda. Bartlett's test can be used to test whether one R_c, or a set of R_cs, is significantly different from zero. As discussed in the section on MANOVA, Wilks' lambda is an index of variance that is *unaccounted* for. In canonical analysis, this statistic is defined as:

$$\lambda = (1 - R^2_{c_1})(1 - R^2_{c_2}). . .(1 - R^2_{c_j})$$

where $R^2_{c_1}$ = square of first canonical correlation
$R^2_{c_2}$ = square of second canonical correlation
j = number of maximum canonical variate pairs

Bartlett's test involves a transformation of lambda that is distributed as a chi-square with pq degrees of freedom (p = number of variables on the left; q = number of variables on the right). The significance of Wilks' lambda can also be evaluated using the F distribution, as it is in SPSS.

After determining whether all the R_cs, taken together, are significantly different from zero, it is usually important to determine whether individual R_cs are significant— that is, whether each dimension identified in the analysis is a reliable one. If the overall test is significant, then it can be concluded that at least the first canonical correlation is significant. A new lambda (λ') can be computed by removing the expression for the first R^2_c:

$$\lambda' = (1 - R^2_{c_2}). . .(1 - R^2_{c_j})$$

If this lambda is statistically significant, it can be concluded that the first *two* canonical correlations are statistically significant. This "peel-away" process continues until a lambda is not significant at the desired level of α, at which point it is concluded that previous R_cs are significant but any remaining ones are not.

Assumptions described previously in connection with other multivariate procedures also apply to significance testing within canonical analysis. These include the assumption of multivariate normality, linearity between pairs of variables, and homoscedacticity. Distributions of canonical variate scores can be examined to evaluate whether these assumptions have been violated. The variables in canonical analysis can be either continuous interval- or ratio-level variables, or dummy-coded categorical variables.

Limitations of Canonical Analysis

Canonical analysis is the most general of the multivariate techniques we have discussed thus far. In fact, multiple regression, ANCOVA, and MANOVA are all special cases of canonical analysis. Yet it is an infrequently used analytic technique—despite the fact that *most* researchers do, in fact, have more than one independent variable and more than one dependent variable in their data set.

One difficulty is that canonical analysis is complex, and the results are usually hard to explain and to effectively communicate, particularly to practicing nurses. Moreover, the results of canonical analysis are not always easy to interpret, even for the researcher. If an underlying dimension in the pattern of structure coefficients cannot be readily identified, it may be problematic to understand what the canonical correlation coefficients mean. A canonical solution is geared to maximizing correlation, not to enhancing interpretability. The requirement that canonical variate pairs after the first R_c is extracted be orthogonal to (uncorrelated with) other canonical variate pairs may make interpretation even more strained.

One further concern is that the canonical solution is highly sensitive to changes in the variables in either set. The canonical variates that are created are based on correlations among variables within a set and on correlations among variables between sets. Changing even one variable in a set can alter the entire analysis. Nevertheless, canonical analysis is an option that researchers should consider in developing their data analysis plan, and it may be especially useful as a descriptive or exploratory technique.

COMPUTER ANALYSIS FOR ANCOVA, MANOVA, AND CANONICAL ANALYSIS

Although the procedures discussed in this chapter were developed nearly 50 years ago, these techniques were rarely used before computers became widely available because the calculations are exceedingly laborious. Virtually no one would consider manually calculating an ANCOVA, MANOVA, or canonical correlation to analyze data, and therefore it is important to understand the printouts from these procedures.

```
          * * *   A N A L Y S I S   O F   V A R I A N C E   * * *

              POSTPAIN
        BY    GROUP
A       WITH  PREPAIN
```

Source of Variation	Sum of Squares	DF	Mean Square	F	Signif of F
Covariates	9703.174	1	9703.174	290.018	.000
PREPAIN	9703.174	1	9703.174	290.018	.000
Main Effects	1343.608	2	671.804	20.080	.000
GROUP	1343.608	2	671.804	20.080	.000
Explained	11046.782	3	3682.261	110.059	.000
Residual	869.885	26	33.457		
Total	11916.667	29	410.920		

```
B   * * *   M U L T I P L E   C L A S S I F I C A T I O N   A N A L Y S I S   * * *

              POSTPAIN
        By    GROUP
        With  PREPAIN


   Grand Mean =       53.333
```

Variable + Category	N	Unadjusted Dev'n	Eta	Adjusted for Independents Dev'n	Beta	Adjusted for Independents + Covariates Dev'n	Beta
GROUP							
1 BEDREST	10	4.17				3.15	
2 EXERCISE	10	-6.33				-9.38	
3 CONTROL	10	2.17				6.23	
			.23				.34

```
   Multiple R Squared                                               .927
   Multiple R                                                       .963
```

FIGURE 11–4. COMPUTER PRINTOUT OF ANCOVA

Computer Example of ANCOVA

Figure 11–4 presents the SPSS printout for the analysis of covariance based on the data presented in Table 11–1.[10] Panel A presents the summary table for the ANCOVA in which POSTPAIN is the dependent variable, PREPAIN is the covariate, and GROUP is the independent variable. The summary table breaks down the total sum of squares in

---

[10]The SPSS/PC command that created the printout in Figure 11–4 is as follows:

ANOVA VARIABLES=POSTPAIN BY GROUP (1,3) WITH PREPAIN
  /STATISTICS=1.

the posttreatment pain scores into several components. The first is the sum of squares due to the covariate. The F statistic for the significance of the covariate PREPAIN is 290.018, significant beyond the .0005 level. (Had there been two covariates, there would have been a significance test for the two combined, and then separate tests for each one.) After the effect of the covariate is removed, the main effect for GROUP is tested. With 2 and 26 degrees of freedom, the F of 20.080 is also significant beyond the .000 level. The next line shows the test for whether the covariate and independent variable, when combined, explain a significant proportion of variance in posttest pain scores. The sum of squares Explained is 11,046.782, which yields an F of 110.059. The remaining sum of squares is the Residual—the amount of unexplained variation, or error. The mean square for this term is the denominator for each of the F tests.

Panel B presents the multiple classification analysis, that is, information for computing adjusted means. The overall sample (grand) mean for POSTPAIN is 53.333. The column labeled Unadjusted Dev'n shows the raw deviations from the grand mean for the three groups. For example, the unadjusted mean of the posttest pain scores for the bedrest group is 53.33 + 4.17 = 57.50, the same as shown in Table 11–1. To the far right, we find the column labeled Adjusted for Independents + Covariates Dev'n. The numbers in this column indicate how far above or below the grand mean each group's *adjusted* mean is:

    BEDREST 53.333 + 3.15 = 56.483
    EXERCISE 53.333 − 9.38 = 43.953
    CONTROL 53.333 + 6.23 = 59.563

Within rounding error, these are the same values we obtained earlier in this chapter when we computed adjusted means manually.

Other pieces of information are also shown in panel B. First, the value of eta is shown as .23. This is *not* the adjusted eta, but rather the unadjusted eta that indicates the relationship between the independent and dependent variables prior to covariate adjustment. Eta, when squared (.0529) is the proportion of *all* of POSTPAIN's variability that is explained by GROUP. To the right of eta is beta (.34), which is the standardized regression coefficient for GROUP after PREPAIN is in the equation. The final numbers at the bottom right show the value of R (.927) and R^2 (.963) for the multiple correlation of POSTPAIN with both PREPAIN and GROUP. Taken together, the covariate and independent variable account for 92.7% of the variance in posttreatment pain scores. This represents the ratio of the Explained sum of squares to the Total sum of squares from Panel A, i.e., 11,046.782 ÷ 11,916.667 = .927.

Computer Example of MANCOVA

Computer programs for MANOVA/MANCOVA typically offer dozens of options for statistical information and displays, including tests of violations of the underlying assumptions. Figure 11–5 presents a portion of a printout for a "bare-bones" MANCOVA, involving the analysis of data presented in Table 11–3, with the pretreatment pain scores from Table 11–1 as the covariate.[11] In this analysis, POSTPAIN and MEDICATE are the dependent variables, PREPAIN is the covariate, and GROUP is the independent variable. We now comment on major features of this printout.

Panel A presents the results of the test of the assumption regarding the homogeneity of the variance-covariance matrices. The Box M statistic is 14.31062. The significance level of this test can be based on either the F distribution or the chi-squared distribution, and this printout shows the M statistic transformed to both an F value (.99710) and a chi-square value (12.01385). Both are nonsignificant ($p = .45$) and thus there is no reason to believe that the assumption of homogeneity has been violated.[12]

Panel B presents MANOVA results for the combined effect of the covariate and independent variable (EFFECT . . . WITHIN CELLS Regression). The four MANOVA statistics indicate that, overall, PREPAIN and GROUP explained a significant proportion of the variance of the composite dependent variable. For example, we see that the value of the Wilks' lambda statistic is .07450 (i.e., about 93% of the variance is explained). No matter which statistic is used, the significance level for the statistics (as transformed to F) is less than .0005.

Panel C presents some "univariate" results—i.e., statistics for each dependent variable separately. This information essentially involves the results of analyses in which each dependent variable is regressed on PREPAIN and GROUP. For example, the R^2 for POSTPAIN regressed on the covariate and independent variable is .92298, while that for the regression of MEDICATE on these two variables is .75055. Both are significant beyond the .001 level.

Panel D (Regression analysis. . .) shows further information regarding the separate regressions of the two dependent variables, POSTPAIN and MEDICATE. For each dependent variable, the printout specifies the following information with regard to the covariate PREPAIN: the unstandardized regression coefficient (b), beta weight, standard error, t statistic for the significance of the b weight, the significance of t, and the 95% confidence interval around the b weight for the covariate *with the GROUP variable also in the equation*. The information in this panel indicates that the covariate is a highly significant predictor of both POSTPAIN ($t = 17.652$, $p < .000$) and MEDICATE ($t = 8.850$, $p < .000$), even when the independent variable is taken into account. Note that the b weight for PREPAIN in the regression of POSTPAIN is 1.01609, the value we noted earlier in this chapter as 1.02 in connection with the manual computation of adjusted mean scores for POSTPAIN.

---

[11]The SPSS/PC command that created the printout in Figure 11–5 is as follows:

```
MANOVA POSTPAIN MEDICATE BY GROUP (1,3) WITH PREPAIN
    /PRINT   = HOMOGENEITY (BOXM)
    /METHOD=NOCONSTANT.
```

[12]To conserve space, Figure 11–5 omits the portion of the printout that displays the determinants of all the variance-covariance matrices; this information is used in the calculation of the Box M test.

Multivariate test for Homogeneity of Dispersion matrices

A
```
Boxs M =                        14.31062
F WITH (12,3532) DF =            .99710, P =   .449 (Approx.)
Chi-Square with 12 DF =        12.01385, P =   .445 (Approx.)
```

- - - - - - - - - -

* * ANALYSIS OF VARIANCE -- DESIGN   1 * *

B
EFFECT .. WITHIN CELLS Regression
Multivariate Tests of Significance (S = 1, M = 0, N = 11 1/2)

Test Name	Value	Approx. F	Hypoth. DF	Error DF	Sig. of F
Pillais	.92550	155.29091	2.00	25.00	.000
Hotellings	12.42327	155.29091	2.00	25.00	.000
Wilks	.07450	155.29091	2.00	25.00	.000
Roys	.92550				

C
- - - - - - - - - -
Univariate F-tests with (1,26) D. F.

Variable	Sq. Mul. R	Mul. R	Adj. R-sq.	Hypoth. MS	Error MS
POSTPAIN	.92298	.96072	.92002	10425.11513	33.45711
MEDICATE	.75077	.86647	.74118	243.02275	3.10297

Variable	F	Sig. of F
POSTPAIN	311.59640	.000
MEDICATE	78.31938	.000

D
- - - - - - - - - -
Regression analysis for WITHIN CELLS error term
Dependent variable .. POSTPAIN

COVARIATE	B	Beta	Std. Err.	t-Value	Sig. of t
PREPAIN	1.01609	.96072	.058	17.652	.000

COVARIATE	Lower -95% CL- Upper	
PREPAIN	.898	1.134

Dependent variable .. MEDICATE

COVARIATE	B	Beta	Std. Err.	t-Value	Sig. of t
PREPAIN	.15514	.86647	.018	8.850	.000

COVARIATE	Lower -95% CL- Upper	
PREPAIN	.119	.191

FIGURE 11–5.   COMPUTER PRINTOUT OF MANCOVA

```
E  * * ANALYSIS   OF   VARIANCE -- DESIGN   1 * *

   EFFECT .. GROUP
   Multivariate Tests of Significance (S = 2, M = -1/2, N = 11 1/2)

   Test Name          Value  Approx. F Hypoth. DF    Error DF  Sig. of F

   Pillais           .62735   5.94144     4.00        52.00     .001
   Hotellings       1.61821   9.70928     4.00        48.00     .000
   Wilks             .37937   7.79443     4.00        50.00     .000
   Roys              .61645


   - - - - - - - - - -

F  Univariate F-tests with (2,26) D. F.

   Variable   Hypoth. SS   Error SS Hypoth. MS    Error MS        F  Sig. of F

   POSTPAIN  1343.60777  869.88487  671.80388    33.45711  20.07955    .000
   MEDICATE    33.25807   80.67725   16.62903     3.10297   5.35907    .011
```

FIGURE 11–5.   (CONTINUED)

Panel E (ANALYSIS OF VARIANCE—DESIGN 1) is the panel of major interest because it presents the test of the independent variable's effect on the composite dependent variable, once variability attributable to the covariate is removed. The values for all four MANOVA statistics are quite different from the values without the covariate, which we reported in the section "Statistical Tests for MANOVA." For example, the value of Pillai's criterion changed from .06 for MANOVA to .63 (.62735) for MANCOVA, and the level of significance changed from .44 (nonsignificant) to .000 (highly significant). Thus, the addition of the covariate alters the conclusions that we can reach concerning the differential effectiveness of the treatment conditions.

With a significant overall MANCOVA, it is meaningful to identify which dependent variable is contributing to the result. Panel F of Figure 11–5 shows the "univariate" ANCOVAs. The results for the first dependent variable, POSTPAIN, are essentially identical to the ANCOVA results shown in Figure 11–4 (e.g., $F = 20.07955$ is comparable to the F of 20.080 in Figure 11–4). The univariate tests indicate that GROUP has a significant effect on *both* dependent variables, when considered separately. For MEDICATE, the F of 5.35907 is significant at the .011 level. Remember, however, that with a desired overall α of .05, each univariate F test must be equal to or less than .025, as previously discussed. Both dependent variables meet this criterion, and thus we can conclude that, after controlling for initial levels of pain, the three treatments had different effects on both posttreatment pain and the use of pain medications.[13] Post hoc comparisons would have to be used to determine which treatment(s) accounted for the significant difference.

---

[13]In this example, the stepdown analysis also resulted in significant F values for both dependent variables. The stepdown results are not shown in the Figure 11–5 due to space constraints.

Computer Example of Canonical Analysis

In Chapter 10, we presented a table (Table 10–10) to illustrate how hierarchical regression results could be displayed for three separate dependent variables—depression, parenting stress, and alcohol abuse. Here we discuss a computer printout for a canonical analysis of the same data set, which involved a sample of nearly 2000 low-income teenage mothers. In this present example, we use the three outcomes from Table 10–10 as the dependent variables for the canonical analysis (PSTRESS, CESD, and ALCOHOL), but to conserve space we use only six independent variables: partner present (PARTNR), number of children (NKIDS), receiving welfare (WELFARE), has a high school diploma (DIPLOMA), Difficult Life Circumstances Scale scores (DLC), and Self-Esteem Scale scores (ESTEEM).

Figure 11–6 presents the most relevant portion of the computer printout for the canonical analysis.[14] Given the complexity of the printout, we will point out only its most important features. Panel A presents the multivariate tests of significance, which are tests of the hypothesis that all R_cs as a set are zero in the population. The value of Wilks' lambda is .68755, which is significant beyond the .001 level. All other multivariate test statistics shown in the printout are similarly significant. We can thus conclude that there is a relationship between the two variable sets in the population.

Panel B shows the eigenvalues and canonical correlations. (Eigenvalues, which are measures of explained variance, are discussed in the next chapter.)[15] Since there are three variables in the smaller of the two sets, there are three pairs of canonical variates, here labeled Roots. The canonical correlation for the first canonical variate pair is .528, and the R^2_c is .279. The correlation for the second pair of canonical variates is .176, while that for the third is .127. Clearly, the first canonical correlation accounts for the greatest proportion of variance between the two sets of variables (88.9% of the explained variance).

Panel C, labeled Dimension Reduction Analysis, presents the results of the "peel-away" procedure in which successive canonical correlations are removed to determine the statistical significance of remaining R_cs. The first line, for roots 1 to 3, repeats statistical information about all canonical correlations (e.g., Wilks' lambda = .68755 here and in Panel A). The second line for roots 2 to 3 shows the value of Wilks' lambda when the first canonical correlation is "peeled away"—i.e., for the second and third R_c only. Although the value of lambda is now dramatically

---

[14]The SPSS/PC command that created the printout in Figure 11–6 is as follows:

    MANOVA PSTRESS DEPRESS ALCOHOL WITH PARTNER NKIDS DIPLOMA WELFARE DLC ESTEEM
       /DISCRIM = STAN COR
       /PRINT SIGNIF (MULTIV EIGEN DIMENR)
       /DESIGN.

[15]The eigenvalues here are computed by dividing R^2_c by $1 - R^2_c$. For example, for the first eigenvalue, .279/(1 − .279) = .387.

A

```
EFFECT .. WITHIN CELLS Regression
Multivariate Tests of Significance (S = 3, M = 1 , N = 948 )
```

Test Name	Value	Approx. F	Hypoth. DF	Error DF	Sig. of F
Pillais	.32594	38.59893	18.00	5700.00	.000
Hotellings	.43500	45.83639	18.00	5690.00	.000
Wilks	.68755	42.24020	18.00	5368.84	.000
Roys	.27883				

- - - - - - - - - -

B Eigenvalues and Canonical Correlations

Root No.	Eigenvalue	Pct.	Cum. Pct.	Canon Cor.	Sq. Cor
1	.387	88.882	88.882	.528	.279
2	.032	7.324	96.205	.176	.031
3	.017	3.795	100.000	.127	.016

- - - - - - - - - -

C Dimension Reduction Analysis

Roots	Wilks L.	F	Hypoth. DF	Error DF	Sig. of F
1 TO 3	.68755	42.24020	18.00	5368.84	.000
2 TO 3	.95339	9.17353	10.00	3798.00	.000
3 TO 3	.98376	7.84051	4.00	1900.00	.000

- - - - - - - - - -

D Univariate F-tests with (6,1900) D. F.

Variable	Sq. Mul. R	Mul. R	Adj. R-sq.	Hypoth. MS	Error MS
PSTRESS	.09501	.30824	.09215	5675.45058	170.71348
CESD	.25909	.50901	.25675	8831.12798	79.74928
ALCOHOL	.04396	.20966	.04094	10.01203	.68767

Variable	F	Sig. of F
PSTRESS	33.24547	.000
CESD	110.73615	.000

E Standardized canonical coefficients for DEPENDENT variables
        Function No.

Variable	1	2	3
PSTRESS	-.244	.423	.943
CESD	-.869	.004	-.607
ALCOHOL	-.130	-.957	.292

FIGURE 11-6.   COMPUTER PRINTOUT OF CANONICAL ANALYSIS

F Correlations between DEPENDENT and canonical variables
        Function No.

Variable	1	2	3
PSTRESS	-.543	.312	.780
CESD	-.962	.049	-.270
ALCOHOL	-.244	-.907	.344

- - - - - - - - -

G Variance explained by canonical variables of DEPENDENT variables

CAN. VAR.	Pct Var DE	Cum Pct DE	Pct Var CO	Cum Pct CO
1	42.633	42.633	11.887	11.887
2	30.727	73.360	.949	12.836
3	26.640	100.000	.433	13.269

- - - - - - - - -

H Standardized canonical coefficients for COVARIATES
        CAN. VAR.

COVARIATE	1	2	3
PARTNR	.086	.243	-.607
NKIDS	-.029	.496	.390
DIPLOMA	.176	-.467	.358
WELFARE	-.060	.028	.482
DLC	-.754	-.503	-.189
ESTEEM	.506	-.467	-.150

- - - - - - - - -

I Correlations between COVARIATES and canonical variables
        CAN. VAR.

Covariate	1	2	3
PARTNR	.117	.295	-.691
NKIDS	-.082	.571	.334
DIPLOMA	.272	-.488	.278
WELFARE	-.130	-.030	.642
DLC	-.836	-.406	-.141
ESTEEM	.596	-.457	-.093

- - - - - - - - -

J Variance explained by canonical variables of the COVARIATES

CAN. VAR.	Pct Var DE	Cum Pct DE	Pct Var CO	Cum Pct CO
1	5.417	5.417	19.428	19.428
2	.528	5.946	17.116	36.545
3	.300	6.246	18.469	55.014

FIGURE 11–6. (CONTINUED)

(.95339), the F of 9.17353 is statistically significant (p = .000), and so we can conclude that the second R_c is significant. The final line shows results for the third canonical variate pair alone (root 3 to 3). Because of the large sample size, even though lambda is as high as .98376, the third R_c is also statistically significant.

Panel D, which we do not discuss in detail, presents the results of multiple regression analyses in which the three dependent variables are separately regressed on the independent variables. Panel E shows the standardized canonical weights associated with the three dependent variables on the three roots. Panel H shows analogous information with regard to the six independent variables. Note than in SPSS, the independent variables are labeled COVARIATES in canonical analysis because it is performed as part of the MANOVA procedure.

Panel F (for the dependent variables) and Panel I (for the independent variables) show the structure coefficients associated with the three canonical variate pairs. These are the coefficients that can be used to help interpret the meaning of the canonical correlations. On the first variate pair, both PSTRESS and, especially, CESD have high loadings (−.543 and −.962) on the dependent variable side, while DLC and ESTEEM have high loadings on the independent variable side. This suggests that, among these young mothers, emotional well-being is related to the stress they experience in their lives. The second canonical correlation involves primarily alcohol abuse (loading of −.907). Several of the demographic variables have high loadings on this second root (number of children, high school diploma status, DLC scores, and self-esteem); on the independent variable side, this second dimension has no single obvious "theme." Finally, the third canonical correlation appears to mainly involve parenting stress (loading = .780). It appears that the financial circumstances of the mother may be especially important in understanding parenting stress, since on the independent variable side, the mother's welfare status (.642) and the presence of a male partner (−.691) have the highest loadings.

Finally, panels G and J contain information on redundancy. Panel G shows the percent of variance in the three linear combinations of the dependent variable explained by, first, the dependent variables themselves, and then by the independent variables (redundancy). For example, the first canonical variate of the dependent variables accounts for 42.633% of the variance in the dependent variable set (Pct Var DE), while redundancy (the percentage of variance explained in the independent variable set) is 11.887% (Pct Var CO). The cumulative redundancy across the three canonical variates of the dependent variables is 13.269 (Cum Pct CO). By contrast, we see in Panel J that the cumulative redundancy of the dependent variables across the three canonical variates of the independent variables is only 6.246% (Cum Pct DE). This means that the independent variables do a better job at explaining the outcome variables than the outcome variables do at explaining the independent variables.

RESEARCH APPLICATIONS OF ANCOVA, MANOVA, AND CANONICAL ANALYSIS

The multivariate procedures discussed in this chapter are not among the most commonly used procedures in nursing research. And yet, many research situations lend themselves to ANCOVA, MANOVA, or canonical analysis. Thus, these techniques most definitely belong in the analytic repertoire of nurse researchers.

The multivariate statistical procedures discussed here are used primarily to test research hypotheses and to address research questions. Table 11–4 presents some recent examples of studies in which the techniques described here were used. The remainder of this section discusses the presentation of results from these techniques.

The Presentation of ANCOVA, MANOVA, and MANCOVA in Research Reports

ANCOVA results are presented in much the same fashion as ANOVA results. When there is only a single one-way ANCOVA to report, it is usually more efficient to simply describe the results in the text. As an example of a narrative presentation, here is how the ANCOVA results from Table 11–2 (also Figure 11–4) might be reported:

> The posttreatment pain scores for the three treatment groups were analyzed by means of AN-COVA, with pretreatment pain scores as the covariate. After controlling for initial levels of pain, group differences in posttreatment pain scores were highly significant (F (2,26) = 20.08, $p <$

TABLE 11–4. RESEARCH EXAMPLES OF ANCOVA, MANOVA, AND CANONICAL CORRELATION

Research Question	Statistical Procedure	Covariate(s)
What is the effect of supplemental dietary calcium on the development of mineralocorticoid hypertension—as measured by blood pressure and total serum calcium levels—in weanling rats? (Perry, 1995)	One-way MANCOVA	Body weight
What is the effect of three common patient events (bed bath, range-of-motion exercises, turning) on transcutaneous oxygen tension in men and women? (Verderber, Gallagher, & Severino, 1995)	Three-way repeated measures ANCOVA	Ambient temperature
What are the differences in arousal levels and stress response among women with three perimenstrual symptom patterns, both premenses and postmenses? (Woods, Lentz, Mitchell, & Kogan, 1994)	Two-way MANOVA	NA
What are the relationships among components of perceived health status on the one hand and positive health practices on the other among adolescents? (Mahon, 1994)	Canonical analysis	NA

.001). The adjusted group means for the bedrest, exercise, and control groups were 56.5, 43.9, and 59.6, respectively. Post hoc tests revealed that, net of pretreatment pain, patients in the exercise group experienced significantly less posttreatment pain than those in both the bedrest group (F (1,26) = 23.20, $p < .001$) and the control group (F = 36.09, $p < .001$). The posttreatment pain levels of the bedrest and control groups were not significantly different from one another (F = 1.42, $p > .05$).

When there is more than one dependent variable, a table with means and SDs—or adjusted means—and significance test results is usually the most efficient way to display ANCOVA. (Of course, if there are multiple dependent variables, a MANCOVA would be appropriate, but the ANCOVA results still could be displayed in the table.) As an example, consider a study in which a researcher examined measures of medication knowledge and compliance in a sample of elderly patients exposed to three different treatments: two innovative teaching conditions and a control condition. Table 11–5 illustrates a table in which ANCOVA results for four dependent variables from this hypothetical study are presented. Note that the table specifies the adjusted group means, F statistic, and p value for each dependent variable. A footnote at the bottom specifies that the covariates used to statistically adjust the means were the subjects' age, medication dosage, and reading levels. According to this table, the results of all four ANCOVAs were statistically significant at or beyond the .01 level.

When the ANCOVA is not based on a one-way design, or when the relationship between the individual covariates and the dependent variable is of substantive interest, then an ANCOVA summary table would probably be needed to supplement a table of means and/or adjusted means. A summary table would be similar to Panel B of Table 11–2, showing the sums of squares and mean squares for all sources of variation, together with all F tests.

TABLE 11–5. EXAMPLE OF ANCOVA RESULTS TABLE

Dependent Variable	Teaching Group 1 ($n = 25$)	Teaching Group 2 ($n = 25$)	Control Group ($n = 25$)	F	p
Medication Knowledge Test	89.2	82.5	75.0	9.04	<.001
Health Locus of Control Scale	48.9	46.4	41.7	10.21	<.001
No. of Days in Compliance, Past Month	23.1	22.5	16.2	12.99	<.001
Attitude Toward Compliance Scale	55.1	56.2	48.5	6.07	<.01

NOTE: The means in this table have been statistically adjusted for the subjects' age, medication dosage, and reading levels.

ANCOVA Results: Adjusted Group Means on Four Outcome Measures, by Intervention Group

MANOVA and MANCOVA results are usually displayed in tables much like those for ANCOVA. In fact, Table 11–5 could easily be adapted to report MANCOVA results. The addition of a footnote indicating the MANCOVA test results would adequately summarize the overall test results (e.g., Wilks' lambda for MANCOVA $= .45$, $F (4,142) = 11.89$, $p < .001$). The ANCOVAs in the table would then be considered post hoc "univariate" tests. With four dependent variables, the significance level for post hoc tests (for the desired alpha of .05) is .013, and thus each individual ANCOVA can be considered statistically significant within the MANCOVA framework.

Table 11–5 could be further adapted to display the results of stepdown analyses within MANCOVA. On the right side, two additional columns would be added, one labeled Stepdown F and another labeled p.[16] Note, however, that if stepdown analysis results are reported, the dependent variables listed in the left-hand column must be ordered according to the order in which they were stepped into the analysis.

The Presentation of Canonical Analysis in Research Reports

Canonical analysis requires a tabular presentation because of the complexity of information involved. Table 11–6 is an example that summarizes the results of the analysis that was used to illustrate computer printouts of canonical analysis (Figure 11–6). All of the variables in the analysis are listed in the left-hand column. The three canonical variate pairs are numbered and indicated in the top row, and for each root there is a heading for the standardized canonical weights and the structure coefficients or loadings. Most researchers present structure coefficients rather than canonical weights if space constraints require the selection of only one index.

The variables in the analysis are designated as being in either the dependent variable set or the independent variable set. In this table, the variables within the set are not ordered in any particular fashion, but an ordered arrangement sometimes makes sense and should be considered if it facilitates interpretation of the underlying dimensions of the canonical variates.

At the bottom of the two sets there is summary information relating to the canonical variates for that set. The table first presents the percentage of variance in the canonical variates accounted for by variables within the set. The next row shows the redundancy coefficient (the *proportion* of variance in the *other set* accounted for by the canonical variates for the designated set). This information is taken from panels G and J of Figure 11–6.

The bottom row of the table presents the canonical correlation (i.e., R_c) for each canonical variate pair. An alternative would be to present R^2_c values. The results of the "peel-away" significance tests are shown by the asterisks next to each coefficient; all coefficients are significant at the .001 level. The overall Wilks' lambda for the set of canonical correlations is designated in a footnote.

---

[16]Alternatively, of course, both columns with p values could be omitted and asteriks could be attached to the F statistics to indicate the level of significance attained.

TABLE 11-6. EXAMPLE OF A TABLE WITH CANONICAL ANALYSIS RESULTS

Variables and Sets	Canonical Variate Pairs					
	1		2		3	
	Weight	Loading	Weight	Loading	Weight	Loading
Dependent Variables						
Parenting Stress Scores	−.24	−.54	.43	.31	.94	.78
CES-D Depression Scale Scores	−.87	−.96	.00	−.05	−.61	−.27
Alcohol Abuse	−.13	−.24	−.96	−.91	.29	.23
Percentage of Variance[a]	42.63		30.73		26.64	
Redundancy of Independent Vars.	0.12		0.01		0.00	
Independent Variables						
Living with Male Partner	.09	.12	.24	.30	−.61	−.69
Number of Children	−.03	−.09	.50	.57	.39	.33
Has High School Diploma	.18	.27	−.47	−.49	.36	.28
Receiving Welfare	−.06	−.13	.03	−.03	.48	.64
Difficult Life Circumstances Score	−.75	−.84	−.50	−.41	−.19	−.14
Self-Esteem Score	.51	.60	−.47	−.46	−.15	−.09
Percentage of Variance[a]	19.43		17.12		18.47	
Redundancy of Dependent Vars.	0.05		0.01		0.00	
Canonical Correlation	.53***		.18***		.13***	

NOTE: The weights are standardized canonical weights; the loadings are the structure coefficients. Overall Wilks' $\lambda = .69$, $p < .001$
[a]Percentage of variance accounted for within the set by the canonical variates for the set.
*** $p < .001$

   Canonical Analysis of Young Mothers' Depression, Parenting Stress, and Alcohol Abuse with Demographic and Psychological Variables (N = 1892)

RESEARCH EXAMPLE

This concluding section summarizes a recent study that used multivariate analysis of covariance, post hoc ANCOVAs, and a stepdown analysis.

Vessey, Carlson, and McGill (1994) tested the effectiveness of a distraction technique for reducing pain and distress in children undergoing a blood draw. A sample of 100 children ages 3 through 12 were randomly assigned to either an experimental or a control group. Those in the control group received standard preparation during venipuncture, while those in the experimental group were encouraged to use a kaleidoscope as a distraction.

The researchers used two dependent variables to assess the effect of the intervention. The first was the Wong-Baker FACES Pain Rating Scale (FACES), which is a self-report measure of children's pain perception. The second was the Children's Hospital of Eastern Ontario Pain Scale (CHEOPS), an observational measure of the intensity of the child's behavioral distress and pain that was completed by a research assistant.

MANCOVA was used to compare the two groups with respect to the two dependent variables. (The authors reported that the assumptions underlying MANCOVA were tested and met.) Age,

TABLE 11–7. UNIVARIATE POST HOC DIFFERENCES OF SCORES OF CONTROL AND INTERVENTION GROUP WITH AGE AS A COVARIATE

	CONTROL			EXPERIMENTAL					Stepdown	
	Observed Mean	(SD)	Adjusted Mean	Observed Mean	(SD)	Adjusted Mean	F^a	p	F^a	p
FACES	3.23	(1.78)	3.26	2.18	(1.61)	2.15	11.50	.001	11.50	.001
CHEOPS	8.73	(2.38)	8.79	7.76	(2.50)	7.70	5.52	.021	0.24	.63

[a]The degrees of freedom for all analyses are 1 and 95.
Adapted from Table 1 of Vessey et al.'s (1994) report.

which was strongly correlated with the two pain measures, was used as the covariate. The overall MANCOVA was highly significant ($p < .004$). To further examine the nature of the experimental effect, the researchers conducted post hoc ANCOVAs. The results were displayed in a table, which is reproduced here as Table 11–7. The table shows both the unadjusted group means and the group means adjusted for the child's age. According to the ANCOVAs, the experimental group and control group differed significantly in terms of both the self-reported measure of pain ($F (1,95) = 11.50, p = .001$) and the observational measure of distress ($F (1,95) = 5.52, p = .021$); children in the experimental group experienced significantly less pain and distress than those in the control group. However, the stepdown analysis indicated that once the effect of self-reported pain was taken into consideration, the CHEOPS measure did not contribute significantly to distinguishing the two groups in MANCOVA ($F (1,95) = 0.24, p = .63$).

SUMMARY

Analysis of covariance (ANCOVA) tests differences in group means after first statistically controlling for one or more **covariates.** In ANCOVA, variability associated with extraneous variables (or a pretest measure of the dependent variable) is removed in a first step, and then group differences in what remains of the variability in the dependent variable are analyzed. *F* tests are used to test the significance of both covariates and independent variables. A procedure known as **multiple classification analysis** can be used to calculate **adjusted means** of the groups, i.e., the means net of the effect of the covariates.

Multivariate analysis of variance (MANOVA) is used to test differences in group means for two or more dependent variables simultaneously. In MANOVA, the dependent variables are linearly combined into a new composite variable whose variance is partitioned into different sources, much as in ANOVA. The two most widely used statistical tests for MANOVA are **Wilks' lambda** (λ) and **Pillai's trace criterion,** both of which can be transformed to an *F* distribution for significance testing. A **stepdown analysis** is one method of evaluating the contribution of individual dependent variables to an overall significant MANOVA. When covariates are used in MANOVA, the analysis is called a **multivariate analysis of covariance (MANCOVA).**

Canonical analysis, an extension of multiple regression, is used to determine the nature and extent of the relationship between two sets of variables, each of which has at least two variables. In canonical analysis, two canonical variates (linear composites) are formed, one for each of the two sets. There are as many *pairs* of canonical variates (roots) as there are variables in the smaller of the two variable sets. Each root differentially weights the X and Y variables to extract the maximum amount of variance, net of what has already been extracted, and each yields a separate canonical correlation (R_c) that corresponds to a dimension of the relationship between the two sets. The dimension can be interpreted by examining the structure coefficients (or loadings) of the original variables on the canonical variate pairing. Wilks' lambda is the statistic usually used to evaluate whether the set of R_cs is significantly different from zero, and a "peel-away" procedure can be used to test the significance of individual R_cs.

EXERCISES

The following exercises cover concepts presented in this chapter. Exercises indicated with a dagger (†) can be checked against answers appearing in Appendix A. Additionally, Chapter 11 of the *Applications Manual* offers supplementary exercises, including ones that require computer analysis of a data set on diskette.

† 1. Indicate which statistical procedure discussed in this chapter would most likely be used in the following circumstances:
    a. Independent variables: age, length of time in nursing home, gender, marital status, number of kin living in 25-mile radius; dependent variables: functional ability, fatigue.
    b. Independent variables: type of stimuli used with infants (visual, auditory, tactile), gender; dependent variables: postintervention heart rate, amount of crying; covariates: baseline heart rate.
    c. Independent variable: presence versus absence of boomerang pillows, with subjects in both conditions in random order; dependent variable: respiratory capacity after treatment; covariate: respiratory capacity before treatment.
    d. Independent variable: receipt versus nonreceipt of an intervention to facilitate coping with unexpected hospitalization; dependent variables: scores on a coping scale, scores on an anxiety scale, scores on a fear of hospitals scale.

2. Suppose you were interested in studying the effect of a person's early retirement (at or below age 62 versus at age 65 or later) on indicators of physical and emotional health. What variables would you suggest using as covariates to enhance the comparability of the groups?

† 3. Use the following information from an SPSS multiple classification analysis to compute unadjusted and adjusted group means on patient satisfaction scale scores:

Grand Mean = 20.521

	Unadjusted Dev'n	Adjusted Dev'n
1 No insurance	−2.56	−3.89
2 Private insurance	3.81	4.97
3 Medicaid	−1.65	−2.47

† 4. Could data used for a one-way MANOVA comparing three groups on four outcome variables be analyzed by canonical analysis? Why or why not?

† 5. In a significant MANOVA with two dependent variables, what is the approximate level of significance that should be used in post hoc ANOVAs to determine the significance of individual dependent variables, if the overall desired alpha is .01?

† 6. In a canonical analysis, the variables are as follows: set 1: adolescents' family structure, number of siblings, family income, gender, academic performance, ever suspended from school, religiosity; set 2: use of marijuana, use of crack/cocaine, use of hallucinogens, use of heroine. How many pairs of canonical variates (roots) would there be in this analysis?

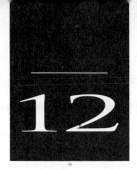

Factor Analysis

Factor analysis[1] is similar to the other multivariate procedures we have described thus far in the sense that factor analysis involves the formation of linear combinations of variables. It is different from most other multivariate procedures, however, because factor analysis is used primarily to determine the structure of a set of variables. Hypothesis testing plays only a small role in factor analysis.

Factor analysis is a powerful and elegant statistical technique, and addresses a key scientific goal—elucidating the underlying meaning of concepts. However, factor analysis is also a somewhat controversial procedure, in large part because it involves a higher degree of subjectivity than is typical in statistical analysis.

BASIC CONCEPTS FOR FACTOR ANALYSIS

Factor analysis is used to capture the underlying dimensionality of a set of measures— that is, to shed light on how variables cluster together to form unidimensional constructs that are of theoretical interest. For example, if we administered 50 questions relating to people's reactions to stress, we might determine through factor analysis that there are four distinct coping styles. Factor analysis would provide information on which of the 50 questions "belong" together on the four dimensions of coping. Researchers often have a priori ideas about which items go together to capture a unidimensional concept, but their ideas are not always correct. Factor analysis provides an *empirical* way to determine the underlying dimensionality of a large set of measures.

---

[1]This chapter deals exclusively with a type of factor analysis that has come to be known as **exploratory factor analysis.** Another type—**confirmatory factor analysis** (CFA)—uses more complex modeling and estimation procedures and more sophisticated computer programs, as briefly discussed in Chapter 14.

Factor analysis determines the structure of a set of variables by analyzing the inter-correlations among them. The underlying dimensions identified in a factor analysis are called **factors.** A factor is a hypothetical entity—a latent variable—that is assumed to underlie the concrete measures administered to research subjects.

Mathematically, a factor is a linear combination of variables in a data matrix. A raw data matrix consists of scores on k variables for N subjects. A factor could be defined by the following equation:

$$F_1 = b_1X_1 + b_2X_2 + \ldots + b_kX_k$$

where F_1 = a factor score for Factor 1
      k = number of original variables
      b_1 to b_k = weights for each k variable
      X_1 to X_k = raw data values on the k variables

Factor analysis solves for the b weights (called **factor loadings**) to yield **factor scores** for the major underlying dimensions.

Information on factors is almost always used in subsequent analyses—that is, most researchers do not perform factor analysis as an end in itself. In our example of coping styles, we might want to determine the characteristics of individuals with different coping styles. Here, the factor scores would become the dependent variables, and individual characteristics would be the independent variables. As another example, we might want to determine if a certain coping style was more effective than others in alleviating stress, and here the coping style factors would be the independent variables and stress would be the dependent variable.

Factor analysis can be viewed as a data reduction technique. That is, rather than having 50 variables to use as independent or dependent variables (i.e., the original items), factor analysis reduces the set to four new variables. Thus, factor analysis is important as a data management strategy that can contribute to analytic parsimony.

Factor Matrices

Matrices play an important role in factor analysis and, indeed, matrix algebra is required in the factor analytic solution. The process begins with the original data matrix (subjects × variables). Many of the operations performed in factor analysis involve manipulations of the correlation matrix (variables × variables, across subjects).

One of the outcomes of a factor analysis is a **factor matrix,** which involves the original variables along one dimension and factors along the other. There are two important types of factor matrix, as we discuss later in this chapter. For now it is important to know that the entries in a factor matrix are factor loadings that convey information about the relationship between the original variables and the underlying factors.

TABLE 12–1. HYPOTHETICAL FACTOR MATRIX FOR SIX APTITUDE TESTS

Tests	Factor I	Factor II	Communality (h^2)
A	.84	.21	.75
B	.90	.24	.87
C	.74	.13	.56
D	.17	.73	.56
E	.22	.80	.69
F	.27	.91	.83
Eigenvalue	2.21	2.12	
% of explained variance	36.8	35.3	

Table 12–1 shows a hypothetical example of a factor matrix. Let us suppose that the variables listed in the left-hand column represent six different aptitude tests (A through F) that were administered to a sample of nursing school applicants. The factors (I and II) are empirically derived factors that might represent, for example, verbal aptitude (Factor I) and quantitative aptitude (Factor II).

Factors loadings can be interpreted in much the same fashion as correlation coefficients.[2] They can range in value from −1.00 through zero for no correlation to +1.00. The first entry in the matrix in Table 12–1 indicates a strong positive correlation between Test A and Factor I (.84). Tests A, B, and C have high loadings on Factor I, while the loadings for Tests C, D, and E on the first factor are more modest—they are all less than .30. Conversely, the first three tests have modest loadings on Factor II, while the last three tests have loadings of .73 or greater on this factor. We would interpret the factors by trying to conceptualize what it is that Tests A, B, and C have in common that they do *not* have in common with Tests D, E, and F. In our example, the Tests A, B, and C might be vocabulary, reading comprehension, and sentence completion tests, respectively, all of which have a strong verbal component. The three other tests might be geometry, math computation, and problem-solving tests—all of which have a quantitative component.

Table 12–1 has two other types of useful information. The **communality** is a measure of a variable's *shared* variance, sometimes referred to as **common factor variance.**

---

[2]Factor loadings following oblique rotations (to be discussed in a subsequent section) *cannot* be interpreted exactly as described here. Most factor analyses involve orthogonal rotations, and therefore this discussion of factor loadings has broad application.

Communality is sometimes labeled h^2, as it is in Table 12–1. The communalities of the original variables in the analysis are equal to the sums of squares of the factor loadings for those variables. Thus, for Test A, the communality is $(.84)^2 + (.21)^2 = .75$.

The common factor variance of a measure indicates the variance that two or more measures share in common. The variability of each of the six tests in Table 12–1 can be expressed as follows:

$$V_{Total} = V_{CommonFactor} + V_{Unique} + V_{Error}$$

where V_{Total} = total variance
$V_{CommonFactor}$ = common factor variance (h^2)
V_{Unique} = variance specific to the measure
V_{Error} = error variance

Using Test A as the example, all of the nursing students' variance in scores on Test A consists of variance that Test A has in common with the other five tests, plus variance that is specific to Test A, plus error variance (e.g., the unreliability of the test). Across the two factors, then, 75% of the variance in Test A is common factor variance, while the remaining 25% is partly unique variance and partly error variance. Table 12–1 indicates that Test F has the highest proportion of common factor variance, while Tests C and D have the lowest. The main problem of factor analysis is the allocation of the total common factor variance (h^2) of a variable to the different factors.

Below the listing of the six tests in Table 12–1 is a row labeled eigenvalue. An **eigenvalue** is the sum of the squared loadings for a specific factor. For Factor I, the eigenvalue is $(.84)^2 + (.90)^2 + (.74)^2 + (.17)^2 + (.22)^2 + (.27)^2 = 2.21$. An eigenvalue is an index of how much variance in the factor solution is explained by a given factor. In this example, the eigenvalues for both factors are about the same (2.21 and 2.12), indicating that both verbal and quantitative aptitude account for a comparable amount of variance in the test scores. The exact percentage of variance is shown in the bottom row, 36.8% for Factor I and 35.3% for Factor II. Together the two factors account for 72.1% of the total variance in the six tests. A subsequent section explains how these percentages are computed.

Requirements and Assumptions for Factor Analysis

Factor analysis uses a correlation matrix as its starting point, and thus the assumptions underlying the use of correlations should be kept in mind. Each pair of variables in a factor analysis should be linearly correlated; curvilinear relationships degrade the analysis. The factor analytic solution is enhanced when the variables are normally distributed, but the solution may be interesting and worthwhile even when normality is not attained for all variables. The discussion in Chapter 9 regarding influences on the value of correlation coefficients (e.g., the presence of outliers, a restricted range of values, and so on) should be kept in mind because things that affect correlations also affect factor analytic solutions.

The variables in a factor analysis are generally measured on a scale that is interval or ratio, or on a scale that approximates interval properties. The variables can be entire scales or tests (as in our example of factor analyzing scores on six aptitude tests) or individual questions or scale items (as in the example of analyzing 50 items that measured reactions to stress).

A basic requirement for a factor analysis is that the correlation matrix be factorable, which means that there should be a number of sizable correlations between the variables in the matrix. If the correlation matrix consists mainly of correlation coefficients with an absolute value less than .30, there is probably nothing to factor analyze.[3]

The correlation matrix for factor analysis should always be based on a rectangular matrix of data values—that is, there should be a valid value on every variable for every subject in the analysis. It is possible to create a correlation matrix based on **pairwise deletion** of missing values—that is, to compute each correlation coefficient for those cases that are not missing for the two variables in question, thereby resulting in coefficients that could be based on a varying number of cases. However, such a correlation matrix should never be used in factor analysis. If there are missing values for some subjects, either the missing values should be estimated or the case should be deleted from the factor analysis (**listwise deletion**).

The sample size for a factor analysis should generally be large, to avoid capitalizing on small random differences in the magnitude of the correlation coefficients. Sample sizes of at least 100 to 200 are usually advisable. Moreover, there should always be *at least* five cases per variable, and 10 cases per variable is vastly preferred. Thus, if there are 50 items being factor analyzed, the sample should ideally be between 250 and 500 cases, if not larger.

Factor analytic solutions almost always require replication. If it is possible to replicate within a single study, this opportunity should be pursued. Thus, with 20 variables and a sample of 500 cases, one alternative is to randomly divide the sample in half, perform a factor analysis with the first subsample, and then cross-validate the results through a factor analysis of the second. If the two analyses reveal similar factor structures, the results will be compelling.

---

[3]Bartlett's test of sphericity, mentioned in the previous chapter, can be used to test the hypothesis that the population correlation matrix is an identity matrix. If the null hypothesis for this test cannot be rejected, factor analysis may not be appropriate. However, Bartlett's test is highly sensitive, and so additional procedures, described in software programs for factor analysis, may be needed as a supplement to determine the factorability of a matrix if visual inspection of the correlation matrix suggests potential problems.

Phases in Factor Analysis

The first step in the factor analysis involves transforming the raw data matrix into a correlation matrix. Researchers should inspect the correlation matrix prior to undertaking a factor analysis to ensure that the correlation matrix is factorable, to determine if there are missing data problems that need to be resolved, and to ascertain that the sample size is adequate.

The next phase is referred to as **factor extraction.** In this phase, the analysis focuses on determining the number of factors that are needed to adequately capture the variance in the set of variables. There are many different approaches to factor extraction, and there are a number of different criteria that can be used to determine the appropriate number of factors. The product from this phase of analysis is an **unrotated factor matrix.**

Factor extraction seeks to maximize variance, but does not result in readily understandable results. Thus, the next phase of factor analysis involves transforming the original factors so that the results are more interpretable, through a process known as **factor rotation.** As with factor extraction, there are alternative methods of factor rotation. The result of this phase of the analysis is a **rotated factor matrix.** The factor matrix in Table 12–1 was a rotated one.

Once the extraction and rotation have been finalized, factor scores for use in subsequent analyses can be computed for each case. As with the other phases, the researcher has some options with regard to the computation of factor scores. Thus, in performing a factor analysis, a researcher must make a number of decisions.

FACTOR EXTRACTION

The goal of factor extraction is to seek clusters of intercorrelated variables within the correlation matrix and to extract as much variance as possible from the common factors. Different statistical criteria and measurement models can be used in the factor extraction stage. Most computer programs for factor analysis offer numerous alternative extraction methods. We explain one method of factor extraction in some detail and then point out the major features of some alternative methods.

The Principal Components Method

A widely used method of factor extraction is the **principal components method.** The principal components (PC) method differs from most other techniques in that it factor analyzes all variance in the observed variables, rather than just common factor variance. The PC method assumes that all measurement error is random and that error variance in one item is not shared with error variance in other items in the analysis. Mathematically, this boils down to what is placed on the diagonal of the correlation matrix prior to matrix operations, because the variance that is analyzed is the sum of the values in the positive diagonal. With the PC method, all of the diagonal values are 1s: there is as much variance to be analyzed as there are variables in the analysis. All variances in the original variables are distributed to the factors, including unique variance and error variance for each variable.

The principal components method creates successive linear combinations of the observed variables. The first factor, or principal component, is the linear combination that accounts for the largest amount of variance, using the least-squares criterion. The second component is formed from residual correlations; it accounts for the second largest amount of variance that is uncorrelated with the first component. Successive components account for smaller and smaller proportions of total variance in the data set, and all are orthogonal to (uncorrelated with) previously extracted components. Thus, the factors (principal components) extracted represent independent sources of variation in the data matrix.

In the PC method, there are as many factors as there are variables, but typically only the first few account for a noteworthy proportion of variance. Table 12–2 presents a summary table from a factor extraction in which the PC method was used. In this analysis, there were 10 items (column 1), and 10 factors were extracted (column 3). All of the variance in the 10 items is accounted for by the 10 factors, and so the communality of each item is 1.00 (column 2). Note that in this table, there is no correspondence between items and factors; they are displayed on the same line for the sake of economy. Columns 1 and 2 show item information and columns 3 through 6 show factor information.

The *amount* of total variance explained by each factor is shown in column 4, labeled Eigenvalue. Each variable in a factor analysis is standardized to have a mean of 0 and an *SD* (and variance) of 1.0. Since there are 10 variables, the sum of all the vari-

TABLE 12–2. SUMMARY OF PRINCIPAL COMPONENTS FACTOR EXTRACTION RESULTS FOR 10 ITEMS

Item (1)	Communality (2)	Factor (3)	Eigenvalue (4)	Percent of Variance (5)	Cum Percent of Variance (6)
1	1.00	1	3.79	37.9	37.9
2	1.00	2	2.70	27.0	64.9
3	1.00	3	1.01	10.1	79.0
4	1.00	4	.51	5.1	80.1
5	1.00	5	.48	4.8	84.9
6	1.00	6	.42	4.2	89.1
7	1.00	7	.39	3.9	93.0
8	1.00	8	.35	3.5	96.5
9	1.00	9	.24	2.4	98.9
10	1.00	10	.11	1.1	100.0

ances accounted for by the factors (i.e., the eigenvalues) is 10.0. To compute the proportion of variance explained by a factor, the eigenvalue associated with the factor must be divided by 10.0. For the first factor in this example, $3.79 \div 10.0 = .379$; that is, 37.9% of the variance in the 10 items is accounted for by the first factor, as shown in column 5 of this table. All subsequent factors account for declining percentages of variance. The final column indicates the cumulative percentage of variance explained by the factor for that row, plus all preceding factors. Thus, the first four factors account for just over 80% of the variance (80.1%) in the 10 variables. Cumulatively, the 10 factors account for 100% of the variance.

Other Methods of Factor Extraction

Other methods of factor extraction use a different measurement model—they assume that measurement error involves both a random component and a systematic component that is not unique to individual items. Consequently, only common factor variance is factor analyzed in these other extraction methods; error and unique variance are excluded.

The **principal factors** (PF) **method** of extraction (sometimes referred to as the **principal-axis factoring method**) is quite similar to the PC method, and is the most popular of the common factor extraction methods. The main difference is that in the PF method, estimates of communality, rather than 1s, are on the diagonal of the correlation matrix. The initial communality estimates are the squared multiple correlation coefficients for the specified variable, with all other variables in the correlation matrix as the predictors. R^2, as we have seen, is an index of shared variance among variables and thus is a reasonable proxy for common factor variance. The communalities are repeatedly reestimated from the factor loadings in an iterative fashion until there are only negligible changes in the communality estimates. As with principal components, the goal of a PF extraction is to extract the largest possible amount of orthogonal variance with successive factors.

The **alpha method** of factoring assumes that the variables in a particular factor analysis are a sample from a hypothetical universe of potential variables. The main concern of alpha factoring is the reliability of the common factors. **Coefficient alpha** (also known as Cronbach's alpha) is the most widely used index of the internal consistency reliability of a measure. In alpha factoring, the communalities are estimated in an iterative process that maximizes coefficient alpha for the factors.

Another option is the **maximum likelihood method.** This method estimates population values for the factor loadings through an estimation process that maximizes the likelihood of yielding a sample with the observed correlation matrix from the population.[4] Again, an iterative algorithm is used to arrive at the factor solution.

Other lesser-used methods of factor extraction include **image factoring, unweighted least-squares (Minres) factoring,** and **generalized least-squares factoring.**

---

[4]Maximum likelihood is a major alternative to least squares as an estimation approach in multivariate analysis, and is discussed in greater detail in the next chapter.

Although there may be sound substantive or methodologic reasons for preferring one method over another, it has generally been found that when there are a fairly large number of variables in the data set and a large sample of subjects, differences in the factor extraction solutions tend to be small.

Number of Factors

In performing a factor analysis, the researcher must make a decision about the number of factors to extract, rotate, and score. There are two competing goals in making the decision. The first is to maximize explained variance. The greater the number of factors, the greater is the percentage of variance explained. We can see in Table 12–2 that we can account for 100% of the variance in the ten items by using 10 factors. However, we then would have as many factors as variables, thereby nullifying the value of the factor analysis. The other competing goal is parsimony; the fewer the factors, the more parsimonious is the factor solution in describing the dimensionality of the data matrix. However, if too few factors are extracted, the proportion of explained variance might be inadequately low and important dimensions within the data set might go unidentified. If we used only the first factor in Table 12–1, for example, we would account for only about 38% of the variance in the data set; moreover, by using only one factor we would miss a sizable percentage of the variance that can be accounted for by the second factor (27%).

The researcher's decision regarding number of factors to use can be based on various criteria. One of the simplest methods is to examine the eigenvalues from an initial run with principal components extraction. A factor with an eigenvalue less than 1 is generally considered unimportant. Since an eigenvalue in a PC analysis represents variance, an eigenvalue of under 1.0 is less important in accounting for variance than an original variable. According to this criterion, we would conclude from Table 12–2 that there should be three factors in this factor analysis, since only factors 1, 2, and 3 have eigenvalues greater than 1.0.

A second approach is to use a **scree test,** which plots successive eigenvalues for the factors. Figure 12–1 shows such a plot in which the eigenvalues from Table 12–2 are graphed along the Y axis and the 10 factors are graphed along the X axis. Scree plots show declining values for the eigenvalues, consistent with the fact that each successive linear combination maximizes extracted variance. What we are looking for is a discontinuity in the steep slope of the plot that separates the larger, more important factors from the smaller, less reliable factors. In this example, an argument could be made that a distinct break occurs between factors 2 and 3, suggesting that two factors should be retained in this example. The scree test has been criticized for its subjectivity, but tends to yield fairly reliable results when the sample size is large and when each factor has several variables with high loadings.

Another criterion that is sometimes used is the proportion of variance accounted for by a factor. It has been argued that a factor is probably not important if it accounts

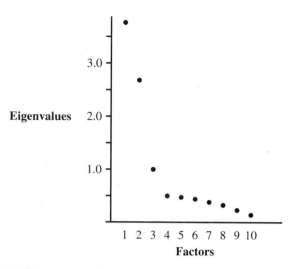

FIGURE 12–1.   SCREE PLOT FOR FACTOR ANALYSIS

for less than 5% of the total variance in a data matrix. In Table 12–2, four factors meet the criterion of accounting for at least 5% of the variance.

Yet another method involves an examination of the **residual correlation matrix,** which can be requested in many factor analysis computer programs. The residual correlation matrix shows partial correlations between variables with the effects of the factors removed. The residual correlation matrix would be requested once a preliminary decision about the number of factors has been made. If there are any sizable residuals (coefficients greater than about .10), another factor may be desirable.

A researcher's decision about the number of factors to retain and interpret is probably more critical than the decision about which factor extraction method to use. Yet, as we have seen in our example, different criteria can lead to different decisions.[5] If the number of important factors is not clear-cut, it may be advisable to inspect more than one rotated factor matrix (which we discuss in the next section) to determine which solution is most sensible. However, it is usually advisable to begin with too many rather than too few factors, and to then "prune" if necessary. For example, if only one variable loads highly on the last factor, that factor would appear to be poorly defined.

FACTOR ROTATION

Regardless of which factor extraction method is used, and regardless of how many factors are extracted, the resulting factor matrix is likely to be very difficult to interpret. For that reason, factor analysis almost always involves a factor rotation phase that helps the re-

---

[5]Significance testing for factors does exist, but there is some controversy regarding the use of such tests (Gorsuch, 1983).

searcher to better understand the meaning of the underlying factors. Factor rotation is performed for those factors that have met an acceptable inclusion criteria, as just described.

Factor rotation is *not* used to improve the quality of the mathematical fit between the variables and the factors. Rotated factors are mathematically equivalent to unrotated ones. Although the factor loadings change after rotation, the communalities and percentage of variance explained remain the same. The objective with rotation is purely to improve the scientific utility of the analysis.

The Principle of Factor Rotation

Factor rotation is a conceptually complex process that can most readily be explained graphically for the situation in which there is a two-factor structure. We will use our earlier example of the six aptitude tests that yielded two factors—which we identified as verbal aptitude and quantitative aptitude—to illustrate factor rotation.

Figure 12–2 (A) presents a graph whose axes are labeled *Y* and *X*. These axes represent Factors I and II, respectively, as they are defined prior to factor rotation. The six dots in this two-dimensional space represent tests A through F. The unrotated factor loadings on the two factors can be read from the appropriate axis. Thus, for example,

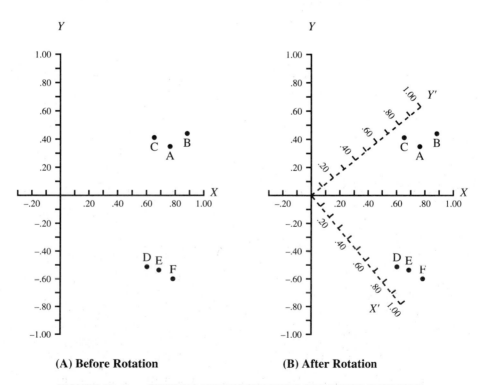

(A) Before Rotation   (B) After Rotation

FIGURE 12–2.   GRAPHIC REPRESENTATION OF FACTOR ROTATION

test A has a loading of about .38 on Factor I (the Y axis) and a loading of about .79 on Factor II (the X axis). As another example, test D has a loading of about $-.50$ on Factor I and .60 on Factor II. In this unrotated factor space, all six tests have high loadings (absolute values above .30) on both factors, making it difficult to identify their underlying dimensionality.

However, when the axes are rotated in such a way that the two variable clusters (A, B, and C versus D, E, and F) align more clearly with the reference axes, the interpretability of the factors is greatly simplified. Figure 12–2 (B) shows the two axes—labeled X' and Y'—after rotation. With the axes turned, the factor loadings are different than they were prior to rotation. The loadings on the rotated factors are the same as those shown in Table 12–1. For example, test A has a loading of .84 on Factor I after rotation, and a loading of .21 on Factor II. As a result of the rotation, tests A, B, and C are aligned with Factor I but not with Factor II, while tests D, E, and F are clustered close to the axis for Factor II but not with that for Factor I. Now, by examining what tests A, B, and C have in common, and what tests D, E, and F have in common, we can determine the meaning of the factors.

The goal in rotating factors is to achieve factors that are as pure as possible. That is, we want a rotation solution such that variables have high loadings on one and only one factor; we also want loadings as close to.1.00 (or -1.00) as possible for the variables aligned with a factor, and loadings as close to 0.00 as possible for variables not aligned with that factor. Ideal factor solutions are difficult to achieve in reality.

Methods of Factor Rotation

Just as there are multiple methods of factor extraction, so too there are multiple methods of factor rotation. The methods fall into two major groupings—orthogonal rotation and oblique rotation.

Orthogonal rotation results in factors that are uncorrelated with one another. During factor extraction, the factors are necessarily orthogonal because each new linear combination is formed such that it is uncorrelated with previously created factors. When factors are orthogonal they are at right angles—they are independent of one another. In Figure 12–2 (A), for example, the unrotated factors are orthogonal. This orthogonality was maintained during rotation, as shown in Figure 12–2 (B).

Oblique rotation, by contrast, results in factors that are correlated with one another. Oblique rotation allows the axes in the rotated factor space to depart from a 90° angle, thereby permitting the variables to more closely align themselves with factors. Figure 12–3 illustrates how an oblique rotation might look for the six aptitude tests. The X' and Y' axes are at an acute angle because they are allowed to pass more closely to the two clusters of variables. Tests A, B, and C now have higher loadings on Factor I but lower loadings on Factor II than they did with orthogonal rotation. Tests D, E, and F now are more closely aligned with Factor II. For example, test F has a loading of about

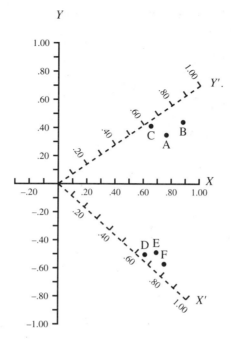

FIGURE 12–3.   OBLIQUE FACTOR ROTATION

.96 on Factor II, but a loading close to zero on Factor I; with orthogonal rotation, the loadings were .91 and .27, respectively.

For those using orthogonal rotation, there are three major types of rotational techniques, which use different statistical criteria for achieving the rotation. The most widely used method of orthogonal rotation is **varimax rotation.** The goal of varimax rotation is to maximize the variance of the loadings within factors, across variables. The varimax method strives to minimize the number of variables that have high loadings on a factor, which facilitates interpretation of the factors. Another method is **quartimax rotation,** which emphasizes the simplification of variables rather than factors. The goal of the quartimax method is to increase the dispersion of the loadings within the variables, across factors. **Equimax rotation** attempts to combine the goals of varimax and quartimax rotation. That is, its goal is to simultaneously simplify factors and variables. In statistical software packages, varimax rotation often is the default—the rotation method used unless there is an explicit instruction to use an alternative.

When oblique rotation is used, the method is usually one called **direct oblimin.** Oblique rotations result in both a **pattern matrix** and a **structure matrix.** A pattern matrix indicates partial regression coefficients, while the structure matrix indicates factor-variable correlations. With orthogonal rotation, the correlations and regression coefficients are identical, and so only one factor matrix is needed to display the results of the rotation. With oblique rotation, the two matrices are not the same because of correlations between factors. The pattern matrix is usually the one used to interpret factors. There is one further product to be considered in oblique rotation: the **factor correlation matrix.** The factor correlation matrix displays the correlation coefficients for each factor with every other factor, much as a correlation matrix.

There is some controversy regarding which rotation approach is preferable. Those who advocate the use of orthogonal rotation claim that it leads to greater theoretical clarity. Moreover, the use of orthogonal rotation makes it easier to compare factor structures across studies. Advocates of oblique rotation point out that in the real world, the underlying dimensions of a construct are, in fact, often correlated. For example, there is a tendency for people who have high scores on verbal aptitude tests to have higher-than-average scores on quantitative aptitude tests. However, oblique rotation sometimes results in peculiarities that are difficult to interpret. One approach is to use oblique rotation first and to inspect the factor correlation matrix. If the correlations are substantial, then orthogonal rotation might not make sense, but if the correlations are more modest (e.g., all under .30), then orthogonal rotation should probably be pursued. In any event, with a good, factorable data matrix, results are often similar regardless of which method of rotation is used.

Interpreting Rotated Factor Matrices

When orthogonal rotation is used, the rotated factor loadings are correlations between the variables and the factors. These loadings, when squared, indicate the amount of variance in a variable that is accounted for by the factor. Clearly, then, the variables with high loadings on a factor are the variables that need to be inspected to help identify the underlying dimension represented by the factor.

Usually, loadings with an absolute value of .30 or greater are considered sufficiently large to attach meaning to them. However, the higher the loading, the better the variable is in capturing the essence of the factor. Loadings in excess of .70 (which means that there is at least 50% overlapping variance between the variable and the factor) are especially desirable for interpretive purposes. Ideally, there will be at least one **marker variable** in each factor. A marker variable is one that is highly correlated with one and only one factor and hence helps to define the nature of the factor. Marker variables tend to be robust—that is, they tend to load on a factor regardless of the method used to extract and rotate factors.

Table 12–3 presents an example of an orthogonally rotated factor matrix for 10 items designed to measure patients' attitudes toward the use of medications. Three factors were extracted and rotated. Four variables (items 2, 5, 7, and 9—whose loadings are underlined in the table) have loadings with absolute values greater than .30 on the first factor. These items seem to capture beliefs about the beneficial effects of medications. For example, the item with the highest loading (.74) is item 5: I've felt better since I

TABLE 12–3. EXAMPLE OF A ROTATED FACTOR MATRIX

Variable	Factor I	Factor II	Factor III
1. Since I started taking medications I feel sleepy.	−.09	.61	.08
2. When I take my medication I feel better.	.63	−.04	−.10
3. I take medication because I am forced to take it.	−.16	.21	.72
4. Sometimes my medication makes me dizzy.	.02	.65	.12
5. I've felt better since I started my medications.	.74	−.06	−.15
6. I get groggy right after taking my medication.	−.04	.50	.19
7. Taking medication makes me feel worse than before.	−.42	.24	.11
8. My medication has been forced on me.	−.07	.03	.59
9. Without my medication, I feel fine.	−.45	.24	.11
10. I only take my medication because I have no choice.	−.13	.06	.48

started my medications. Note that two of the high-loading items directly express the belief that medications are beneficial and have positive loadings (items 2 and 5), while the other two high-loading items express the belief that the medications are *not* helpful and have negative loadings.

There are three variables that have loadings with absolute values greater than .30 on the second factor: items 1, 4, and 6. The main thrust of these items appears to concern the side effects of medication. For example, the item with the highest loading (.65) is item 4: Sometimes my medication makes me dizzy.

Three items have high loadings on the third factor: items 3, 8, and 10. The theme underlying these items concerns coercion and the nonvoluntary nature of medication use. Item 3 has the highest loading (.72): I take medication because I am forced to take it. Thus, although all 10 items express attitudes toward medication, the factor analysis indicates that there are three separate, unitary constructs that need to be considered to fully understand patients' attitudes. All 10 items have high loadings on one (and only one) of the three factors—a highly desirable, but not always attainable, result.

The process is similar for oblique rotation, although the interpretation of the coefficients is less straightforward. The loading in the pattern matrix is not a correlation, but rather an index of the unique relationship between the variable and the factor (i.e., a partial regression coefficient). The coefficients in the structure matrix *are* correlations between variables and factors, but they are inflated by the overlap between the factors. For example, a variable may correlate with one factor *through* its correlation with another related factor, rather than directly. For this reason, the pattern matrix is usually more readily interpretable than the structure matrix.

FACTOR SCORES

Factor scores are the subjects' scores on the abstract dimension defined by a factor. They represent estimates of the scores the subjects would have received if it were possible to measure the constructs directly. Factor scores are often very useful as independent or dependent variables in subsequent analyses, especially if the factors are robust and readily interpretable.

There are a number of alternative procedures for computing factor scores, ranging from highly sophisticated techniques to very simple ones. One relatively simple procedure is to use the factor loadings to weight the individual variables and then add the weighted values together. Let us suppose, for example, that for the 10 items relating to medication attitudes (Table 12–3), respondents answered on a 5-point scale from strongly agree (5) to strongly disagree (1), and that we obtained the following data for our first two subjects:

Item:	1	2	3	4	5	6	7	8	9	10
Subject 1:	2	5	1	4	5	2	2	1	2	3
Subject 2:	5	2	5	5	1	5	4	5	4	4

The factor loadings in Table 12–3 can be used to weight each raw score, through multiplication. Then, separate scores on each of the three factors can be computed by adding the weighted values together. For the first subject, the three factor scores would be as follows:

Factor I: $(-.09)(2) + (.63)(5) + (-.16)(1) + (.02)(4) + (.74)(5) + (-.04)(2)$
$+ (-.42)(2) + (-.07)(1) + (-.45)(2) + (-.13)(3) = \mathbf{4.31}$

Factor II: $(.61)(2) + (-.04)(5) + (.21)(1) + (.65)(4) + (-.06)(5) + (.50)(2)$
$+ (.24)(2) + (.03)(1) + (.24)(2) + (.06)(3) = \mathbf{5.70}$

Factor III: $+ (.08)(2) + (-.10)(5) + (.72)(1) + (.12)(4) + (-.15)(5) + (.19)(2)$
$(.11)(2) + (.59)(1) + (.11)(2) + (.48)(3) = \mathbf{2.96}$

Although we do not show the computations, the factor scores for the second subject would be -3.70, 12.02, and 10.95 for factors I, II, and II, respectively. Thus, the first subject had higher scores than the second subject on the Benefits of Medication factor, but lower scores on the Side Effects and Medication Coercion factors. This scoring method should only be used if all the variables in the analyses are measured on the same scale—or with standard scores for the variables if they are not.

A popular and even simpler method of estimating factor scores is to create scales using only those items with high loadings on the factor. For example, a Benefits of Medication scale would be created by adding together items 2, 5, 7, and 9, with equal weighting for all items. If this method is adopted, attention needs to be paid to the sign of the loadings; items with negative loadings are usually reversed prior to addition to avoid total scores that are negative. **Item reversals** can be accomplished by subtracting a subject's raw score from the maximum possible score value, plus 1. In the first factor, items 7 and 9 had negative loadings, and thus would be reversed by subtracting the sub-jects' original scores from 6. The two subjects' scores on the first factor, using this unit-weighting method, would be:

Subject 1:   5 + 5 + (6 − 2) + (6 − 2) = 18
Subject 2:   2 + 1 + (6 − 4) + (6 − 4) = 7

If this process were also applied to the next two factors, we would find that on the Side Effects scale the subjects' scores would be 10 and 15, and on the Medication Coercion scale their scores would be 5 and 14 for subjects 1 and 2, respectively. This scoring method would lead us to the same conclusion as with the previous one; subject 1 feels that the medications are more beneficial than subject 2, who perceives more side effects and less autonomy in the use of medications than subject 1.

Factor analysis computer programs typically use other, more complex estimation methods for estimating factor scores. The most widely used computer procedure is to use multiple regression to predict factor scores—an approach that results in the highest possible correlation between factors and factor scores.

COMPARISONS AMONG FACTOR ANALYSIS SOLUTIONS

Factor analyses provide information about the underlying structure of the concepts in which we are interested. Often, our research question is addressed by the simple perfor-mance of the factor analysis, but in other situations we might be interested in making comparisons. This section presents a brief overview of some procedures for making fac-tor analytic comparisons.

Types of Factor Comparisons

There are several situations in which researchers may be interested in making compar-isons between the factor analysis solutions from different data matrices. First, a re-searcher may be interested in knowing if the underlying dimensionality of a complex construct is similar for different groups of people. For example, are the health beliefs of men structured similarly to those of women? Are the dimensions of hope similar for can-cer patients and for patients with AIDS? This type of comparison is often done within the context of a single study, by dividing the sample into the groups of interest and then per-forming separate factor analyses for each group. If such a comparison is anticipated, it is important to use a sufficiently large sample to support multiple factor analyses.

A second reason for comparing factor structures involves determining the stability of results from a factor analysis. A researcher might be interesting in knowing whether the factor structure from a previously published study can be replicated with a new sam-ple. Or a researcher might want to perform two factor analyses with random subsamples from a single study to ascertain whether the factor structure can be cross-validated. Both theoretically and methodologically, it is useful to have evidence that a proposed factor structure is a reliable one.

A third reason for a comparative analysis is for testing theory. That is, an obtained factor analysis solution can be compared to a structure hypothesized on the basis of theory. In undertaking such a comparison, the researcher uses theory to predict the number of factors in the solution and to estimate loadings on the factors. These estimates do not need to be very precise. For example, 1s could be used as the hypothesized loadings for variables that are expected to load on a factor, and 0s could be used for other variables in the analysis.

Procedures for Factor Analysis Comparisons

When a goal of the researcher is to compare factor solutions, care should be taken to make the analyses as similar as possible. This means that the same variables should be in the analyses, with comparable rules for coding, missing data, and transformations. The same methods should be used to extract factors and to rotate them, and the criteria for the number of factors to be extracted should also be the same.

Factor analysis comparisons can involve several aspects of the results, and can involve both informal visual inspections or more formal statistical procedures. Several different approaches to making formal comparisons are available and are more fully described in Rummel (1970) and Gorsuch (1983). Here we discuss only the simplest of techniques.

Factor comparisons typically focus on the *configuration* of variables in the factor solution—that is, on the pattern and the magnitude of the loadings in the factor matrix. However, other aspects of the solution may also be important. These include the number of factors, the amount of variance accounted for, the communalities of the variables, and (for oblique rotations) the correlations among the factors.

Informal procedures are sometimes adequate to determine the comparability (or dissimilarity) of factor solutions. Tabachnick and Fidell (1989) suggest that three preliminary questions be answered on the basis of a visual inspection of the two factor analyses before a decision is made to pursue formal procedures: (1) Is the number of factors the same for the two analyses?,(2) Are the variables that load highly on the different factors for the two analyses approximately the same?, and (3) Is it reasonable to use the same descriptive labels to name the factors for both analyses? Statistical comparisons are probably unnecessary if the answers to these three questions are either all negative or all positive. Consider, for example, the two factor analysis results in Table 12–4, which presents hypothetical factor matrices for men and women on the six aptitude tests we used in previous examples. Both solutions yielded two factors, and the pattern of factor loadings is quite similar on both factors (which we would continue to label verbal and quantitative aptitude based on the tests that load on the factors). In this example, statistical procedures are not necessary to conclude that men and women's performance on the six tests is similarly patterned. In many cases, however, the similarities are not so clear-cut.

The simpler statistical procedures typically involve comparisons between pairs of factors (e.g., between Factor I for men and Factor I for women). One relatively easy pro-

TABLE 12–4. FACTOR MATRICES FOR SIX APTITUDE TESTS: MEN VERSUS WOMEN

Tests	MEN Factor		WOMEN Factor	
	I	II	I	II
A	.84	.21	.79	.25
B	.90	.24	.88	.16
C	.74	.13	.61	.31
D	.17	.73	.15	.88
E	.22	.80	.27	.79
F	.27	.91	.19	.81

cedure is to compute a correlation coefficient between the factor loadings for the two sets. In the example in Table 12–4, the correlations between men's and women's loadings are .98 for the first factor and .94 for the second, both of which are substantial. However, this approach can be problematic if there are many variables in the analysis. The correlation coefficient may be artificially high by virtue of many low loadings on the factor in both sets rather than because there are similar high loadings on the factor.

An index known as Cattell's **salient similarity index** (*s*) can be computed to compare patterns of loadings. This index requires the creation of a 3 × 3 contingency table (one dimension for each set) in which tallies are made of the number of positively **salient loadings** (those above some criterion, such as +.30), negatively salient loadings (e.g., those at least −.30), and those that are neither (called the **hyperplane**). In our example, Factor I would yield three loadings that are positively salient for both men and women, and three that are in the hyperplane. This information would be used in a formula to compute the *s* statistic, which would then be compared to a table to determine the statistical significance of the similarity. We will illustrate this procedure in a subsequent section of this chapter.

Researchers are beginning to use a complex modeling procedure referred to as confirmatory factor analysis (CFA) for making factor comparisons. CFA is a promising approach for testing theory and for establishing the construct validity of instruments. CFA is briefly discussed in Chapter 14, but the interested reader should consult Long (1983) for a further description of CFA.

THE COMPUTER AND FACTOR ANALYSIS

This section focuses primarily on a computer printout from a principal components factor analysis with orthogonal rotation. A printout that we use to illustrate factor comparisons is also presented. In both cases, we use data from a sample of women who reacted to a se-

TABLE 12–5. ITEMS USED IN FACTOR ANALYSIS COMPUTER EXAMPLE: CHILDREN'S POSITIVE BEHAVIORS*

Variable Name	Item: MY CHILD. . . .
PBI@A	Is cheerful, happy.
PBI@B	Waits his or her turn in games or other activities.
PBI@C	Is warm, loving.
PBI@D	Is curious and exploring, likes new experiences.
PBI@E	Thinks before he or she acts, is not impulsive.
PBI@G	Usually does what I tell him or her to do.
PBI@I	Is admired and well liked by other children.
PBI@J	Tries to do things for himself or herself, is self-reliant.
PBI@K	Shows concern for other people's feelings.
PBI@L	Can easily find something to do on his or her own.
PBI@O	Is able to concentrate or focus on an activity.
PBI@P	Is helpful and cooperative.
PBI@R	Tends to give, lend, and share.
PBI@S	Is obedient, follows rules.
PBI@T	Is calm, easy-going.
PBI@U	Sticks with an activity until it is finished.
PBI@V	Is eager to please.
PBI@W	Is patient if I am busy and he or she wants something.
PBI@X	Sticks up for himself or herself, is self-assertive.
PBI@Y	Tries to be independent, to do things himself or herself.

*Responses to items were from 0 ("not at all like my child") to 10 ("totally like my child").

ries of items describing desirable behaviors of children. The women were asked to rate the extent to which the item described their child, on a scale from 0 (not at all like my child) to 10 (totally like my child). The 20 items used in the factor analysis are listed in Table 12–5.[6]

Example of a Principal Components Analysis

Figure 12–4 presents the main portions of a printout from a principal components factor analysis based on the responses of 575 women with young children (ages 3 to 7) to the 20 positive behavior items (PBI) concerning their child's behavior.[7] To conserve space,

---

[6]Note that there are gaps in the item list (e.g., there is no item PBI@F) because some items were removed from the data matrix for various reasons (e.g., high amounts of missing data, low variability, and so on) prior to the factor analysis.

[7]The SPSS/PC command used to create this printout is as follows:
    FACTOR VARIABLES = PBI@A TO PBI@E, PBI@G, PBI@I to PBI@L, PBI@O, PBI@P, PBI@R TO PBI@Y
        /PRINT = INITIAL EXTRACTION ROTATION UNIVARIATE CORRELATION
        /FORMAT = SORT.

A Extraction 1 for Analysis 1, Principal-Components Analysis (PC)

Initial Statistics:

Variable	Communality	*	Factor	Eigenvalue	Pct of Var	Cum Pct
PBI@A	1.00000	*	1	8.27840	41.4	41.4
PBI@B	1.00000	*	2	1.64723	8.2	49.6
PBI@C	1.00000	*	3	1.09774	5.5	55.1
PBI@D	1.00000	*	4	.89848	4.5	59.6
PBI@E	1.00000	*	5	.85118	4.3	63.9
PBI@G	1.00000	*	6	.71628	3.6	67.4
PBI@I	1.00000	*	7	.68091	3.4	70.9
PBI@J	1.00000	*	8	.62349	3.1	74.0
PBI@K	1.00000	*	9	.59180	3.0	76.9
PBI@L	1.00000	*	10	.58361	2.9	79.8
PBI@O	1.00000	*	11	.57690	2.9	82.7
PBI@P	1.00000	*	12	.52238	2.6	85.3
PBI@R	1.00000	*	13	.46414	2.3	87.7
PBI@S	1.00000	*	14	.43915	2.2	89.9
PBI@T	1.00000	*	15	.40085	2.0	91.9
PBI@U	1.00000	*	16	.38708	1.9	93.8
PBI@V	1.00000	*	17	.35816	1.8	95.6
PBI@W	1.00000	*	18	.34966	1.7	97.3
PBI@X	1.00000	*	19	.29112	1.5	98.8
PBI@Y	1.00000	*	20	.24143	1.2	100.0

PC Extracted 3 factors.

B Factor Matrix:

	FACTOR 1	FACTOR 2	FACTOR 3
PBI@S	.76940	-.31756	-.01179
PBI@P	.73955	.11471	-.08627
PBI@T	.72401	-.31847	-.15617
PBI@V	.70466	-.14994	.02885
PBI@G	.69768	-.23077	.01716
PBI@I	.69617	.14055	-.12576
PBI@R	.68193	-.07122	-.08713
PBI@K	.65628	.18973	-.12669
PBI@O	.65257	-.08221	.08947
PBI@U	.64620	-.25075	.29232
PBI@C	.64556	.18634	-.46945
PBI@B	.64540	-.24273	-.07138
PBI@A	.63554	.14231	-.35711
PBI@W	.62389	-.37526	.21478
PBI@J	.61003	.52635	.18294
PBI@L	.56362	.25913	.08111
PBI@Y	.56214	.44495	.45746
PBI@E	.53181	-.38016	.12442
PBI@D	.51506	.46612	-.23646
PBI@X	.47729	.25873	.46031

FIGURE 12–4. COMPUTER PRINTOUT OF A PRINCIPAL COMPONENTS FACTOR ANALYSIS WITH ORTHOGONAL ROTATION

C Final Statistics:

Variable	Communality	*	Factor	Eigenvalue	Pct of Var	Cum Pct
		*				
PBI@A	.55170	*	1	8.27840	41.4	41.4
PBI@B	.48055	*	2	1.64723	8.2	49.6
PBI@C	.67185	*	3	1.09774	5.5	55.1
PBI@D	.53846	*				
PBI@E	.44282	*				
PBI@G	.54031	*				
PBI@I	.52023	*				
PBI@J	.68264	*				
PBI@K	.48276	*				
PBI@L	.39140	*				
PBI@O	.44062	*				
PBI@P	.56754	*				
PBI@R	.47769	*				
PBI@S	.69297	*				
PBI@T	.65000	*				
PBI@U	.56590	*				
PBI@V	.51987	*				
PBI@W	.57619	*				
PBI@X	.50664	*				
PBI@Y	.72326	*				

Varimax   Rotation 1, Extraction 1, Analysis 1 - Kaiser Normalization.

D   Varimax converged in   7 iterations.

Rotated Factor Matrix:

	FACTOR 1	FACTOR 2	FACTOR 3
PBI@S	.75864	.31892	.12540
PBI@W	.73352	.05198	.18825
PBI@T	.70363	.39353	.00575
PBI@U	.67577	.06275	.32449
PBI@E	.65734	.06012	.08434
PBI@G	.65292	.29366	.16664
PBI@B	.60989	.32053	.07640
PBI@V	.60381	.32341	.22513
PBI@O	.53028	.27930	.28533
PBI@R	.51429	.42460	.18140
PBI@C	.24766	.77961	.05216
PBI@A	.28955	.67664	.10011
PBI@D	.00059	.65843	.32394
PBI@I	.37140	.54875	.28490
PBI@K	.30917	.54702	.29655
PBI@P	.42626	.53525	.31518
PBI@Y	.16235	.19041	.81280
PBI@J	.09458	.44458	.68996
PBI@X	.23206	.06133	.67009
PBI@L	.23016	.37705	.44301

FIGURE 12–4.   (Continued)

we have omitted the portion of the printout that shows the item means and standard deviations, and the item-to-item correlation matrix.

Panel A, labeled Extraction 1 for Analysis 1, Principal-Components Analysis, shows the initial statistics for the 20 items. This panel is formatted in a similar fashion to Table 12–2, which we discussed earlier. The first two columns list the items in the analysis and show that the communality is 1.00 for every item (as it always must be in a principal components analysis). On the right side of panel A is information on the 20 factors that are extracted in the extraction phase. The first factor has a large eigenvalue (8.27840) and accounts for 41.4% of the variance. The next two factors have eigenvalues of 1.64723 and 1.09774, respectively. All remaining factors have eigenvalues less than 1.00. A scree plot might suggest that only one factor should be used, inasmuch as there is a considerable discontinuity between the first and second factors. However, since the first three factors have eigenvalues greater than 1.00 and all three account for at least 5% of the variance, three factors are used in subsequent phases of the analysis.

The initial, unrotated factor matrix for the three factors is shown in panel B. The first column lists the 20 items, sorted such that the item with the highest loading on the first factor is listed first (PBI@S) and the item with the lowest loading is listed last (PBI@X). This matrix is difficult to interpret. For example, all of the items have reasonably high loadings on the first factor, and most have loadings greater than .30 on two factors.

Panel C shows the "final statistics" for the 20 items and the three factors. First, on the left side of the panel, the communality of each item is specified. As noted earlier, these communalities indicate the proportion of common factor variance for each item. If we squared an item's factor loadings (panel B) and then summed across the three factors, we would have the item's communality. For example, for PBI@S, the communality is:

$$h^2_{PBI@S} = (.76940)^2 + (-.31756)^2 + (-.01179)^2$$
$$h^2_{PBI@S} = .59198 + .10084 + .00014 = .69296$$

Within rounding error, this is the same communality value shown in panel C for PBI@S. The item with the lowest amount of common factor variance is item L, while the item with the highest common factor variance is item Y. Panel C also shows that the three retained factors cumulatively account for 55.1% of the variance in the 20 items.

Panel D presents the rotated factor matrix from a varimax rotation. This panel is formatted to show, in order of descending factor loadings, the items with high loadings on the first factor (PBI@S to PBI@R), then the items with high loadings on the second factor (PBI@C to PBI@P), followed by the items with high loadings on the third factor (PBI@Y to PBI@L). Thus formatted, we can readily identify the items that "belong" to each factor.

Before using the information in panel D to interpret the three factors, we should point out that the loadings in the rotated factor matrix are not the same as the loadings in the original factor matrix. Take, for example, item PBI@C, the first item in the second grouping of items in Panel D. This item's loadings were .646, .186, and −.469 for factors 1 through 3, respectively, before rotation, but the loadings became .248, .780, and .052 after rotation. However, in both cases the squared factor loadings, when totaled, equal the communality:

$$h^2_{PBI@C\text{-unrotated}} = (.646)^2 + (.186)^2 + (-.469)^2 = .672$$
$$h^2_{PBI@C\text{-rotated}} = (.248)^2 + (.780)^2 + (.052)^2 = .672$$

This confirms that rotation does not alter the factors mathematically; the same amount of variance is accounted for before and after rotation, but rotation distributes the common factor variance across the factors in a manner that makes them easier to understand.

Returning to panel D, we see that there are 10 items that have loadings greater than .50 on the first factor. Reviewing the content of these 10 items in Table 12–5, we can see that the recurrent themes concern the child's compliance and self-control (e.g., My child is obedient, follows rules [item S] and My child is patient if I am busy . . . [item W]). We will call this our Compliance Factor. The second factor has six items with high loadings. The content of these six items suggest the child's likability and sensitivity to others (e.g., My child is warm, loving [item C] and My child is admired and well liked by other children [item I]). We label this our Social Competence Factor. Finally, the four items on the third factor suggest a dimension concerned with independence and self-reliance (e.g., My child tries to do things for himself . . . [item J] and My child tries to be independent, to do things for himself or herself [item Y]). We call this dimension the Autonomy Factor.

An inspection of panel D reveals that the three factors are not as "pure" as we might like. Several of the items have loadings above .30 on two factors, and one item (P) has a loading above .30 on all three factors. However, this overlap is not too surprising, given the content of the items. For example, consider item R: My child tends to give, lend, and share. A child who is compliant and self-controlled would likely exhibit such behaviors—as would a child who is socially sensitive. Thus, the underlying constructs that the three factors represent are not totally unique and independent of one another. It might be surmised, then, that we could have used oblique rotation. Although we do not show the printout, the results from an oblique rotation are highly similar to those shown in Figure 12–4; the same variables have high loadings on the same factors, although there are fewer instances in which an item has a loading of .30 on more than one factor. The factor correlation matrix for the oblique rotation indicated the following correlations between factors:

	Factor 1	Factor 2	Factor 3
Factor 2	.44		
Factor 3	.39	.38	

These correlations have two possible interpretations: (1) children with positive behavior on one dimension tend to have positive behavior on the other two dimensions as well, or (2) mothers who see their children in positive terms tend to rate their children highly, regardless of the content of the item.

We have noted that the three dimensions identified in the factor analysis are robust regardless of which rotation method is used. We might also note (although we do not show the printouts) that the three factors are robust with regard to extraction method. Highly similar factors emerge when the other extraction methods available within SPSS/PC are used, and in all cases the three rotated factors account for just over 50% of the variance in the items.

Example of a Cross-Validation Factor Analysis

A total sample of 1151 women rated their children on the positive behavior items described in the previous section, only half of whom ($N = 575$) were used in the initial factor analysis as described. A second factor analysis was performed using the remaining 576 cases; the two subsamples were divided in half at random. In this section we present a portion of the printout from the cross-validation analysis. In performing the cross-validation, care was taken to use the same decision rules. For example, no cases with missing data were allowed in either analysis; the principal components method and varimax rotation methods were used in both cases; and a minimum eigenvalue of 1.0 was used as the criterion for rotating factors.

Figure 12–5 presents the two main panels of interest from the cross-validation analysis. We have labeled them panels C and D to match the corresponding panels in Figure 12–4. Panel C indicates that the crossvalidation analysis also yielded three factors, and that the first factor was quite sizable, accounting for about 41% of the variance in both analyses. The cumulative amount of variance extracted by these three factors was 55.1% for the initial analysis and 54.3% for the cross-validation analysis. We can also see considerable consistency in the item's communalities across the two analyses. In both cases, for example, the item with the highest amount of common factor variance is item Y.

Panel D of Figure 12–5 presents the rotated factor matrix for the cross-validation sample. For the most part, the rotated factor matrix is highly similar to that for the initial sample. For example, items S, W, and T have especially high loadings on the first factor, items C and D clearly load on the second factor, and items Y and J load on the third factor in both analyses. We can readily label the three factors in the cross-validation analysis Compliance, Social Competence, and Autonomy. There is only one difference of note in Figure 12–5: item P, which loaded more highly on factor 2 than on factor 1 initially, is now more clearly associated with factor 1 in the cross-validation. In both analyses, however, item P straddled all three factors. This item (My child is helpful and cooperative) does suggest overlapping constructs; a helpful child is sensitive to others'

C   Final Statistics:

Variable	Communality	*	Factor	Eigenvalue	Pct of Var	Cum Pct
		*				
PBI@A	.48001	*	1	8.09053	40.5	40.5
PBI@B	.51466	*	2	1.64740	8.2	48.7
PBI@C	.54471	*	3	1.13052	5.7	54.3
PBI@D	.50562	*				
PBI@E	.40078	*				
PBI@G	.51204	*				
PBI@I	.55664	*				
PBI@J	.67385	*				
PBI@K	.42564	*				
PBI@L	.42163	*				
PBI@O	.47392	*				
PBI@P	.57317	*				
PBI@R	.48738	*				
PBI@S	.68853	*				
PBI@T	.65869	*				
PBI@U	.65031	*				
PBI@V	.45290	*				
PBI@W	.58101	*				
PBI@X	.51762	*				
PBI@Y	.74935	*				

Varimax   Rotation 1, Extraction 1, Analysis 1 - Kaiser Normalization.

D   Varimax converged in   6 iterations.

Rotated Factor Matrix:

	FACTOR 1	FACTOR 2	FACTOR 3
PBI@T	.76974	.19813	.16410
PBI@S	.76769	.25143	.18964
PBI@W	.74272	-.04049	.16653
PBI@U	.71695	.09663	.35630
PBI@G	.67845	.20109	.10632
PBI@E	.58081	.24416	.06190
PBI@B	.56476	.44194	.01996
PBI@V	.53484	.35715	.19821
PBI@O	.52694	.24825	.36692
PBI@R	.48153	.45234	.22561
PBI@P	.45957	.42960	.42121
PBI@D	-.01031	.67964	.20881
PBI@C	.29050	.67062	.10289
PBI@I	.27634	.65826	.21672
PBI@A	.15902	.63678	.22189
PBI@K	.36785	.48794	.22856
PBI@Y	.16900	.21521	.82126
PBI@J	.08217	.35921	.73353
PBI@X	.21403	.07854	.68238
PBI@L	.29345	.31533	.48589

FIGURE 12–5. COMPUTER PRINTOUT OF FACTOR ANALYSIS FOR CROSS-VALIDATION SUBSAMPLE

necds, is likely to be obedient and controlled, and—in terms of the third factor—may be self-reliant and thus less personally in need of help from others.

Visual inspection strongly suggests, then, that the factor structures for the two factor analyses are highly similar.[8] We can determine the similarity more precisely through further analysis. First, we can calculate correlation coefficients between the loadings for the two sets of three factors. When we do this we find the following:

		Initial Analysis		
		Factor 1	Factor 2	Factor 3
	Factor 1:	.97		
Cross-validation	Factor 2:		.91	
	Factor 3:			.95

The correlations between the two sets of loadings are high for all three factors, further corroborating the similarity of the factor structures.

We can also use Cattell's salient similarity index to ascertain the probability that the factors from the two analyses are similar. We use in this example a very strict criterion for salience: .50. Table 12–6 illustrates how the statistic is computed, using Factor 2 from the two analyses as an example. The table shows the crosstabulation of positively salient, hyperplane, and negatively salient items from the initial and cross-validation analyses. Each cell is labeled. For example, cell 1 (C1) is for items that were positively salient (items with loadings above .50) in both analyses; cell 4 (C4) is for items that were positively salient in the initial analysis but that were in the hyperplane in the cross-validation. Each item is allocated to one of the nine cells. Then, the following formula is used to compute s:

$$s = \frac{C1 + C9 - C3 - C7}{C1 + C9 + C3 + C7 + .5\,(C2 + C4 + C6 + C8)}$$

where each element in the formula is the number of items in the designated cell.

In our example, we find that item S has a loading of .32 on Factor 2 in the initial analysis (Figure 12–4), and a loading of .25 on Factor 2 in the cross-validation (Figure 12–5). Thus, item S is allocated to cell 5 (hyperplane for both analyses). Using this system, five items (C, A, D, I, and K) are in allocated to cell 1, one item is in cell 4, and the remaining 14 items are in cell 5, as shown in Table 12–6. We can now compute s for comparing the similarity of Factor 2 in the two analyses:

$$s = \frac{5 + 0 - 0 - 0}{5 + 0 + 0 + 0 + .5\,(0 + 1 + 0 + 0)} = .91$$

---

[8]Similar structures were also obtained when oblique rotation was used with both subsamples. The pattern of factor correlations was also similar, with all correlations between factors in the vicinity of .40 for both the initial and cross-validation samples.

TABLE 12–6. CATTELL'S SALIENT SIMILARITY INDEX (s): COMPARISON OF FACTOR 2 FROM INITIAL AND CROSS-VALIDATION ANALYSES

		Initial		
		Positively Salient ($\geq$.50)	Hyperplane ($> -.50, <.50$)	Negatively Salient ($\leq-.50$)
Cross-Validation	Positively Salient	C1 C A D I K	C2	C3
	Hyperplane	C4 P	C5 S W T U E G B V O R Y J X L	C6
	Negatively Salient	C7	C8	C9

To determine the significance of s, we consult a table[9] that takes into account the number of variables in the analysis, and the percentage of cases in cell 5. With 20 variables and 70% of the cases in cell 5 (i.e., $14 \div 20 = 70\%$), the table informs us that $p = .000$ when $s = .63$. Since our computed value of $s = .91$, there is a very high probability (i.e., $p < .0005$) that the two factors are similar, even though a very strict criterion for salience was used.

RESEARCH APPLICATIONS OF FACTOR ANALYSIS

Factor analysis, once considered a sophisticated technique used primarily by highly experienced investigators, has come to be a standard analytic tool used by many researchers. This section discusses the major applications of factor analysis and discusses methods of reporting factor analytic results.

The Uses of Factor Analysis

Factor analysis is used as an important methodological and substantive tool by researchers. Although factor analysis requires researchers to make many decisions and involves some subjectivity in the decision-making and factor interpretation process, it represents an important avenue for understanding quantitatively measured constructs.

---

[9]We do not include the relevant tables in Appendix B. The reader can consult Fidell and Tabachnick (1989), Table C.7, or Cattell et al. (1969).

1. *Data Reduction.* If a researcher has multiple measures of key variables (often the dependent variables), factor analysis is a convenient way to streamline the primary analyses. For example, suppose that we wanted to compare children with minimal brain dysfunction and children without this disorder in terms of their social behavior. If we administered the 20 "positive behavior" items that we used to illustrate printouts of factor analyses (Table 12–5), the 20 items could be used as dependent variables in a series of 20 *t*-tests (or in a complex MANOVA). However, by computing factor scores for the three factors that emerged in the factor analysis, a much cleaner, more efficient, and probably more comprehensible analysis would result.

2. *Instrument Development.* One of the primary applications of factor analysis is in the development of instruments to measure constructs of interest to researchers. Researchers often begin with a large pool of items that are derived on the basis of theory, adaptations from other instruments, or in-depth, qualitative interviews. The item pool is then administered to a sample of subjects and the responses are factor analyzed to determine which items should be discarded and which should be used to create summated scales. After appropriate psychometric analyses are performed, the scales are generally used by other researchers in subsequent investigations of the factor analytic constructs.

3. *Instrument Validation.* Factor analysis is also used to validate previously developed instruments. This often involves factor analytic comparisons—for example, the cross-validation of a factor structure in a replication study or a confirmatory study to ascertain that the factor structure of an instrument is appropriate for different groups than the group used to develop the instrument. Factor analysis has come to be used frequently as a method of construct validation.

4. *Theory Development and Theory Testing.* Factor analysis can play an important role in the development and evolution of theory. When an area of inquiry is new, factor analysis can contribute to the conceptualization of underlying dimensions of a construct. Factor analysis can be used to describe phenomena of interest, to disentangle complex relationships among interrelated variables, and to examine the adequacy of a researcher's preliminary conceptualizations—all of which are integral to theory development.

The Presentation of Factor Analysis in Research Reports

When reporting the results of a factor analysis, the researcher must pay careful attention to communicating not only the results of the analysis, but also the various analytic decisions that produced the results. The following aspects of the analytic procedures usually should be documented in the text of the report:

- Variables in the analysis
- Number of cases in the analysis
- Any limitations that might exist and how they were addressed (outliers, missing data problems, low intervariable correlations)

- Method used to extract factors (and a rationale if an unusual method was used)
- Criteria used to determine the number of factors
- Method used to rotate factors (and a rationale for that decision)
- Minimum value of loadings used to interpret factors
- Method used to create factor scores, if applicable
- Method used to compare factor structures, if applicable

Tables are usually used to summarize the results of factor analyses. The tables typically indicate the variables, number of cases in the analysis, number of factors, factor loadings, eigenvalues, and percentages of variance explained by each factor. Some researchers also present the communalities.

Table 12–7 presents a table that could be used to present the results of the factor analysis of the 20 positive behavior items (i.e., from the computer printout shown in

TABLE 12–7. EXAMPLE OF A FACTOR ANALYSIS TABLE FOR A REPORT

Variable: My child. . .	Factor Loadings			Communality
	1	2	3	
Is obedient, follows rules	**.76**	.32	.13	.69
Is patient if I am busy	**.73**	.05	.19	.58
Is calm, easy-going	**.70**	.39	.01	.65
Sticks with an activity	**.68**	.06	.32	.57
Is not impulsive	**.66**	.06	.08	.44
Does what I tell him/her	**.65**	.29	.17	.54
Waits his/her turn	**.61**	.32	.08	.48
Is eager to please	**.60**	.32	.23	.52
Is able to concentrate	**.53**	.28	.29	.44
Tends to give, lend, share	**.51**	.42	.18	.48
Is warm, loving	.25	**.78**	.05	.67
Is cheerful, happy	.29	**.68**	.10	.55
Is curious, exploring	.00	**.66**	.32	.54
Is well liked by children	.37	**.55**	.28	.52
Shows concern for others	.31	**.55**	.30	.48
Is helpful, cooperative	.43	**.54**	.32	.57
Tries to be independent	.16	.19	**.81**	.72
Is self-reliant	.09	.44	**.69**	.68
Is self-assertive	.23	.06	**.67**	.51
Can find things to do on own	.23	.38	**.44**	.39
Eigenvalue	8.28	1.65	1.10	
% of Variance Explained	41.4	8.2	5.5	

Rotated Factor Matrix for Principal Components Analysis of Positive Behavior Items (N = 575)

Figure 12–4). This table lists all 20 items, shown in abbreviated form to conserve space. Variables are listed in the order that facilitates interpretation of the factors, not in the order the items were presented to respondents. All of the loadings from the computer printout are presented, to two decimal places. Most tables use a convention to highlight the important loadings. Here, we have put in bold print those loadings that are greater than .40. Some authors underline or italicize the important loadings (as in Table 12–3), others completely omit loadings below a cutoff value, and still others use boxes to surround a cluster of variables loading highly on a factor. The point is to use a method that will help the reader to understand the basis for interpreting the factor.

The text is used to highlight the important features of the table, and then to offer the researcher's interpretation of the factors. Here is an illustration of how the results from this factor analysis might be presented in the text:

> The 20 positive behavior items were factor analyzed with a sample of 575 mothers, using the principal components method of factor extraction. Using a minimum eigenvalue of 1.0 as the criterion for factors, three factors that accounted for a total of 55.1% of the variance were extracted. The factors were orthogonally rotated using the varimax procedure, and the results are presented in Table 12–7. (Oblique rotation yielded virtually identical results and thus orthogonal rotation was retained because of conceptual simplicity and ease of description.) The items are ordered and blocked by size of loading to facilitate interpretation of the factor matrix.
>
> Overall, the factor structure that emerged was reasonably clear and interpretable. The first factor, which accounted for 41.4% of the variance, had 12 items with loadings above the cutoff of .40. This factor appears to capture the child's ability to be disciplined, self-controlled, and obedient; this factor is called the Compliance Factor. Eleven of the 12 items had loadings in excess of .50 on the factor; only two (My child tends to give, lend, and share, and My child is helpful, cooperative) also had high loadings on another factor.
>
> The second factor had eight items with loadings above .40, and six of these items loaded most distinctly on Factor 2. The theme of this factor involves the child's social interactions—his or her tendency to show warmth and concern for other people. This factor has been labeled the Social Competence Factor.
>
> Four items had high loadings on the third factor. Although this factor accounted for only 5.5% of the variance, it was relatively well defined, with a clear-cut marker variable that had a loading of .81 on the factor. This factor captures a dimension of independence and self-reliance, and has been named the Autonomy Factor.
>
> For subsequent analysis, factor scores were created by summing together the items most clearly associated with the factors, with unit weighting. Thus, the sum of responses to the first block of 11 items formed the scores on the Compliance Factor (alpha reliability = .88); the second block of 6 items was used to compute scores on the Social Competence Factor (alpha = .86); and the third block of four items was used to compute scores on the Autonomy Factor (alpha − .76).

RESEARCH EXAMPLE

Detailed results from a factor analysis are most likely to be reported in the context of a methodological study focused on instrument development or instrument validation. For example, Algase and Beel-Bates (1993) presented factor analysis results from a study designed to develop a new screening scale to identify everyday indicators of impaired cognition. As another example, Lowe (1993) summarized factor analysis results in her project to develop and validate the Childbirth Self-Efficacy Inventory. Here we summarize the results from a study in which factor analysis was used primarily as a data reduction tool.

Kocher and Thomas (1994) used survey data from a random sample of 158 female junior nurse-officers in the Army to examine the factors that might explain the nurses' turnover behavior. The dependent variable in their analysis was nurse retention—whether or not nurses remained on active duty 3 years after the survey was completed. The predictor variables available for the analysis included a range of demographic characteristics (e.g., race/ethnicity, age, marital status), as well as 10 items relating to the nurses' satisfaction with various aspects of their jobs.

The 10 job satisfaction items were factor analyzed "to minimize multicollinearity and for purposes of parsimony" (p. 62). The principal factors method was used to extract factors, and varimax was used as the rotation method.

The results of the factor analysis are presented in Table 12–8, which is an adaptation of the report's Table 1. This table indicates that the 10 job satisfaction items could be reduced to four factors, which are labeled in the left-hand column. The first factor, labeled Work/military life, consists of three items that describe various aspects of the nurses' work and working conditions. The second factor, labeled Location/assignment stability, involves two items that relate to Army reassignments. The third factor, called Advancement opportunities, involves three items (promotions, job training, job security). The fourth factor is called Economic benefits. This factor falls just short of achieving an eigenvalue of 1.0 (i.e., .95), but is nevertheless interpretable, consisting of

TABLE 12–8. FACTOR ANALYSIS OF NURSE JOB SATISFACTION ITEMS

Composite Dimension and Item	Factor Loadings				Communality
	F1	F2	F3	F4	
Work/Military Life					
Current job	**.84**	.17	.26	.03	.80
Personal freedom	**.68**	.14	.09	.15	.51
Work conditions	**.67**	.01	.36	.10	.58
Location/assignment stability					
Reassignment policy	.01	**.86**	.01	.05	.74
Frequency of moves	.24	**.73**	.16	−.04	.62
Advancement opportunities					
Promotions	.29	.36	**.70**	.18	.75
Job training	.41	.04	**.58**	−.02	.57
Job security	.17	.04	**.46**	.10	.25
Economic benefits					
Pay	.21	.09	.06	**.84**	.76
Retirement	−.02	−.08	.34	**.41**	.29
Eigenvalues	2.05	1.47	1.39	.95	5.86

Notes: Extraction of factors by principal factors with varimax rotation (N = 158). Level of satisfaction with items reported from 1 = very satisfied to 5 = very dissatisfied.

Adapted from Table 1 of Kocher & Thomas' (1994) report.

two items that have an economic theme. The communality values for most items are high, and the pattern of loadings is fairly clear-cut. Each factor has a variable that can be described as a marker variable, and overlap among the factors (i.e., high loadings on more than one factor) is minimal. The factor analysis appears to have been successful in delineating the major dimensions of nurses' job satisfaction.

Factor scores on the four factors were used in an analysis designed to predict retention of Army nurses. The results revealed that two of the satisfaction dimensions (satisfaction with work/military life and satisfaction with location/assignment stability) were significant predictors of retention of nurses in the Army.

SUMMARY

Factor analysis is a statistical technique used to determine the underlying structure and dimensionality of a set of variables. By analyzing the intercorrelations among variables, factor analysis determines which variables cluster together to form unidimensional constructs.

Mathematically, factor analysis creates **factors** that are linear combinations of variables. Factor analysis begins with **factor extraction,** which involves the extraction of as much variance as possible through the successive creation of linear combinations that are orthogonal to previously created combinations. A widely used factor extraction procedure is the **principal components method,** an approach that analyzes *all* variance in the variables. Other methods of factor extraction, which analyze **common factor variance** (i.e., variance that is shared with other variables), include the **principal factors method,** the **alpha method,** and the **maximum likelihood method.**

Various criteria can be used to determine how many factors account for a reliable amount of variance in the data set. One criterion is to use only factors with an **eigenvalue** equal to 1.0 or greater. An eigenvalue is a standardized index of the amount of variance each factor extracts. Another approach is to use a **scree test** to identify sharp discontinuities in the eigenvalues for successive factors.

Factor extraction results in a **factor matrix** that indicates, through the **factor loadings,** the relationship between original variables and the factors. The factor loadings, when squared, indicate the proportion of variance accounted for in the variable by the factor. Across the factors, the sum of the squared loadings for the variable indicate the variable's **communality** (shared variance). The sum of a factor's squared loadings for all variables indicates the factor's eigenvalue.

Since the initial factor matrix is usually difficult to interpret, most factor analyses involve a **factor rotation** phase. Factor rotation moves the reference axes within the factor space such that variables more clearly align with a single factor. **Orthogonal rotation** keeps the reference axes at right angles and results in factors that are uncorrelated. Orthogonal rotation is usually performed through a method known as **varimax,** but other methods (**quartimax** and **equimax**) are also available. The product of an orthogonal rotation is a **rotated factor matrix. Oblique rotation** allows the reference axes to rotate into acute or oblique angles, thereby resulting in correlated factors. When oblique rotation is used, there are two resulting matrices: a **pattern matrix** that indicates partial regression coefficients between variables and factors, and a **structure matrix** that indicates variable-factor correlations.

Factors are interpreted by examining the pattern and magnitude of the factor loadings in the rotated factor matrix (orthogonal rotation) or pattern matrix (oblique rotation). Ideally, there are one or more **marker variables**—variables with a very high loading on one and only one factor. Generally, loadings of .30 and higher are sufficiently large to be meaningful. Once a factor is interpreted and labeled, researchers usually create **factor scores,** which are scores on the abstract dimension defined by the factor.

Researchers sometimes want to make comparisons between two factor analytic solutions. Although comparisons are often done by visual inspection of the results, formal statistical procedures (such as the computation of Cattell's **salient similarity index** and the use of **confirmatory factor analysis**) are available.

EXERCISES

The following exercises cover concepts presented in this chapter. Exercises indicated with a dagger (†) can be checked against answers appearing in Appendix A. Additionally, Chapter 12 of the accompanying *Applications Manual* offers supplementary exercises, including ones that require computer analysis of a data set on diskette.

† 1. What are the eigenvalues for the three factors displayed in Table 12–3? Assuming the principal components methods was used to extract the factors, what percentage of variance does each factor account for? What is the *total* (cumulative) percentage of variance accounted for by the three factors?

† 2. What are the communalities for the 10 variables displayed in Table 12–3?

† 3. Suppose that a seventh test (Test G) was added to the factor analysis graphed in Figure 12–2. This test has the following coordinates on the unrotated axes: Y $(-.40)$, X $(.45)$. Plot this test on graph (B) of this figure. What would the coordinates be on the new (rotated) reference axes? Is it more likely that Test G is a measure of verbal aptitude (Factor I) or of quantitative aptitude (Factor II)?

† 4. The following are scores for two subjects on Tests A through F (Table 12–1). Compute factor scores for both subjects on both factors, weighting each score by the appropriate factor loading:

	Subject 1	Subject 2
Test A	115	82
Test B	109	80
Test C	120	90
Test D	90	89
Test E	100	91
Test F	97	86

† 5. In the factor analysis presented in Table 12–8, what is the total percentage of variance (of the 10 satisfaction items) accounted for by the four factors? How much variance would have been accounted for cumulatively if the fourth factor had not been retained?

Discriminant Analysis and Logistic Regression

The majority of multivariate techniques we have discussed thus far involve analyses in which the dependent variable is measured on an interval- or ratio-level scale. Examples include multiple regression, analysis of covariance, MANOVA, and MANCOVA. This chapter reviews two techniques that are used when there are multiple independent variables and a categorical dependent variable—discriminant analysis and logistic regression.[1]

DISCRIMINANT ANALYSIS

Discriminant analysis (sometimes referred to as **discriminant function analysis**) is a multivariate technique that has much in common with other multivariate procedures we have examined. Discriminant analysis uses a least-squared criterion for analyzing relationships among variables. Like multiple regression, discriminant analysis involves the development of a predictive equation that is a linear combination of the predictors in the analysis. However, in discriminant analysis, the dependent variable is a categorical index of *group membership*. For example, we could use discriminant analysis to predict compliant versus noncompliant diabetics, cancer patients who survive versus those who die within 5 years of diagnosis, and infants who do versus those who do not develop sudden infant death syndrome. Discriminant analysis is thus like MANOVA turned around[2]; in MANOVA the independent variable is group membership (e.g., experimen-

---

[1]Another statistical technique that can be used to analyze relationships between multiple independent variables and a dichotomous dependent variable is **probit analysis.** This technique is not frequently used by nurse researchers and so is not described here. In most cases, probit analysis results are similar to logistic regression results.

[2]Mathematically, MANOVA and discriminant analysis are the same. In both, the major question is whether a linear combination of variables is reliably associated with group differences.

tal versus control) with multiple dependent variables. However, discriminant analysis also has some similarities with factor analysis and canonical analysis. When there are more than two groups, separate linear combinations—called **discriminant functions**—are formed to maximally separate the groups, and the loadings on the discriminant functions can be used to interpret the dimensionality that separates the groups. Given the overlap between discriminant analysis and other multivariate techniques we have already discussed, we present only a brief overview of this technique.

Basic Concepts for Discriminant Analysis

In Chapter 10 we illustrated multiple regression with an example in which we wanted to predict graduate nursing students' grade point average on the basis of GRE scores, undergraduate grades, and scores on a motivation scale. Suppose that instead of predicting graduate GPA we wanted to predict whether or not the student would complete graduate training and receive a graduate degree. Some fictitious data are shown in Table 13–1, which is identical to Table 10–1 except for the data in the last column (the dependent variable). According to this table, 8 of the 20 students who entered the graduate program did not finish it (code 0), while 12 earned a graduate degree (code 1). Discriminant analysis can be used to determine whether students who finished the program can be reliably discriminated from those who did not on the basis of the four predictor variables.

Discriminant Equations

Discriminant analysis forms a linear combination of the independent variables to predict group membership. The linear discriminant equation is similar to the multiple linear regression equation. In unstandardized form, the equation is:

$$D = a + b_1X_1 + b_2X_2 + . . .+ b_kX_k$$

where D = predicted discriminant score
     a = intercept constant
     k = number of independent variables
     b_1 to b_k = discriminant coefficients for the k predictor variables
     X_1 to X_k = values on the k predictor variables

The discriminant analysis solves for the values of a and b so as to maximize the separation of the groups, using the least-squares criterion. The **discriminant scores** (D scores) are such that the ratio of the between-group sum of squares to the within-group sum of squares is a maximum. Although we do not show the actual calculations, the discriminant equation for the data shown in Table 13–1 is:

$$D = -13.414 + 1.584(X_1) + .010(X_2) - .007(X_3) + .094(X_4)$$

TABLE 13–1. FICTITIOUS DATA FOR DISCRIMINANT ANALYSIS EXAMPLE

| Subject | Independent Variables | | | | Dependent Variable |
	Undergrad GPA X_1	GRE-Verbal X_2	GRE-Quant X_3	Motivation X_4	Finished Grad School Y 1 = yes 0 = no
1	3.4	600	540	75	1
2	3.1	510	480	70	1
3	3.7	650	710	85	1
4	3.2	530	450	60	0
5	3.5	610	500	90	1
6	2.9	540	620	60	0
7	3.3	530	510	75	1
8	2.9	540	600	55	0
9	3.4	550	580	75	0
10	3.2	700	630	65	1
11	3.7	630	700	80	1
12	3.0	480	490	75	1
13	3.1	530	520	60	0
14	3.7	580	610	65	1
15	3.9	710	660	80	1
16	3.5	500	480	75	1
17	3.1	490	510	60	0
18	2.9	560	540	55	0
19	3.2	550	590	65	0
20	3.4	600	550	70	1

Based on this equation, D scores could be computed for each case in Table 13–1. For example, the D score for case 1 would be 1.26 and the D score for case 4 would be $-.53$.

As in multiple regression, the discriminant equation can also be standardized, providing a better means for comparing the relative contribution of the predictors. In standardized form, all predictor variables have a mean of 0 and an SD of 1. The equation for the data in Table 13–1 in standardized form is:

$$D = .38(z_{x1}) + .56(z_{x2}) - .57(z_{x3}) + .71(z_{x4})$$

We can now readily see from the standardized coefficient values that the motivation scores (X_4) contribute especially heavily to the discrimination of the two groups (completers and noncompleters) in this particular sample. However, as in multiple regression, caution must be used in interpreting the coefficients since the predictor variables are correlated.

The mean of the discriminant scores for a function over all cases is 0, and the *SD* is 1. Since we can compute a *D* score for each individual case, we can also compute a mean value of *D* for each group. The group mean, usually called the **centroid,** indicates the distance of the group in *SD* units from the overall mean of 0 on the discriminant function. In our example, the centroid for the noncompleters is -1.42, while that for the completers is .95.

When the dependent variable involves more than two groups, there is more than one discriminant function, and each has a separate equation for predicting discriminant scores. *The number of discriminant functions is either the number of groups minus 1 or the number of predictor variables, whichever is smaller.* For example, suppose that we wanted to use the predictors in Table 13–1 to predict whether a graduate student would earn a degree, voluntarily drop out of the program, or "flunk out." In this case, there would be two discriminant functions (i.e., three groups minus 1). When more than one discriminant function is derived, the first function extracts the maximum amount of variance possible. The second function has the second highest ratio of between-group to within-group sums of squares, but is subject to the constraint that it must be uncorrelated with the first function.

Classification in Discriminant Analysis

Based on the discriminant scores, it is possible to use statistical criteria for classifying cases into groups. When the classification process is done for the subjects in the original sample, the percentage of correct classifications versus misclassifications can be determined by comparing actual group membership with projected group membership for each case. If the classification process is successful (i.e., a high percentage of correct classifications), the discriminant function equation can then be used to classify new cases for which group membership is unknown. In our example, nursing school administrators might want to use the four predictor variables to predict which applicants would not complete the program.

As part of the classification process, a classification equation is developed for each group.[3] Then the raw data for a case are inserted into each equation, and this yields that case's classification probability for each group. The case is assigned to the group for which it has the highest classification probability. The researcher can adjust the classification probabilities based on knowledge of the groups' relative proportions in the population. For example, if we knew that 25% of the graduate students failed to complete the program (despite the fact that in our sample 40% were noncompleters), the classification could be adjusted to take this information into account by the establishment of a **prior probability.**

Computer programs for discriminant analysis can be instructed to list classification information for each case in the sample, but it is usually sufficient simply to examine the summary table. The summary classification table for the data in Table 13–1 is presented

---

[3]If there are only two groups, discriminant scores can be used directly to classify cases into groups; a case is classified into one group if his or her *D* score is above zero, and into the other group if the *D* score is below zero.

TABLE 13-2. SUMMARY CLASSIFICATION TABLE FOR GRADUATE STUDENT EXAMPLE*

		Predicted Group Membership	
Actual Group Membership	N	0 = Did Not Finish	1 = Finished
0 Did Not Finish	8	7 (87.5%)	1 (12.5%)
1 Finished	12	1 (8.3%)	11 (91.7%)

*Overall rate of successful classification = 90.0% (18 ÷ 20).

in Table 13–2. This table shows that of the eight students who actually did not finish the graduate school program, seven (87.5%) were correctly classified, but one (12.5%) was misclassified as finishing the program. Among the 12 students who actually *did* finish their graduate program, 1 (8.3%) was misclassified as a noncompleter but 11 (91.7%) were correctly classified. Altogether then, 18 of the 20 students (90.0% of the sample) were correctly classified on the basis of the discriminant function.

To be useful, the classification should be substantially better than what could be achieved by chance alone. In the example in Table 13–2, the classification was performed without specifying any prior probability, and so the classification proceeded under an assumption of equal probability for membership in the two groups (i.e., a 50-50 chance of being assigned to either group). The obtained 90% correct classification rate is much greater than the chance probability of 50%.[4]

Classification rates are generally higher in the sample used to generate the discriminant function than in other samples from the same population, and so the percentage of correctly classified cases is usually an inflated estimate of actual performance in the population. Cross-validation of the discriminant function is highly recommended, and can be achieved within a single sample—by dividing it in half—if the sample is sufficiently large. When the sample is smaller, **jackknifing** can be used to obtain a better estimate of the true classification rate. Jackknifing involves omitting a case to develop the discriminant function and then classifying the omitted case.[5] When this is done for each of the cases in turn, the overall estimated classification rate is less biased.

Structure Coefficients

The relationship between discriminant scores and individual predictor variables can be evaluated by computing a Pearson correlation. These correlations are referred to as

[4]When the prior probability is established as 40% noncompleters and 60% completers (i.e., the same distribution as achieved in the sample), only one case is misclassified by the discriminant function, for an overall correct classification rate of 95.0%. With a 40-60 split, the percentage of cases that would have been correctly classified by chance alone is 52.0%.

[5]Jackknifed classification is available as an option in some computer programs for discriminant analysis, such as some versions of Biomedical Programs (BMD-P).

structure coefficients, as in canonical analysis (or loadings, as in factor analysis). Structure coefficients are useful for interpreting the results of a discriminant analysis. The **structure matrix** (or loading matrix) for our fictitious example is:

Variable	D
X_1 (Undergraduate GPA)	.64
X_2 (Verbal GRE)	.38
X_3 (Quantitative GRE)	.11
X_4 (Motivation)	.86

These loadings tell us that motivation scores were strongly correlated with discriminant scores, but that GRE-Quantitative scores had a negligible relationship with the composite D scores. Structure coefficients, when squared, indicate the proportion of variance in the variable that is accounted for by the discriminant function. Thus, 74% of the variance in motivation scores is accounted for by this function.

Structure coefficients are particularly useful for interpreting discriminant analysis results when there are two or more functions. Different underlying dimensions may contribute to discrimination among multiple groups, and the structure coefficients help us to understand the pattern. For example, suppose that we wanted to use the four predictors from our graduate program example to discriminate between completers, dropouts, and "flunkouts." A hypothetical structure matrix for this example is shown in Table 13–3. This table indicates that motivation scores, and to a lesser extent undergraduate grades, have a high loading on the first function (D_1). By contrast, verbal and quantitative GRE scores have high loadings on the second function (D_2). Thus, the two separate dimensions captured in this analysis might be motivation on the one hand and cognitive skills on the other.

TABLE 13–3. STRUCTURE MATRIX AND GROUP CENTROIDS FOR THREE-GROUP GRADUATE STUDENT EXAMPLE

	D_1	D_2
Predictor Variable		
X_1 (Undergraduate GPA)	.44	.33
X_2 (Verbal GRE)	.28	.61
X_3 (Quantitative GRE)	.13	.48
X_4 (Motivation)	.66	.14
Group Centroids		
Group 1 (Completers)	.71	.26
Group 2 (Dropouts)	−.24	.20
Group 3 (Flunkouts)	.11	−.33

To understand how the groups are differentiated on these two dimensions, we must examine the pattern of group centroids, i.e., the overall group means of the D scores on the two functions. As indicated in the bottom panel of Table 13–3, the centroid for the first function (which captures motivation) is quite high for the completers (.71), and lower for the flunkouts (.11) and, especially, the dropouts ($-.24$). Thus, it appears that the motivation function mainly distinguishes completers from the two groups that did not complete the program. The second function (cognitive skills) differentiates the flunkouts, whose centroid of $-.33$ is especially low, from the completers and dropouts.

Most computer programs allow researchers to compute discriminant scores on all functions for each case, and these scores can be used in subsequent analyses. When there is more than one function, these scores are analogous to factor scores produced in a factor analysis.

Significance Tests in Discriminant Analysis

The main significance test in discriminant analysis is the test of the null hypothesis that the discriminant functions reflect chance sampling fluctuations (i.e., that groups cannot be reliably distinguished on the basis of the predictors in the analysis). A test of the null hypothesis can be based on Wilks' lambda,[6] and the significance level of the lambda statistic is based on a transformation that approximates a chi-square or F distribution.

When there are two groups, as we have in our example, Wilks' lambda is the ratio of SS_W to SS_T—i.e., the proportion of total variance in the discriminant scores *not* explained by group differences. A lambda of 1 would be obtained if the mean of the discriminant scores were the same for both groups and there were no between-group variability. In our example, the value of Wilks' lambda is .40 ($\chi^2 = 14.63$), which is significant at the .01 level. Thus, 60% of the total variance in discriminant scores is accounted for by group differences in the four predictor variables (($1 - .40) \times 100 = 60\%$).

When there is more than one discriminant function, it is useful to evaluate whether each function contains discriminatory information that is reliable. Typically, computer programs use a "peel-away" process to successively test discriminatory power as functions are removed. For example, if there were two functions, the first test would evaluate whether, overall, both functions significantly discriminated groups. In the next step, the first function would be removed to determine whether the Wilks' lambda for the second function was statistically significant—i.e., whether the second function contributes significantly to group differences.

It should be kept in mind that a significant Wilks' lambda does not necessarily imply successful classification. When large samples are used, small group differences can result in a significant Wilks' lambda without resulting in good discrimination among groups.

---

[6]SPSS uses Wilks' lambda for evaluating the statistical significance of the discriminant functions, but other computer programs use other criteria, such as Hotelling's trace and Pillai's criterion.

Strategies for Entering Predictors in Discriminant Analysis

Like multiple regression, discriminant analysis has several options for entering predictors into the analysis. The analyses we have described thus far have involved the direct entry of all predictors as one block, often referred to as **direct discriminant analysis.** This is analogous to simultaneous multiple regression.

Discriminant analysis can also be performed in a hierarchical manner. That is, the researcher can specify the order of entry of the predictor variables, and can assess improvements to classification as each predictor or set of predictors is added to previously entered predictors. A hierarchical approach might be used for theoretical reasons—for example, to test for the incremental discriminatory power of variables that are conceptualized as belonging in a specified sequence. It might also be used to control extraneous variables—for example, entering demographic variables first to make the groups being compared as similar as possible before entering the independent variables of primary interest.

Discriminant analysis can also be performed in a stepwise fashion, whereby variables are stepped into the discriminant function in the order in which they meet certain statistical criteria. This approach is especially useful for exploratory work. For example, the researcher might want to identify a reduced set of variables from a pool of potential predictors. In stepwise discriminant analysis, predictors are evaluated one at a time. The first variable included is the one with the largest value for the selection criteria, and then at each step the value of the criterion is reassessed for each predictor not yet entered. When further variable entry results in a nonsignificant improvement, the analysis ceases.

Computer programs usually offer several options for the statistical criterion to be used in entering predictors in stepwise discriminant analysis. One criterion is the minimization of Wilks' lambda, whereby the variable that results in the smallest Wilks' lambda is selected for entry at each step. Other criteria include the **Mahalanobis distance** (D^2), a generalized measure of the distance between groups, and **Rao's V,** a statistic that captures differences between group means. The results are often the same regardless of which statistical criterion is used. In our graduate school example, all three criteria yielded the same outcome; after entering the motivation scores into the discriminant analysis predicting students' completion versus noncompletion of the graduate program, no other variable made a statistically significant contribution. For example, when the motivation variable was the only predictor in the analysis, the value of Wilks' lambda was .47. Using the lambda criterion, the variable that would have most reduced lambda after taking motivation scores into account was GRE-Verbal scores, which would have resulted in a lambda of .45—a nonsignificant improvement ($F = 0.91$).

As in multiple regression, the researcher can control the probability level used to control the entry of predictors in discriminant analysis. The researcher can also adjust the tolerance level, the criterion that is used to identify multicollinearity problems.

Assumptions and Requirements for Discriminant Analysis

In discriminant analysis, the dependent variable is always a categorical variable measured on a nominal scale (or on an ordinal scale with a small number of values). The independent variables can be either continuous interval- or ratio-level variables or dummy-coded dichotomous variables. However, when the predictor variables are all dichotomous, the discriminant function is not optimal.

It is generally wise to have, *at a minimum*, 5 cases for each predictor in the analysis, and 10 to 20 cases per predictor is definitely advantageous. When stepwise discriminant analysis is used, an even greater number of cases is desirable to avoid capitalizing on small chance fluctuations. Another guideline relating to sample size is that the number of cases in the smallest group should always be greater than the number of predictor variables.

The assumptions underlying the use of discriminant analysis are the same as for MANOVA. When using statistical inference, multivariate normality is assumed, but this assumption is usually robust to violation when there are more than 20 cases in the smallest group, or if the overall sample is greater than 20 *and* the groups are of equal size. Discriminant analysis also assumes a linear relationship among all pairs of predictors within each group, as well as homogeneity of the variance-covariance matrix. As with MANOVA, the Box M test can be used to assess the equality of the group covariance matrices, but this test is highly sensitive. When the sample size is large and groups are of approximately equal size, the homogeneity assumption is fairly robust.

Classification is generally less demanding than tests of statistical significance in discriminant analysis. If the primary goal of the analysis is classification, violation of the assumptions is less worrisome. The exception is violation of the homogeneity assumption; cases are more likely to be misclassified into groups with greater variability.

LOGISTIC REGRESSION

Logistic regression is a statistical technique that is becoming more common among nurse researchers. Logistic regression (sometimes referred to as **logit analysis**) is similar to multiple linear regression in that it analyzes the relationship between multiple independent variables and a single dependent variable, and yields a predictive equation. As in discriminant analysis, logistic regression is used when the dependent variable is categorical. However, logistic regression is based on an estimation procedure that has less restrictive assumptions than multiple regression and discriminant analysis, both of which are based on least-squares estimation criteria. For example, logistic regression does not assume multivariate normality. Since multivariate normality is almost impossible to achieve in reality, logistic regression is often a more statistically appropriate technique than discriminant analysis for predicting a categorical outcome.

Basic Concepts for Logistic Regression

In logistic regression, estimation of parameters is based on the **maximum likelihood method,** a major alternative to least-squares estimation. Maximum likelihood estimators are ones that estimate the parameters that are most likely to have generated the observed data. Maximum likelihood estimation can be used in several multivariate statistical techniques, including factor analysis (see Chapter 12) and structural equation modeling (see Chapter 14).

Logistic regression develops models for estimating the probability that an event occurs. For example, we might be interested in modeling the factors that affect the probability of being HIV positive, the probability of a woman practicing breast self-examination, or—to continue with our earlier example—the probability of completing a nursing school graduate program. We will use the graduate school example again in discussing logistic regression, but we will make one change to the data shown in Table 13–1 so that we can better illustrate some features of logistic regression. Instead of using the original motivation scores, we will substitute a dummy code to signify high motivation; students with a score over 70 are coded 1 (highly motivated) and students with a score of 70 and below are coded 0 (not highly motivated). Thus, in Table 13–1, nine students would be coded as highly motivated and 11 would be coded as not highly motivated.

Logistic regression transforms the probability that an outcome will occur (e.g., the probability of completing the graduate program) into its odds. The **odds** of an event is defined as the ratio of two probabilities: the probability of an event occurring to the probability that it will not occur. For example, if 40% of all entering graduate students completed the program, the odds would be:

$$\text{Odds}_{\text{completing}} = \frac{\text{Prob (completing)}}{\text{Prob (not completing)}} = \frac{.40}{.60} = .667$$

In a logistic regression analysis, the dependent variable is transformed to be the natural log of the odds, which is called a **logit** (short for *log*istic probability un*it*). As a result of the transformations, the dependent variable ranges from minus to plus infinity. Maximum likelihood is then used to estimate the coefficients of the independent variables, with the logit as a continuous dependent variable.

The logistic regression model can be written as:

$$\log\left[\frac{\text{Prob (event)}}{\text{Prob (no event)}}\right] = b_0 + b_1 X_1 + \ldots + b_k X_k$$

where b_0 = constant
  k = number of independent variables
  b_1 to b_k = coefficients estimated from the data
  X_1 to X_k = values of the k independent variables

In other words, the logit (log of the odds) is predicted from a weighted combination of the independent variables, plus a constant. In our graduate school example, the logistic regression equation is:

$$\log\left[\frac{\text{Prob (completing)}}{\text{Prob (not completing)}}\right] = -19.695 + 4.600X_1 + .030X_2 - .022X_3 + 2.306X_4$$

The right-hand side of the logistic regression equation essentially takes the same form as the equation for multiple regression. The interpretation, however, is different because we are no longer predicting actual values of the dependent variable. In logistic regression, a b coefficient can be interpreted as the change in the log odds associated with a one-unit change in the associated independent variable. For example, a b of 2.306 for X_4 (high motivation) means that when the variable changes from 0 to 1 (from not highly motivated to highly motivated), the log odds of completing graduate school increase by 2.306. A b of 4.600 for X_1 (undergraduate grades) means that when grade point average increases by one point (e.g., from 2.0 to 3.0), the log odds of completing the program increase by 4.600.

The Odds Ratio

It is difficult to comprehend what the logistic regression equation means because we are not used to thinking in terms of log odds. However, we can transform the equation so that the left-hand expression is the odds rather than the log odds:

$$\frac{\text{Prob (event)}}{\text{Prob (no event)}} = e^{b_0 + b_1X_1 + \ldots + b_kX_k}$$

where e = the base of natural logarithms (approximately 2.7183)

Written to solve for the odds, the equation tells us that e raised to the power of, say, b_4 is the factor by which the odds change when X_4 increases by one unit, after controlling for all other variables in the model. When the coefficient is positive, the odds increase, and when the coefficient is negative, the odds decrease. In our example, when X_4 (high motivation) changes from 0 to 1 and all other predictors are the same, the odds of completing the graduate program are increased by a factor of about 10.0 ($e^{2.306} = 10.03$).

The factor by which the odds change is usually referred to as the **odds ratio.** To fully convey what the odds ratio represents, we must present the logistic regression equation in yet another form, this time solving for the probability of an event:

$$\text{Prob (event)} = \frac{e^{b_0 + b_1X_1 + \ldots + b_kX_k}}{1 + e^{b_0 + b_1X_1 + \ldots + b_kX_k}}$$

Written in this fashion, we can use the logistic equation to estimate the probability that a student will complete the graduate program. Suppose that we had a highly motivated student ($X_4 = 1$) with an undergraduate grade point average of 3.0 and scores of 600 for both verbal GRE and quantitative GRE. Using the coefficients we obtained earlier, the probability of this student completing the graduate program would be:

$$\text{Prob (completing)} = \frac{e^{(-19.695)+(4.6)(3.0)+(.03)(600)-(.022)(600)+(2.306)(1)}}{1 + e^{(-19.695)+(4.6)(3.0)+(.03)(600)+(.022)(600)+(2.306)(1)}}$$

$$\text{Prob(completing)} = 0.77$$

The estimated probability that this student would complete the program is, thus, .77 and the estimated probability of *not* completing it is .23 (i.e., $1 - .77 = .23$). The *odds* of completion for this student are then estimated as 3.35 (i.e., $.77 \div .23 = 3.35$).

Suppose now that this same student had been classified as *not* highly motivated ($X_4 = 0$), but that all other independent variables stayed the same. Inserting 0 instead of 1 for X_4 in the previous formula, we would now estimate that the student's probability of completing is .251, and the probability of not completing is .749. If the student were not highly motivated, the *odds* of completion are $.749 \div .251 = .334$. We can now calculate the *odds ratio* for the motivation predictor as follows:

$$\text{Odds ratio}_{X_4} = \frac{\text{odds}_{\text{IfMotivated}}}{\text{odds}_{\text{IfNotMotivated}}} = \frac{3.35}{.334} = 10.03$$

By changing the value of motivation from 1 to 0 with all else constant, the odds changed from 3.35 to .334. That is, the odds ratio changed by a factor of 10.03. This is the same value we obtained earlier by raising e to the power of 2.306, the value of the logistic coefficient for the motivation variable X_4.

The odds ratio provides an estimate of **relative risk**—the risk of the event occurring given one condition, versus the risk of it occurring given a different condition. In our example, we would estimate that the risk of not finishing graduate school is about 10 times greater if a student is not highly motivated than if he or she is motivated.

Classification in Logistic Regression

As in discriminant analysis, logistic regression can be used to classify cases with respect to the categorical dependent variable, thereby providing a mechanism for evaluating the success of the model. For the purposes of classification, each subject's probability is computed based on the logistic regression equation. If prob (event) is greater than .50, the case is classified as a positive case. In the example we just worked through, the motivated student would be classified as completing the graduate program (prob = .77) but the unmotivated student would be classified as a noncompleter (prob = .25).

TABLE 13–4. PREDICTED CLASSIFICATION FOR GRADUATE STUDENT EXAMPLE USING LOGISTIC REGRESSION

Case	Actual Status C = Completed N = Not Completed	Estimated Probability of Completing	Predicted Status C = Completed N = Not Completed
1	C	.98	C
2	C	.29	N*
3	C	.96	C
4	N	.70	C*
5	C	.99	C
6	N	.02	N
7	C	.90	C
8	N	.02	N
9	N	.85	C*
10	C	.87	C
11	C	.94	C
12	C	.45	N*
13	N	.14	N
14	C	.73	C
15	C	.97	C
16	C	.95	C
17	N	.10	N
18	N	.16	N
19	N	.15	N
20	C	.83	N

*Misclassification

Classification information for the 20 students whose data are shown in Table 13–1 (with, however, X_4 dichotomized to be coded 1 for motivation scores above 70 and 0 otherwise) is presented in Table 13–4. This table shows the students' *actual* completion status in the second column. For example, the first student, who completed the graduate school program, has a code of C (completed) for actual completion status. The probability estimate based on the logistic regression is then presented for each case. The first student's probability of completion is quite high—.98. This student's predicted classification, shown next, is completed (C), which is correct. The asterisks in the last column indicate that there were four misclassifications: students 2 and 12 actually finished graduate school but were predicted to be noncompleters, while students 4 and 9 failed to complete the program but were predicted to be completers. Overall, then, 80.0% of the 20 cases were correctly classified.[7]

[7]When logistic regression is performed on the data as they are actually presented in Table 13–1 (i.e., with continuous rather than categorical motivation scores), 95.0% of the cases are correctly classified.

In practical applications, a researcher might want to establish a different rule for classifying probabilities if the consequences of making a mistake in one direction were more severe than misclassification in the other direction. For example, a graduate program might be more willing to accept students with a risk of not completing than to reject students who would have finished. In such a situation, a different probability value can be used as the cutoff value for classification.

Entering Predictors in Logistic Regression

Predictor variables in logistic regression can be continuous variables or coded dichotomous variables. In logistic regression, unlike discriminant analysis, the solution is not compromised even when *all* the variables are dichotomous. Dichotomous variables for logistic regression can be coded in a variety of ways, including dummy coding, effect coding, and several other alternative methods. The manuals for the main computer programs for logistic regression offer guidance on the coding options that are available.

As with multiple regression and discriminant analysis, there are alternative methods of entering predictors into the logistic regression equation. In our graduate school example, we used simultaneous entry of all predictors as a block. Hierarchical and stepwise entry are alternative methods that are available in most logistic regression programs.

Associated Statistics and Significance Tests in Logistic Regression

Several statistics are available for assessing the performance of the logistic regression. One index is known as the **likelihood index,** which is the probability of the observed results, given the parameters estimated from the analysis. If the model fits the data perfectly, the likelihood is 1.00. Since the likelihood index is almost always a small decimal number, it is customary to transform the index by multiplying -2 times the log of the likelihood. The transformed index $(-2LL)$ is a small number when the model fit is good; when the model is perfect, $-2LL$ equals zero.

The chi-square statistic is used to test the null hypothesis that all the b_1 to b_k coefficients are zero. The overall model chi-square test is the analog of the overall F test in multiple regression. The chi-square value is derived by computing the difference between $-2LL$ for the model with only the constant term and $-2LL$ for the model being tested. In our graduate school example, the values are as follows:

$-2LL$, model with only a constant $= 26.920$
$-2LL$, full model with 4 predictors $= \underline{13.383}$
Model chi-square $= 13.537$ $p = .0089$

In our example, then, the overall logistic model is statistically significant.

In a hierarchical or stepwise logistic regression, another chi-square test would be performed to assess the significance of the *improvement* to $-2LL$ between successive steps. The improvement chi-square test, which tests the null hypothesis that the coefficients for the variables added at the last step are zero, is comparable to the F-change test in multiple regression.

It is also possible to test the significance of individual predictor variables in the model (just as the t statistic is used to test the significance of individual predictors in multiple regression). The statistic that is usually used in logistic regression is the **Wald statistic,** which is distributed as a chi-square.[8] When the predictor variable has 1 degree of freedom, the Wald statistic is:

$$\left[\frac{b}{SE_b} \right]^2 = \text{Wald statistic}$$

In our graduate school example, the value of b for the dichotomous motivation variable was 2.306 and the standard error of the coefficient was 1.66, which yields a Wald statistic of 1.93. With 1 df, this is not statistically significant at the .05 level ($p = .16$). In this example, none of the predictors is statistically significant, even though the overall model attained significance.

A statistic that is useful for interpreting the magnitude of the contribution of individual predictors is the **R statistic** (which is *not* the same as the R in multiple linear regression). The R statistic, which ranges from -1.00 to $+1.00$, is an index of the partial correlation between the dependent variable and each predictor. When R is greater than zero, it indicates that as the variable increases so does the likelihood of the event occurring; when R is negative, increases to the variable are associated with a decreased likelihood of the event occurring. The smaller the absolute value of R, the smaller is its partial contribution to the model. In our example, the value of R for the X_4 (high motivation) variable is .00.

Logistic Regression, Discriminant Analysis, and Multiple Regression Compared

Logistic models are based on the assumption that the underlying relationship among variables can be represented as an S-shaped probabilistic function—an assumption that is generally much more tenable than the least-squares assumptions of linearity and multivariate normality. Logistic regression is thus more appropriate than discriminant analysis when the data are not distributed multivariate normally. When all the predictors are dichotomous, there is inevitably a violation of multivariate normality.

In practice, logistic regression and discriminant analysis often yield similar results, particularly if the sample is large. In fact, when the mean of a dichotomous dummy-

---

[8]When the absolute value of the coefficient is large, the Wald statistic has a tendency to lead to Type II errors. If the Wald statistic leads you to retain the null hypothesis for a coefficient that is large, an alternative way to test the predictor is to enter that variable in a later step and to use the improvement chi-square test to determine the significance of its contribution.

coded dependent variable lies between .25 and .75,[9] even multiple linear regression generally yields the same assessments of significance as logistic regression. Multiple linear regression has a desirable feature that is lacking in logistic regression—the computation of the R^2 statistic, which has immediate descriptive value as an index of the strength of a relationship among variables. Thus, when the dependent variable being modeled is not a rare event (i.e., when there is between a 25% and 75% rate of occurrence), some researchers actually prefer to use multiple regression. However, multiple regression (and also discriminant analysis) provide poorer estimates of probabilities for events in the extreme ranges than logistic regression.

When the sample is large and when the mean of a dichotomous dependent variable has a midrange value, the choice of a statistical technique for predicting the dependent variable may depend on the type of information the researcher is seeking, and the manner in which the researcher has conceptualized the problem. If the researcher's main interest is classification, then either logistic regression or discriminant analysis can be used. If the researcher is interested in relative risks and probabilities, then logistic regression will yield the desired information. However, if the dependent variable is conceptualized more as group membership than as the occurrence versus nonoccurrence of an event, discriminant analysis might be preferred.

One final consideration[10] involves the number of categories represented by the dependent variable. When there are only two categories, the researcher may have flexibility in selecting a statistical technique (including multiple regression) if the sample size is large and the mean is close to .50. However, when there are three or more categories, discriminant analysis might be the only available choice. Although **multinomial logistic regression** does exist for situations in which there are more than three categories of the dependent variable, not all major software packages perform such analyses.

COMPUTER ANALYSIS FOR DISCRIMINANT ANALYSIS AND LOGISTIC REGRESSION

In this section we review and discuss the computer printouts for a discriminant analysis and a logistic regression analysis of the same data set and the same variables. This will enable us to more directly compare the types of information that these two analyses typically yield.

The data for these analyses were from a longitudinal study of about 2000 low-income teenage mothers—the same data set used in Chapter 10 to illustrate the presentation of hierarchical regression results (Tables 10–10 and 10–11). In this chapter, we use eight independent variables to predict a repeat pregnancy by the time of the follow-

---

[9]When the average of a dummy variable is .25, it means that 75% of the sample had a code of 0 and 25% had a code of 1.

[10]If a mainframe computer is being used and computer time must be paid for, cost might be an additional consideration. Logistic regression is generally more expensive than linear specifications because the maximum likelihood solution requires multiple iterations. In such a situation, a linear model might be used for exploratory analyses, followed by maximum likelihood estimation.

up interview, which was scheduled 18 months after an initial (baseline) interview. The young mother typically had given birth to her first child 3 to 9 months prior to the baseline interview. The dependent variable—named NEWPREG in the printouts—was coded 0 if the young mother had not had a pregnancy between the baseline and follow-up interviews and was coded 1 if the mother had had one or more repeat pregnancies in the 18-month interval. The eight predictor variables were:

ASPIREHI   Whether mother had high aspirations at baseline (0 = no; 1 = yes)
BASEAGE   Age at baseline
BASECESD   Scores on the CES-D Depression Scale at baseline
BCBASE   Whether mother used birth control at baseline (0 = no; 1 = yes)
DIPLOMA   Whether mother had a high school diploma (0 = no; 1 = yes)
PARTNR   Whether mother was living with a male partner (0 = no; 1 = yes)
PREGCNT   Total number of pregnancies at baseline
WELFARE   Whether mother was on welfare (0 = no; 1 = yes)

As this list suggests, the predictors were a mix of dichotomous dummy-coded variables and continuous variables.

In both the discriminant analysis and the logistic regression analysis, an option available in SPSS was used to divide the research sample roughly in half for the purposes of cross-validation. The first subsample was used to develop the predictive equation and to run the tests of statistical significance. Then, the classification procedure was run for both subsamples to determine the reliability of the predictive equation.

Computer Example of Discriminant Analysis

Discriminant analysis was used to determine whether the eight independent variables could be used to predict group membership in the repeat-pregnancy versus no-repeat-pregnancy groups. Figure 13–1 presents the most relevant portions of a computer printout for this analysis.[11]

Panel A indicates that the total sample consisted of 2106 cases, 1063 of which were excluded from the main analyses. No case was excluded because of missing information on the dependent variable, but 26 cases were dropped due to missing

---

[11]The SPSS/PC commands that created the printout in Figure 13–1 are as follows:

```
DSCRIMINANT GROUPS=NEWPREG (0,1)
  /VARIABLES=PREGCNT PARTNR BCBASE DIPLOMA WELFARE BASECESD BASEAGE ASPIREHI
  /SELECT SUBGROUP (1)
  /PRIORS=SIZE
  /STATISTICS=10,11,13.
```

- - - - - - - -   D I S C R I M I N A N T   A N A L Y S I S   - - - - - - - -

On groups defined by NEWPREG   PREGNANT AFTER BASELINE

A

2106 (unweighted) cases were processed.
1063 of these were excluded from the analysis.
    0 had missing or out-of-range group codes.
   26 had at least one missing discriminating variable.
1037 were excluded by the SELECT= variable.
1043 (unweighted) cases will be used in the analysis.

Number of Cases by Group

NEWPREG	Number of Cases Unweighted	Weighted	Label
0	467	467.0	
1	576	576.0	
Total	1043	1043.0	

Analysis number   1
Direct method: All variables passing the tolerance test are entered.
    Minimum Tolerance Level................. .00100

Canonical Discriminant Functions

Maximum number of functions.............   1
Minimum cumulative percent of variance... 100.00
Maximum significance of Wilks' Lambda.... 1.0000

Prior Probabilities

Group	Prior	Label
0	.44775	
1	.55225	
Total	1.00000	

B

Canonical Discriminant Functions

Fcn	Eigenvalue	Pct of Variance	Cum Pct	Canonical Corr	After Fcn	Wilks' Lambda	Chisquare	DF	Sig
					: 0	.9532	49.728	8	.0000
1*	.0491	100.00	100.00	.2164	:				

* marks the   1 canonical discriminant functions remaining in the analysis.

C Standardized Canonical Discriminant Function Coefficients

	FUNC 1
PARTNR	.54062
BCBASE	-.33469
DIPLOMA	-.28976
WELFARE	.17413
ASPIREHI	.15203
PREGCNT	.61314
BASECESD	.22362
BASEAGE	-.65999

FIGURE 13–1.   COMPUTER PRINTOUT OF A DISCRIMINANT ANALYSIS

D Structure Matrix:

Pooled-within-groups correlations between discriminating variables
and canonical discriminant functions
(Variables ordered by size of correlation within function)

	FUNC 1
PARTNR	.40688
PREGCNT	.39203
BASEAGE	-.38315
DIPLOMA	-.35172
BCBASE	-.31715
BASECESD	.26966
WELFARE	.08677
ASPIREHI	.02185

E Unstandardized Canonical Discriminant Function Coefficients

	FUNC 1
PARTNR	1.316288
BCBASE	-.7419925
DIPLOMA	-.6030127
WELFARE	.5073446
ASPIREHI	.3221122
PREGCNT	.6377245
BASECESD	.2189009E-01
BASEAGE	-.5222676
(constant)	8.289179

F Canonical Discriminant Functions evaluated at Group Means (Group Centroids)

Group	FUNC 1
0	-.24591
1	.19937

G Classification Results for cases selected for use in the analysis -

Actual Group	No. of Cases	Predicted Group Membership 0	1
Group 0	467	187 40.0%	280 60.0%
Group 1	576	155 26.9%	421 73.1%

Percent of "grouped" cases correctly classified: 58.29%

Classification Results for cases not selected for use in the analysis -

Actual Group	No. of Cases	Predicted Group Membership 0	1
Group 0	461	200 43.4%	261 56.6%
Group 1	576	159 27.6%	417 72.4%

Percent of "grouped" cases correctly classified: 59.50%

Classification Processing Summary
   2106 Cases were processed.
      0 Cases were excluded for missing or out-of-range group codes.
     26 Cases had at least one missing discriminating variable.
   2080 Cases were used for printed output.

FIGURE 13-1. (CONTINUED)

information on at least one predictor and 1037 cases were omitted for the purposes of the cross-validation. Thus, a total of 1043 cases were used to estimate the discriminant function: 467 in the no-repeat-pregnancy group and 576 in the repeat-pregnancy group. The prior probabilities, as shown at the bottom of Panel A, were set equal to the distribution of cases in the sample (e.g., $576 \div 1043 = .55225$).

Panel B presents various pieces of information relating to the overall discriminant function. Since there are only two groups, there is only one function, which has an eigenvalue of .0491. The extracted variance always totals 100%, and if there were two or more functions, the printout would tell us how the extracted variance was distributed across the functions. The canonical correlation—the correlation between all predictors on the one hand and the dependent variable on the other—is .2164, indicating that the predictors accounted for about 5% of the variance in group membership ($.2164^2 = .047$).

The right-hand portion of Panel B indicates that the Wilks' lambda, which is used to test the overall significance of the discriminant function, is .9532. This is consistent with the canonical correlation, since lambda is an index of variance *un*accounted for (i.e., $1.0 - .047 = .953$). The chi-square statistic for the Wilks' lambda is 49.728, which is significant beyond .00005. Thus, the eight predictors, as a set, can reliably be used to discriminate young mothers who did and did not have a post-baseline pregnancy. Note that this information is associated with After Fcn 0. This means that the Wilks' lambda is the value after zero functions have been removed—i.e., for all functions taken together. If there had been three groups, yielding two functions, there would be another line for the Wilks' lambda computed after removing the first function. In other words, the second line would be used to test the significance of the second function.

Panel C shows the standardized discriminant function coefficients for each predictor. (Panel E presents the *un*standardized discriminant function coefficients). Panel D shows the structure coefficients—the correlations between the predictors and the linear discriminant function. The predictors are listed in order of the structure coefficients' magnitude. Thus, the predictor that contributed most to the discrimination of the two groups was whether the young mother was living with a male partner, followed by the number of pregnancies she had had in total at the outset of the study. The young mother's aspiration level had the lowest correlation with the discriminant function. Care must be taken in interpreting the directionality of the structure coefficients. In this example, the *dependent variable* is coded such that the larger value (1) is associated with occurrence of a repeat pregnancy while the smaller value (0) indicates the absence of a repeat pregnancy. The direction of the *discriminant function* may occasionally be reversed—although this is not the case in this example.

Panel F indicates that the centroid (group mean on the discriminant function) for the norepeat-pregnancy group is $-.24591$, compared to the centroid of .19937 for the pregnancy group. Thus, a positive structure coefficient (panel D) indicates a predictor variable that is associated with repeat pregnancy, while a negative coefficient is associated with avoidance of another pregnancy during the follow-up period. For example, the structure coefficient for DIPLOMA is −.35172, indicating that mothers who had graduated from high school were *less* likely to have had another pregnancy than those who had not graduated. Higher levels of depression at baseline, by contrast, were associated with greater risk of a subsequent pregnancy (.26966).

The final panel (G) shows the results of the classification analysis. The first classification table is for the 1043 cases used in the discriminant analysis. Of the 467 cases whose actual group membership was 0 (no repeat pregnancy), 187 (40.0%) were correctly predicted to be in that group on the basis of the discriminant function, but 280 (60.0%) were misclassified. Of the young mothers who had actually had a subsequent pregnancy, 73.1% were correctly predicted to be in that group. Overall, 58.29% of the actual sample was correctly classified. Thus, since prior probabilities were set to roughly a 45-55 split, the classification was only about 3 percentage points higher than what we would expect if we had made predictions at random. Nevertheless, the statistically significant results suggest that we could *consistently* improve on random classification, and this is confirmed by the cross-validation. The bottom portion of Panel G indicates that the percentage of correctly classified cases for the 1037 cases not selected for the creation of the discriminant function was 59.50%.

Computer Example of Logistic Regression

The printout for the logistic regression analysis of the same data is presented in Figure 13–2.[12] The first panel is similar to Panel A of the discriminant analysis; it shows that of the 2106 cases in the sample, 1059 were selected to create the logistic regression equation, 16 of which had missing data. Thus, the analysis is based on the same 1043 cases as for the discriminant analysis.

Panel B has only one piece of information: the value of $-2LL$ when only the constant is in the logistic regression analysis. In this example, $-2LL$ for the constant is 1434.493. Panel C shows the names of the eight predictor variables, followed by information on the adequacy of the overall model. The value of $-2LL$ for the entire model is 1384.381, a value that is lower than $-2LL$ for the constant by 50.112 (1434.493 − 1384.381 = 50.112). This corresponds to the value for the model chi-square, which is statistically significant beyond .00005. Note that the chi-square of

---

[12]The SPSS/PC commands that created the printout in Figure 13–2 are as follows:

```
LOGISTIC REGRESSION
  /VARIABLES = NEWPREG WITH PARTNR BCBASE
   DIPLOMA WELFARE ASPIREHI PREGCNT BASECESD BASEAGE
  /SELECT SUBGROUP EQ 1.
```

```
A   Total number of cases:      2106 (Unweighted)
    Number of selected cases:   1059
    Number of unselected cases: 1047

    Number of selected cases:                       1059
    Number rejected because of missing data:        16
    Number of cases included in the analysis: 1043


B   Dependent Variable..   NEWPREG     PREGNANT AFTER BASELINE

    Beginning Block Number  0.  Initial Log Likelihood Function

    -2 Log Likelihood    1434.493

    * Constant is included in the model.


    Beginning Block Number  1.  Method: Enter

C   Variable(s) Entered on Step Number
    1..        PARTNR     LIVING W A PARTNER
               BCBASE     USED BC AT BASELINE
               DIPLOMA    HAS HS DIPLOMA
               WELFARE    AFDC RECEIPT
               ASPIREHI   HI ASPIRATIONS BASELINE
               PREGCNT    NO OF PREGS AT BASELINE
               BASECESD   BASELINE DEPRESSION SCORE
               BASEAGE    AGE AT BASELINE

    Estimation terminated at iteration number 3 because
    Log Likelihood decreased by less than .01 percent.

     -2 Log Likelihood        1384.381
     Goodness of Fit          1042.326
                              Chi-Square    df Significance
     Model Chi-Square          50.112       8      .0000
     Improvement               50.112       8      .0000

         Classification Table for NEWPREG

D        Selected cases SUBGROUP EQ 1.00

                              Predicted
                             .00   | 1.00      Percent Correct
                              0    |   1
                 Observed        +-------+-------+
                   .00      0   | 187   | 280   |     40.04%
                                +-------+-------+
                   1.00     1   | 154   | 422   |     73.26%
                                +-------+-------+
                                       Overall  58.39%

         Classification Table for NEWPREG
         Unselected cases SUBGROUP NE 1.00

                              Predicted
                             .00   | 1.00      Percent Correct
                              0    |   1
                 Observed        +-------+-------+
                   .00      0   | 199   | 262   |     43.17%
                                +-------+-------+
                   1.00     1   | 159   | 417   |     72.40%
                                +-------+-------+
                                       Overall  59.40%
```

FIGURE 13–2.   COMPUTER PRINTOUT OF A LOGISTIC REGRESSSION

E

```
---------------------- Variables in the Equation ----------------------
```

Variable	B	S.E.	Wald	df	Sig	R	Exp(B)
PARTNR	.5948	.1653	12.9502	1	.0003	.0874	1.8126
BCBASE	-.3335	.1440	5.3655	1	.0205	-.0484	.7164
DIPLOMA	-.2679	.1362	3.8670	1	.0492	-.0361	.7650
WELFARE	.2309	.1934	1.4256	1	.2325	.0000	1.2597
ASPIREHI	.1415	.1383	1.0456	1	.3065	.0000	1.1520
PREGCNT	.2846	.0731	15.1440	1	.0001	.0957	1.3292
BASECESD	.0097	.0063	2.3613	1	.1244	.0159	1.0098
BASEAGE	-.2328	.0553	17.7107	1	.0000	-.1047	.7923
Constant	3.9137	1.0490	13.9204	1	.0002		

```
------------------------------------------------------------------------
```

FIGURE 13–2. (CONTINUED)

50.112 is very close to the value of chi-square obtained in the discriminant analysis (49.73). In a stepwise logistic regression, the value for the improvement chi-square would tell us whether newly stepped-in variables resulted in a significant improvement to the model. Panel C contains one other statistic, the **goodness-of-fit statistic,** which in this example is 1042.326. This statistic is based upon the residuals for all of the cases in the analysis which, in logistic regression, is the difference between the observed probability of the event and the predicted probability. This goodness-of-fit statistic also has a chi-square distribution and thus is an alternative mechanism for evaluating the fit of the predictive model.

The classification results are shown in Panel D. The overall rate of correct classification is 58.39% for the cases selected for the analysis, and 59.40% for those not selected (i.e., those in the cross-validation subsample). Note that the overall rate of correct classification is very similar for the logistic regression and the discriminant analysis in this example.

Information on the logistic regression equation is presented in Panel E. The logistic regression coefficients (b weights) associated with each predictor are listed in the column labeled B. The last row of this first column indicates the value of the constant (3.9137). Thus, the full logistic equation for predicting the log of the odds of a repeat pregnancy can be constructed from the information in the first column. The next column shows the standard error of each b (S.E.), followed by a column indicating the value of the Wald statistic for each predictor variable. After the column showing degrees of freedom (df), the significance level associated with each predictor is presented (Sig). According to this printout, the variables that were significantly associated with the probability of having a repeat pregnancy were PARTNR, BCBASE, DIPLOMA, PREGCNT, and BASEAGE. The next column indicates the partial correlation of the predictor with the dependent variable (R). Net of other factors, a young mother had the greatest likelihood of a subsequent pregnancy if she had not finished high school, if she was living with a male partner, if she was not using birth control at baseline, if she had had multiple pregnancies at baseline, and if she was younger. The final column, labeled Exp(B), is the odds ratio. For example, the odds ratio for living with a partner (versus not living with a partner) is 1.81.

Overall, the conclusions we can reach are similar regardless of whether we used logistic regression or discriminant analysis with these data.[13] Both analyses yielded models that were highly significant statistically, a fact that is not surprising given the large sample size. The classification results for the two analyses were also very similar, with a successful classification rate in the vicinity of 60%. However, each analysis yields somewhat different information, so the investigator's research aims and information needs would likely determine which analysis to use.

With its modest assumptions, logistic regression is clearly suitable for the data in this example. Discriminant analysis also is justifiable here because of the large sample size, the inclusion of both continuous and dummy-coded predictors, and groups of roughly equal size, yielding a mean value of the dependent variable near the midrange (55.2% of the cases were coded 1 and thus the mean of NEWPREG was .552). Moreover, it is equally sensible to conceptualize the dependent variable as membership in a repeat pregnancy status group *or* as the occurrence of an event (repeat pregnancy) whose likelihood can be predicted.

RESEARCH APPLICATIONS OF DISCRIMINANT ANALYSIS AND LOGISTIC REGRESSION

Although the two techniques discussed in this chapter are not as widely used as multiple regression and factor analysis, discriminant analysis and logistic regression are becoming more popular among nurse researchers—particularly now that appropriate software has become available for personal computers. This section examines some of the major applications of discriminant analysis and logistic regression and discusses methods of effectively displaying the results from such analyses in a research report.

The Uses of Discriminant Analysis and Logistic Regression

Discriminant analysis and logistic regression can be used for several purposes by nurse researchers, as described below.

1. *Answering Research Questions.* The primary use of the two techniques described in this chapter is substantive—i.e., to answer questions about the relationships among

---

[13]Multiple regression applied to these data also yields similar results. The R^2 of .047 is highly significant ($p = .0000$).

research variables when the dependent variable is categorical. Discriminant analysis is especially valuable when the researcher is interested in assessing the magnitude of the relationship, because the canonical correlation coefficient and Wilks' lambda provide information on magnitude. Logistic regression, on the other hand, is especially useful if the researcher wants to estimate the probability of an event occurring, and the relative risk associated with one status on a predictor variable as opposed to another. Table 13–5 presents some examples of studies that involved either discriminant analysis or logistic regression.

2. *Prediction and Classification.* Both techniques described here offer an excellent vehicle for making predictions about a person's classification when there is information on a set of predictor variables. Classification predictions can be very important for decision making and resource management—for example, predicting which discharged patients are most in need of follow-up or projecting which patients would most benefit from a costly intervention. As an actual example, Metheny and her colleagues (1993) used both discriminant analysis and logit analysis to classify gastric versus intestinal tube (and gastric versus respiratory tube) placement based on pH values of aspirates from feeding tubes.

3. *Validity Assessments.* Instruments are sometimes developed with the specific aim of classifying people—for example, there are psychological tests that are used in the diagnosis of different types of mental illness. Both discriminant analysis and logistic regression can be used to determine the validity of such instruments—i.e., to assess the extent to which the instrument makes accurate classifications. For example, Glick and Swanson (1995) used discriminant analysis to examine the validity of the Motor Performance Inventory, an instrument designed to predict functional dependence and independence.

4. *Assessing Bias.* In earlier chapters we discussed how *t*-tests and ANOVA could be used to assess various types of bias, such as selection bias, nonresponse bias, or attrition bias. These assessments involve comparing groups (e.g., those who continue in a longitudinal study versus those who drop out) in terms of various background characteristics *one variable at a time.* Both logistic regression and discriminant analysis can be used to determine whether the groups can be reliably differentiated on the basis of a set of characteristics taken as a whole. In effect, this involves an effort to model the biasing process—for example, to model the attrition process or the selection process. When multivariate techniques such as logistic regression and discriminant analysis are used and no biases are detected, the conclusion that the results are unbiased is considerably more compelling than when univariate tests are used.

The Presentation of Discriminant Analysis and Logistic Regression in Research Reports

Like all other multivariate statistics, results from the techniques described in this chapter almost always require the use of tables because of the complexity of the analyses and the wealth of information they yield. Often, two or more tables are needed—for example, when classification is an important research objective.

TABLE 13–5. EXAMPLES OF STUDIES USING DISCRIMINANT ANALYSIS OR LOGISTIC REGRESSION

Research Question	Analytic Technique
What are the predictors of mortality among ICU patients? (Kollef, 1995)	Stepwise logistic regression
What are the factors that predict parents' level of involvement (nonattendance versus low attendance versus high attendance) in a Head Start alcohol and drug prevention program? (Hahn, 1995)	Direct discriminant analysis
What are the factors that differentiate women with three perimenstrual severity patterns: premenstrual syndrome, premenstrual magnification, and low symptom? (Mitchell, Woods, & Lentz, 1994)	Stepwise discriminant analysis
Are selected clinical and functional status measures useful in distinguishing need for home health services among patients ready for hospital discharge? (Prescott, Soeken, & Griggs, 1995)	Direct discriminant analysis
What are the predisposing husband and wife factors associated with the occurrence of an unplanned pregnancy? (Zotti & Siegel, 1995)	Direct logistic regression

Discriminant Analysis Results. A summary table for a discriminant analysis normally includes the following information: sample size, names of the predictor and dependent variables, structure coefficients, value of the canonical correlation and/or Wilks' lambda, value of the test statistic for testing the overall discriminant function (chi-square or *F,* depending on the software used), and significance level. Table 13–6 presents an example of a table that displays information from our computer printout example (Figure 13–1). The title of this table indicates the dependent variable and sample size. All predictors are listed in the first column of the table, in the order of the structure coefficients' magnitude. An acceptable alternative ordering would be to list the predictors either in alphabetical order or in some theoretically relevant order. For each predictor two pieces of information are shown: the *un*standardized discriminant function coefficient and the structure coefficient. The unstandardized coefficient is not essential, but it provides information that could be used for scoring new cases. Information on the overall function—the strength of association and statistical significance—is shown at the bottom of the table. The rate of correct classification in the analysis sample is presented in the last line.

When there is more than one function, researchers usually omit the discriminant function coefficients, displaying only the structure coefficients for each predictor on all functions. With multiple functions, group centroids should also be included in the table so that readers can interpret the dimensionality of the functions. If a stepwise analysis

TABLE 13–6. EXAMPLE OF A TABLE FOR DISCRIMINANT ANALYSIS RESULTS

Predictor Variable	b^*	Structure Coefficient
Living with partner/husband	1.32	.41
Number of pregnancies at baseline	.64	.39
Age at baseline	−.52	−.38
Has high school diploma	−.60	−.35
Used birth control at baseline	−.74	−.32
Depression scores at baseline	.02	.27
Receiving welfare	.51	.09
High aspirations at baseline	.32	.02
Constant	8.29	
Canonical correlation	.22	
Wilks' lambda	.95	
Chi-square ($df = 8$)	49.73	
p	.0000	
Overall rate of correct classification	58.3%	

*Unstandardized discriminant function coefficients.
Discriminant Analysis: Prediction of a Post-Baseline Pregnancy (N 5 1043)

has been performed, the table should indicate the order of entry of variables into the model, the level of significance of entered variables, and the names of variables not entered into the equation in a footnote.

Classification results are often presented in a separate table that is arrayed like a contingency table. By convention, actual group membership is listed in the left-hand column and predicted group membership is displayed along the top row, as in Table 13–2. With such an arrangement, readers can readily determine correct classification by examining the positive diagonal (i.e., reading from the upper left cell to the lower right cell) and misclassifications by examining off-diagonal entries. Each cell of the table usually includes information on both the n and % for that cell. The overall rate of correct classification should always be displayed at the bottom of the table.

The text of a research report should be used to summarize the most salient features of the table. Here is an example of how the results presented in Table 13–6 could be described:

A direct discriminant analysis was performed to predict which young mothers had a repeat pregnancy during the follow-up period on the basis of eight predictor variables, most of which were measured at the outset of the study. The analysis was performed with half the research sample ($N = 1043$), selected at random; the second half was used to cross-validate the classification results ($N = 1037$). As shown in Table 13–6, the eight predictors significantly discriminated women who did and women who did not have a post-baseline pregnancy ($\chi^2 = 49.73$, $p < .00005$). Women who were living with a partner or husband were especially likely to have had a subsequent pregnancy, as indicated by the structure coefficient (.41). Women who had had multiple pregnancies at baseline, who were younger, who had not completed high school, and who were not using birth control at baseline were also more likely to become pregnant during the follow-up period. Interestingly, welfare receipt and baseline aspiration levels were not highly correlated with discriminant scores. Although significant, the discriminant function only accounted for about 5% of the variance in repeat pregnancy status (canonical correlation = .22), suggesting that factors other than those used in this analysis need to be identified. The classification results indicate modest success, with an overall rate of correct classification of 58.3% in the analysis sample and a similar rate (59.5%) in the cross-validation sample.

Logistic Regression Results. A summary table for a logistic regression analysis normally includes the following information: sample size, names of the predictors, name of the event whose probability is being predicted, logistic regression coefficients, odds ratio, value of -2 log likelihood (or the goodness-of-fit statistic), value of the chi-square statistic for testing the overall model, and the significance level. An example of a logistic regression table is presented in Table 13–7, which summarizes the results from the printout shown in Figure 13–2. This table is quite similar to the table used to display discriminant analysis results; the eight predictor variables are listed in the left-hand column, followed by their associated *b* weights. This table includes the odds ratio rather than the structure coefficients, and also displays information on the significance level of each predictor via the Wald statistic and its associated probability. The bottom portion displays the test of the overall model: $-2LL$, chi-square, and the overall significance. The table also shows the rate of correct classification. If more detail on classification errors were desired, a supplementary table with the classification contingency table could be included.

The following paragraph is an example of how the results could be described in the text:

Logistic regression was used to estimate the probability of a repeat pregnancy during the 18-month follow-up period. Eight predictor variables, most of which were measured at the outset of the study, were used in the analysis. The regression was performed with half the research sample ($N = 1043$), selected at random; the second half was used to cross-validate the classification results ($N = 1037$). As shown in Table 13–7, the overall predictive model was statistically significant (model $\chi^2 = 50.11$, $p < .00005$). Five of the predictor variables were significantly related to the likelihood of having a repeat pregnancy: women who were living with a partner or husband, who had had multiple baseline pregnancies, who were younger, and who were not using birth control at baseline had a higher-than-average risk of a subsequent pregnancy. The risk of a repeat pregnancy was nearly twice as great among those living with a male partner in comparison with those who were not (odds ratio = 1.81). Although the model was significant, the classification results indicate only modest success, with an overall rate of correct classification of 58.4% in the analysis sample and a similar rate (59.4%) in the cross-validation sample.

TABLE 13–7. EXAMPLE OF A TABLE FOR LOGISTIC REGRESSION RESULTS

Predictor Variable	b§	Wald	Odds Ratio
Living with partner/husband	.59	12.95***	1.81
Number of pregnancies at baseline	.28	15.14***	1.33
Age at baseline	−.23	17.71***	0.79
Has high school diploma	−.27	3.87*	0.77
Used birth control at baseline	−.33	5.37*	0.72
Depression scores at baseline	.01	2.36	1.01
Receiving welfare	.23	1.43	1.26
High aspirations at baseline	.14	1.05	1.15
Constant	3.91	13.92***	
−2 Log Likelihood	1384.38		
Model Chi-square ($df = 8$)	50.11		
p	.0000		
Overall rate of correct classification	58.4%		

§Unstandardized logistic regression coefficients.
*$p < .05$ ***$p < .001$
Logistic Regression: Prediction of the Likelihood of a Repeat Pregnancy During 18-Month Follow-Up Period (N 5 1043)

RESEARCH EXAMPLE

This section describes an interesting recent study that used discriminant analysis.

Hanneman (1994) used discriminant analysis to determine the interdependent contributions of various clinical measures to the prediction of cardiac surgery patients' success or failure from early weaning from mechanical ventilation. The sample consisted of 162 patients, 134 of whom were successfully weaned and extubated within 24 hours of admission to the cardiovascular critical care unit (the success group), and 28 of whom were not weaned within 24 hours (the failure group). The sample was divided in half at random, with 82 cases used in the analysis phase to develop the discriminant function equation, and the remaining half used as a cross-validation subsample.

Various variables capturing three dimensions of physiological status (pulmonary mechanics, gas exchange, and hemodynamic function) were measured at two points postoperatively: 2 hours after critical care unit admission while on mechanical ventilation and during a spontaneous ventilation trial (SVT). Variables that significantly differentiated the two groups at the .01 level using a univariate t-test and that were nonredundant and normally distributed were used as the predictors in a direct discriminant analysis. The predictor variables included the following: pH of the arterial blood during mechanical ventilation and SVT, mean arterial blood pressure on mechanical ventilation, vital capacity during SVT, and ratio of arterial oxygen tension to fraction of inspired oxygen at both points in time.

The discriminant analysis revealed a fairly strong relationship between the six predictors and membership in the success versus failure groups. The canonical correlation was .733, which was highly significant. The predictor variables that had the highest structure coefficients ($>.30$) were pH during both SVT and mechanical ventilation, and mean arterial pressure during mechanical ventilation.

The classification results, adjusting prior probabilities equal to the actual distribution of cases to the groups, indicated a high level of accurate predictions based on the discriminant analysis: 95% and 92% of the cases were correctly classified in the analysis and cross-validation samples, respectively. Of the 162 patients in the entire sample, only 11 cases (7%) were misclassified.

SUMMARY

Discriminant analysis is a multivariate technique that is used to predict a categorical dependent variable on the basis of several predictor variables. Using a least-squares criterion and with least-squares assumptions, discriminant analysis involves the formation of linear combinations of the predictors—called **discriminant functions**—to predict group membership. There are either as many functions as there are groups, minus one, or as many as there are predictors, whichever is smaller. **Discriminant scores** can be computed for each function based on its discriminant equation; each group's mean discriminant score is called its **centroid.** Discriminant scores can be used to classify cases into groups, and thus predicted and actual classifications can be compared to evaluate the adequacy of the discriminant model. Cross-validation and **jackknifing** can be used to obtain a better estimate of the true classification rate. **Structure coefficients,** which indicate the correlation between the independent variables and discriminant scores, are useful in assessing the contribution of individual predictors and in interpreting results. The test of the null hypothesis that the discriminant functions reflect chance sampling fluctuations is usually based on Wilks' lambda. As is true with multiple regression, discriminant analysis allows direct, hierarchical, or stepwise entry of predictors.

Logistic regression is also a multivariate technique for predicting a categorical dependent variable, but logistic regression uses the **maximum likelihood method** of estimation rather than least-squares estimation and thus has less stringent assumptions than discriminant analysis. Logistic regression develops a model for estimating the odds that an event will occur. The **odds** of an event is the ratio of the probability that it will occur to the probability that it will not. The dependent variable is further transformed to be the natural log of the odds, which is called a **logit.** The logit is predicted from a combination of predictors, weighted by logistic coefficients, plus a constant. For each predictor, the logistic regression analysis yields an **odds ratio,** which is the factor by which the odds change for a unit change in the predictors. The odds ratio provides an estimate of **relative risk**—the risk of the event given one condition versus the risk of the event given an alternative condition. Predicted probabilities based on the logistic regression equation can be used to classify cases, as in discriminant analysis. The overall logistic model can be evaluated using the **likelihood index**—the probability of the observed results—which is usually reported as -2 times the log of the likelihood ($-2LL$). An alternative is the **goodness-of-fit** statistic which, like $-2LL$, has a chi-square distribution.

The **Wald statistic** is used to assess the significance of individual predictors in the logistic model. The **R statistic** is an index of the partial correlation between the dependent variable and the predictor.

Logistic regression is often the most statistically appropriate procedure when the dependent variable is categorical, but if the sample is large and the groups are roughly equal in size, discriminant analysis is robust to violation of the underlying assumptions. When the mean of a dummy-coded dependent variable is between .25 and .75, multiple regression analysis often yields results that are similar to logistic regression.

EXERCISES

The following exercises cover concepts presented in this chapter. Exercises indicated with a dagger (†) can be checked against answers appearing in Appendix A. Additionally, Chapter 13 of the accompanying *Applications Manual* offers supplementary exercises, including ones that require computer analysis of a data set on diskette.

† 1. Using the following discriminant function equation, which was presented earlier in this chapter, calculate the D scores for the last five students in Table 13–1:

$$D = -13.414 + 1.584(X_1) + .010(X_2) - .007(X_3) + .094(X_4)$$

† 2. Based on the D scores calculated in Exercise 1, how would each student be classified (finished graduate school versus did not)? What percentage of the five students were correctly classified?

† 3. How many discriminant functions would be formed in the following situations?
   a. Groups: Completely dependent; needs assistance; completely independent. Predictors: Age; motor performance test scores; living at home versus in a nursing home.
   b. Groups: Nondrinkers; moderate drinkers; heavy drinkers; alcoholics. Predictors: Family history of alcoholism; level of depression.
   c. Groups: Completed second wave of study; did not complete second wave. Predictors: Gender; race/ethnicity; age; educational attainment; income; length of residence in community.

† 4. a. Write out the full discriminant function equation from Figure 13–1 in unstandardized form. Round to two decimal places.
   b. Write out the logistic regression equation from Figure 13–2. Round to two decimal places.

† 5. Assume that the probability of developing lung cancer is .37 for smokers and .11 for nonsmokers. Calculate the odds ratio.

6. Read one of the studies cited in Table 13–5. Was the researcher justified in using the chosen analytic technique (discriminant analysis or logistic regression)? Could the alternative procedure have been used? Why or why not?

The **Wald statistic** is used to assess the significance of individual predictors in the logistic model. The ***R* statistic** is an index of the partial correlation between the dependent variable and the predictor.

Logistic regression is often the most statistically appropriate procedure when the dependent variable is categorical, but if the sample is large and the groups are roughly equal in size, discriminant analysis is robust to violation of the underlying assumptions. When the mean of a dummy-coded dependent variable is between .25 and .75, multiple regression analysis often yields results that are similar to logistic regression.

EXERCISES

The following exercises cover concepts presented in this chapter. Exercises indicated with a dagger (†) can be checked against answers appearing in Appendix A. Additionally, Chapter 13 of the accompanying *Applications Manual* offers supplementary exercises, including ones that require computer analysis of a data set on diskette.

† 1. Using the following discriminant function equation, which was presented earlier in this chapter, calculate the D scores for the last five students in Table 13–1:

$$D = -13.414 + 1.584(X_1) + .010(X_2) - .007(X_3) + .094(X_4)$$

† 2. Based on the D scores calculated in Exercise 1, how would each student be classified (finished graduate school versus did not)? What percentage of the five students were correctly classified?

† 3. How many discriminant functions would be formed in the following situations?

    a. Groups: Completely dependent; needs assistance; completely independent. Predictors: Age; motor performance test scores; living at home versus in a nursing home.

    b. Groups: Nondrinkers; moderate drinkers; heavy drinkers; alcoholics. Predictors: Family history of alcoholism; level of depression.

    c. Groups: Completed second wave of study; did not complete second wave. Predictors: Gender; race/ethnicity; age; educational attainment; income; length of residence in community.

† 4. a. Write out the full discriminant function equation from Figure 13–1 in unstandardized form. Round to two decimal places.

    b. Write out the logistic regression equation from Figure 13–2. Round to two decimal places.

† 5. Assume that the probability of developing lung cancer is .37 for smokers and .11 for nonsmokers. Calculate the odds ratio.

6. Read one of the studies cited in Table 13–5. Was the researcher justified in using the chosen analytic technique (discriminant analysis or logistic regression)? Could the alternative procedure have been used? Why or why not?

Causal Modeling: Path Analysis and Linear Structural Relations Analysis

Although the concept of causality is a controversial one in scientific circles, causal thinking is a fundamental feature of scientific research. Researchers do not always use terms like cause and effect, causation, and causality, yet they generally are interested in the influences on the phenomena they study; those influences often involve the notion of causation. The researcher who studies the risk factors for a disease, for example, is interested in learning what *causes* the disease. This chapter provides a brief introduction to two sophisticated methods for testing causal hypotheses. We begin with a discussion of causality.

CAUSALITY

There are three conditions that must be met to make an inference that variable X (e.g., cigarette smoking) causes variable Y (e.g., lung cancer): (1) temporal ordering, (2) existence of a relationship, and (3) absence of spuriousness. The first condition simply means that if smoking is a cause of lung cancer, smoking must precede the development of the disease. The second condition is that there must be an association between the two variables; smokers must be more likely than nonsmokers to develop lung cancer if there is, indeed, a causal connection. The third condition stipulates that the relationship between the two variables must not be spurious—i.e., must not be the result of a third variable that is related to both. This essentially means that the relationship between smoking and lung cancer must persist even when the effects of confounding variables are controlled. For example, if smokers were systematically different genetically from nonsmokers and the genetic differences were also linked to lung cancer, the relationship between smoking and lung cancer should not disappear when genetic differences are controlled if smoking is a cause of the disease.

Causality and Research Design

In a true experimental design in which research participants are randomly assigned to conditions, the three requirements for causality usually are met. For example, suppose children were randomly assigned to a smoking group (required to smoke) or a non-smoking group (prohibited from smoking). If the smokers eventually had a higher rate of lung cancer than the nonsmokers, the causal effect of smoking on cancer could be inferred because all three conditions for causality have been met: the smoking preceded the disease, the association between the two variables exists, and no other factor could have influenced the outcome, since random assignment presumably equalized the two groups with respect to an infinite number of biological, social, psychological, and economic factors.

Scientists could not, of course, ethically conduct such an experiment. Most research with humans is nonexperimental, and because of this fact scientists cannot readily draw causal inferences from their results. In nonexperimental research, the first two conditions for causality are often easy to attain, but the third—ruling out potentially confounding factors—is not. It is the third condition that is the basis for the widely repeated admonition: *Correlation does not prove causation.* That is, the existence of a relationship between two variables, no matter how strong, does not in itself provide evidence that one variable caused the other. Nevertheless, researchers who undertake nonexperimental research often *do* have an interest in unraveling causes and effects, and these researchers are increasingly relying on methods of causal modeling.

Causal Modeling and Theory

Causal modeling involves the development of a hypothesized causal explanation of a phenomenon of interest on the basis of other phenomena, and the application of statistical procedures for testing the model. In a causal model, the researcher posits a set of linkages among three or more variables. Correlation-based procedures are used to test whether the hypothesized pathway from the causes to the effect is consistent with the data.

Causal modeling is *not* a method for discovering causes. Rather, it is an approach to testing a hypothesized causal pathway that is developed on the basis of prior knowledge or theory. Theories and accumulated knowledge form the underpinnings for the connection among variables in the model—not statistical technique. The researcher who undertakes an analysis such as the ones we discuss in this chapter should begin with a carefully formulated and defensible hypothesized scheme. Without such a scheme, causal modeling techniques can be easily misused.

PATH ANALYSIS

Path analysis is a widely used approach to studying patterns of causation among a set of variables. Path analysis, which relies on multiple linear regression, attempts to isolate the separate contributions to a dependent variable (the effect) made by a set of interrelated predictor variables (the causes). Path analysis is a highly sophisticated technique about which many books have been written. Here we present only an overview of path analytic concepts. The interested reader should consult more detailed presentations in such books as those by Pedhazur (1982), Kenny (1979), Li (1975), or Blalock (1964).

Path Diagrams

Researchers use path diagrams to specify their causal hypotheses. A **path diagram** is a visual representation of the hypothesized linkages and sequencing among variables in a causal network. Three simple path diagrams are illustrated in Figure 14–1. All three diagrams represent hypothesized explanations of the causes of variable 3 (V_3) on the basis of two predictor variables (V_1 and V_2).

In the first diagram (A), there is a hypothesized causal path leading from the presumed causes (V_1 and V_2) to the effect (V_3), as indicated by the straight lines and arrows. V_1 and V_2 are hypothesized to be independent causes—that is, they are not correlated with one another, and so there are no lines or arrows connecting these two variables to each other. In the context of a path analysis, V_3 is an **endogenous variable**—a variable that is affected by other variables within the model. Endogenous variables are ones that have arrows leading to them from other variables. By contrast, V_1 and V_2 are **exogenous variables;** they are presumed not to be caused by or influenced by any other variable in

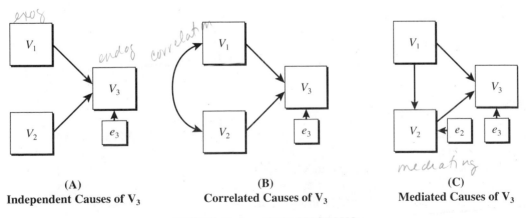

(A)
Independent Causes of V_3

(B)
Correlated Causes of V_3

(C)
Mediated Causes of V_3

FIGURE 14–1.   PATH DIAGRAMS

the model. There is one other box represented in this diagram, labeled e_3. In a path diagram, the es are the residual or error terms that represent the factors not included in the model that affect the endogenous variables.[1] The subscript for e_3 indicates that it is the error term for variable 3.

Figure 14–1 (B) is similar to the first diagram in that V_1 and V_2 are again the hypothesized causes of V_3. Here, however, there is a curved line between V_1 and V_2, which signifies that the two variables are presumed to be correlated. Despite a correlation between V_1 and V_2, there is no hypothesized *causal* connection. That is, V_1 is not a hypothesized cause of V_2, nor vice versa. In this diagram, as in diagram A, V_1 and V_2 are exogenous variables and V_3 is endogenous.

Figure 14–1 (C) presents a diagram for a more complex model in which V_3 is hypothesized to be caused directly by both V_1 and V_2, as before, but here V_2 is also hypothesized to be caused by V_1. In this model, V_2 is known as a **mediating variable** because one path of influence of V_1 on V_3 is *through* the influence of V_1 on V_2. The line connecting V_1 and V_3 indicates the hypothesized *direct* causal link between the two variables, but V_1 also affects V_3 indirectly through its effect on V_2. In this model, both V_2 and V_3 are endogenous, and there are e terms associated with each of these variables.

All of the diagrams in Figure 14–1 represent was is known as recursive models. A **recursive model** is one in which the causal flow is in one direction. Variable 3 is *not* presumed to be a cause of V_1 or V_2—it is assumed that reciprocal causation does not occur. All of our discussion relating to path analysis concerns recursive models.

Path Coefficients

Path analysis solves for **path coefficients,** which are the weights that represent the impact of one variable on another. Path analysis yields weights for each path in a path diagram.

Our discussion of path coefficients will be easier to follow if we use a simple illustration of a path analysis. We draw once again on the data that we presented in Table 10–1 in connection with multiple regression. It may be recalled that the regression analysis example involved the prediction of nursing students' graduate grade point average (GPA) on the basis of undergraduate grades, scores on the verbal and quantitative portions of the GRE, and scores on a motivation scale. To keep our illustration of path analysis simple, we will test a three-variable mediated-cause model. Figure 14–2 shows that our model predicts that graduate GPA (V_3) is caused by motivation (V_1) and undergraduate GPA (V_2); undergraduate grades are also hypothesized to be affected by the student's motivation, and V_2 mediates the relationship between motivation and graduate GPA. This path diagram indicates the bivariate correlations between all variables in the model. The subscripts associated with each r indicate which two variables are being correlated. Thus, the correlation between V_1 and V_2 (r_{12}) is .708. The correlation coefficients tell us that the three variables are highly interrelated, but they shed no light on the validity of the hypothesized causal model.

---

[1]The e term sometimes is referred to as the R (residual) term or the U (unexplained) term by different authors.

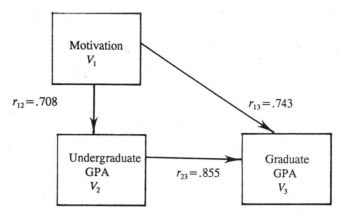

FIGURE 14–2.   THREE-VARIABLE PATH DIAGRAM FOR PREDICTING GRADUATE GPA

In path analysis, the researcher solves for a set of **structural equations.** Each endogenous variable in the model is represented by an equation in which that variable is predicted on the basis of the variables upon which it is presumed to depend, plus a residual term. In these equations, each predictor variable is weighted by a path coefficient that indicates the amount of change expected in the equation's dependent variable for a unit change in the predictor variable. Exogenous variables, which are not explained by variables in the model, are represented by a residual term only. Structural equations are conventionally expressed in standardized form—i.e., variables are represented as standard scores. For our model presented in Figure 14–2, the structural equations are:

$$z_1 = e_1$$
$$z_2 = p_{21}z_1 + e_2$$
$$z_3 = p_{31}z_1 + p_{32}z_2 + e_3$$

In these equations, the zs are the standard scores for motivation (z_1), undergraduate GPA (z_2), and graduate GPA (z_3). The ps are the path coefficients, and the associated subscripts indicate the variables involved. By convention, the first subscript indicates the dependent variable (the effect) and the second subscript indicates the independent variable (the cause). Thus, p_{21} in our example is the path coefficient representing the effect of motivation on undergraduate grades. Motivation (z_1) is exogenous and is represented by the residual term e_1. Undergraduate grades (z_2) are hypothesized to be affected by motivation, plus other factors not in the model (e_2). Finally, graduate GPA (z_3) is affected by both motivation and undergraduate grades, as well as by other factors (e_3).

Path analysis solves for the path coefficients through a series of multiple regression analyses.[2] The path coefficients are, in fact, the standardized regression coefficients (βs) from linear regression. Each endogenous variable must be regressed on the variables upon which is it hypothesized to depend. Thus, to solve for the ps in our example, two regression analyses must be run: one predicting z_2 from z_1 and the second predicting z_3 from z_1 and z_2. The first regression involves the straightforward calculation of a correlation coefficient, i.e., $r_{12} = \beta_{12} = p_{21}$. Thus, we can see from Figure 14–2 that $r_{12} = p_{21} = .708$. When a multiple regression analysis is performed to predict graduate GPA from the two other variables, the following standardized regression equation is obtained:

$$z_3 = .277z_1 + .659z_2$$

where $.277 = \beta_{13} = p_{31}$
$.659 = \beta_{23} = p_{32}$

We now have all values for the path coefficients, which are presented on the path diagram in Figure 14–3. We can also solve for the residual terms by computing the amount of unexplained variation. For e_2, where only two variables are involved, the calculation is simply:

$$e_2 = \sqrt{1 - r_{12}^2}$$
$$e_2 = \sqrt{1 - (.708)^2} = .706$$

This indicates that the correlation between undergraduate GPA and its residuals (e_2) is .706. The proportion of variance in undergraduate grades accounted for by motivation is 50.2% ($.708^2$), while that *un*accounted for by variables in the model is 49.8% ($.706^2$).

To solve for e_3, the r^2 in the above equation becomes the squared multiple correlation coefficient, and R in our example is .877:

$$e_3 = \sqrt{1 - R^2_{3 \cdot 12}}$$
$$e_3 = \sqrt{1 - .877^2} = .480$$

Thus, we have completely solved for all path coefficients and residual terms in our model.

Decomposition of Correlations among Variables

Through path analysis, the correlations among independent variables and dependent variables in the model can be decomposed into different effects. It is through such a

---

[2]Since multiple regression is the basis for path analysis, the assumptions that apply to multiple regression also apply to path analysis (see Chapter 10).

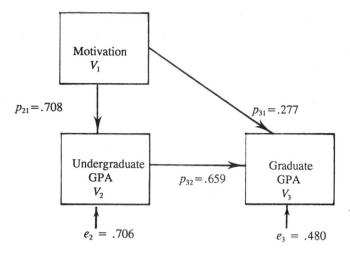

FIGURE 14–3. THREE-VARIABLE PATH DIAGRAM FOR PREDICTING GRADUATE GPA, WITH PATH COEFFICIENTS

decomposition that the researcher can interpret the causal connection among the variables. **Direct effects** are the effects of an independent variable on a dependent variable represented by a direct path between the two variables. In our example, there is a direct effect of both undergraduate GPA and motivation on graduate GPA. Direct causal effects are equal to the path coefficients connecting the variables. **Indirect effects** are effects on the dependent variable that occur *through* a mediating variable. Motivation has, in addition to a direct effect on graduate GPA, an indirect effect through its effect on undergraduate GPA. The calculation of indirect effects is discussed later in this section. When indirect and direct causal effects for a predictor are added together, we obtain the **total effect** of the predictor, which is sometimes referred to as its **effect coefficient.**

While correlations associated with the dependent variable can be decomposed into direct and indirect effects, not all correlations among variables in the model are causal effects. There are two types of **noncausal effects.** One involves correlations among correlated exogenous variables, such as V_1 and V_2 in Figure 14–1 (B), and is referred to as the **unanalyzed** component of a correlation. The second, called the **spurious effect,** occurs with endogenous variables that are not the dependent variable. In our example, there is a direct effect of undergraduate GPA (an endogenous variable) on graduate GPA, but there is also a spurious effect between these variables that arises because they both share a common cause, namely motivation.

There are different approaches to calculating the decomposed effects, some of which are elegant and convenient for complex path diagrams, but involve the use of matrix algebra. For relatively simple path analyses, an algorithm called the **tracing rule** can be used to decompose correlations by tracing the paths in path diagrams. The tracing rule stipulates that a correlation between variables can be decomposed into the sum of products of all path tracings from one variable to another *except* (1) the same variable cannot be entered twice on a tracing, and (2) a variable cannot be entered *and* left on a tracing through the arrowheads.

We can best explain the tracing rule by applying it to our model of graduate GPA (Figure 14–3). From the path coefficients, we are trying to decompose effects on the dependent variable and to recreate the correlations among all variables, i.e., r_{12}, r_{13}, and r_{23}. The first correlation (r_{12}) is that between motivation and undergraduate GPA. From the figure we see that there is a tracing from V_1 to V_2. We cannot count the tracing from V_2 to V_3 to V_1, because that would involve a violation of the second condition of the tracing rule, namely entering and leaving V_3 through an arrowhead. Thus, r_{12} cannot be further decomposed, and $r_{12} = p_{21} = .708$. This is perfectly sensible; since no other variable in the model affects V_1, its correlation cannot be decomposed into different contributing components. In general, correlations for exogenous variables are treated as "givens" and are not subject to further decomposition.

With regard to the correlation between motivation and graduate GPA (r_{13}), there are two tracings that qualify under the tracing rule: the direct path between V_1 and V_3, and the indirect path from V_1 to V_2 to V_3. (No variable is entered twice on a tracing, and no variable is entered and left through arrowheads.) As indicated by the tracing rule, we can calculate the indirect effect as the product of the path coefficients involved in the tracing. In this case, the indirect effect from V_1 to V_3 through V_2 is the product of p_{21} and p_{32}:

$$p_{21}p_{32} = (.708)(.659) = .466$$

As noted earlier, the direct effect equals the path coefficient between two variables, and thus the direct effect between V_1 and $V_3 = p_{31} = .277$. We have now totally decomposed the correlation between motivation and graduate GPA into direct and indirect effects:

    total effect = direct effect + indirect effect
    total effect =   .277   + .466
    total effect =   .743   = r_{13}

The path analysis suggests that, although motivation is strongly related to graduate grades, its direct causal effect is small relative to the indirect causal effect it has on graduate GPA *through* undergraduate GPA.

Only one correlation remains to be decomposed, namely, the correlation between undergraduate and graduate grades (r_{23}). Part of the correlation can be attributed to the direct effect of V_2 on V_3; i.e., $p_{32} = .659$. We can see from our model in Figure 14–3 that there is no other *causal* connection between V_2 and V_3—for example, undergraduate grades are not hypothesized to affect graduate grades *through* motivation. Thus, the dif-

TABLE 14-1. DECOMPOSITION OF CORRELATIONS

r	Direct Effect	Indirect Effect	Total Effect	Noncausal Covariation	All Effects
r_{12} (.708)	p_{21} (.708)	—	p_{21} (.708)	—	p_{21} (.708)
r_{13} (.743)	p_{31} (.277)	$p_{21}p_{32}$ (.466)	$p_{31} + p_{21}p_{32}$ (.743)	—	$p_{31} + p_{21}p_{32}$ (.743)
r_{23} (.855)	p_{32} (.659)	—	p_{32} (.659)	$p_{21}p_{31}$ (.196)	$p_{32} + p_{21}p_{31}$ (.855)

ference between the value of the correlation coefficient r_{23} (.855) and the path coefficient p_{32} (.659) must be a spurious, noncausal effect. We can calculate the spurious effect through the tracing of V_2 to V_1 to V_3. Clearly, this is a noncausal path, since V_2 is not a hypothesized cause of V_1. But this tracing does not violate the tracing rule—no variable is entered twice and no variable is entered *and* left through an arrowhead. The spurious effect from V_2 to V_3 through V_1 is the product of p_{21} and p_{31}:

$$p_{21}p_{32} = (.708)(.277) = .196$$

This spurious effect, .196, accounts for the difference between r_{23} and p_{32}; i.e., $.855 - .659 = .196$. The total decomposition of effects in the path diagram shown in Figure 14–3 is summarized in Table 14–1. As this table shows, the three values for All Effects, shown in the last column, correspond exactly to the three correlations coefficients in this example.

Identification

One of the ways that researchers can evaluate the validity of their causal models is to examine the extent to which the correlation matrix (i.e., intercorrelations among all variables in the model) can be reproduced or closely approximated on the basis of path coefficients. In our example, despite the fact that we were able to reproduce all correlations perfectly, we are unable to draw conclusions about model validity because the model is what is called a just-identified model. **Identification** refers to the existence of sufficient information to estimate the parameters of a causal model. A **just-identified model** is one in which the number of known parameters[3] (correlation coefficients) is equal to the number of unknown parameters (path coefficients) being estimated. In our example, there were three correlations (r_{12}, r_{13}, and r_{23}) and three path coefficients. A recursive model in which all variables are interconnected is always just-identified. Just-identified models *always* fit the data perfectly and therefore cannot be tested.

---

[3]The number of known parameters is calculated as $[k\,(k - 1)]/2$, where k is the total number of exogenous and endogeneous variables in the model.

When paths are dropped from a just-identified model, the result is an overidentified model. An **overidentified model** is one in which there are more known parameters— and more structural equations—than there are paths to be estimated. For example, suppose that in Figure 14–3 we dropped path p_{31}—the direct path between motivation and graduate GPA. This model, shown in Figure 14–4, hypothesizes that all of the effect of motivation on graduate GPA can be accounted for through motivation's effect on undergraduate GPA. The structural equations for this new model are:

$$z_1 = e_1$$
$$z_2 = p_{21}z_1 + e_2$$
$$z_3 = p_{32}z_2 + e_3$$

Thus, there are now only two unknown parameters to be estimated from three equations, based on three known parameters. Overidentification is the result of a constraint that we have placed on the model—namely, our presumption that the path coefficient between V_1 and V_3 is zero. In this new model, the path coefficient between V_1 and V_2 remains the same, but the path coefficient between V_2 and V_3 is now simply the correlation between the two variables, i.e., .855. For the overidentified model, then, the path coefficients are:

$$p_{21} = .708 \qquad p_{31} = .000 \qquad p_{32} = .855$$

We can assess the adequacy of this overidentified model by examining the extent to which the path coefficients reproduce the correlation matrix. The calculations are shown in Table 14–2. A comparison of the values in the first column (rs) and the last column (All Effects) indicates that our new model did not perfectly reproduce the correlation between motivation and graduate GPA ($r_{13} = .743$, all effects $= .605$). In other words,

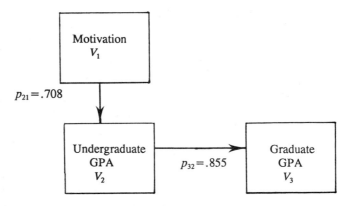

FIGURE 14–4.   OVERIDENTIFIED MODEL FOR PREDICTING GRADUATE GPA

TABLE 14–2. DECOMPOSITION OF CORRELATIONS IN OVERIDENTIFIED MODEL

r	Direct Effect	Indirect Effect	Total Effect	Noncausal Covariation	All Effects
r_{12} (.708)	p_{21} (.708)	—	p_{21} (.708)	—	p_{21} (.708)
r_{13} (.743)	p_{31} (.00)	$p_{21}p_{32}$ (.605)	$p_{31} + p_{21}p_{32}$ (.605)	—	$p_{31} + p_{21}p_{32}$ (.605)
r_{23} (.855)	p_{32} (.855)	—	p_{32} (.855)	$p_{21}p_{31}$ (.00)	$p_{32} + p_{21}p_{31}$ (.855)

the effect of motivation on graduate grades cannot be accounted for totally by motivation's effect on undergraduate grades. The decomposition in this case suggests a need to modify the model.

Theory Trimming

The process of dropping paths from a causal model is often referred to as **theory trimming.** A researcher may begin with a just-identified model in which all variables are interconnected, and then trim the theory on the basis of one or more criteria. (Of course, paths can also be trimmed from a model that was originally overidentified as well.)

One criterion for trimming the model involves the statistical significance of individual paths. Multiple regression analyses provide information on the significance of individual βs, which are the path coefficients, via t statistics. Using the criterion of statistical significance, paths would be deleted from the model if the associated βs were not significantly different from zero. Another criterion is the meaningfulness of the path. With a large sample size, almost all βs are statistically significant, even though the magnitude of the path coefficient may be very small. Researchers may establish their own criterion for how large the β must be in order to make a meaningful contribution to the causal theory. A β less than .05 has been suggested as one possible cutoff value for trimming a path (Pedhazur, 1982).

It is important to remember than once paths have been deleted, the regressions must be rerun, using only paths that have been retained. Deletion of paths will result in changes to the βs for the retained paths. For example, when we changed the just-identified model (Figure 14–3) to an overidentified model (Figure 14–4), the path coefficient p_{32} increased from .659 to .855. After a path model has been trimmed and new regressions have been run, correlations should be decomposed to determine their reproducibility.

Theory trimming offers several advantages, including the development of a parsimonious causal explanation for phenomena of interest. Additionally, when a just-identified model is trimmed to an overidentified one, its statistical significance can be tested and the reproduction of correlations can be used to assess the adequacy of the model. However, theory trimming suffers from the fact that paths are trimmed after the fact on a statistical rather than theoretical basis. Nevertheless, theory trimming remains an important analytic tool and is especially useful at the exploratory stage of model development.

Evaluating Path Models

The reproducibility of the correlation matrix is an important means of assessing the validity of the path model. As noted earlier, however, just-identified models cannot use this criterion because the correlation matrix invariably can be reproduced, no matter how absurd the model. For example, suppose that we interchanged V_2 and V_3 in Figure 14–3. Such a model would test the hypothesis that motivation and graduate grades *caused* undergraduate grades—a temporal impossibility. The regression analyses, however, are agnostic with regard to the plausibility of the model and would faithfully give us path coefficients that could be used to exactly reproduce the correlation matrix.[4]

An important point to remember is that *it is possible for alternative causal models to be consistent with the same data,* in both just-identified and overidentified models. This is precisely why it is important for a model to be theoretically driven rather than empirically driven. It is also important to build a model that takes into account the criteria for causality discussed at the beginning of the chapter. In particular, careful thought needs to be paid to the issue of temporal sequencing—a thorny issue when the data for a path model are from a cross-sectional design (i.e., when the data are all collected at one point in time). For example, suppose we proposed a mediated model such as the one in Figure 14–3 for a sample of cancer patients, in which V_1 was pain level, V_2 was hopefulness, and V_3 was coping ability—all measured at the same time. This model postulates that cancer patients' ability to cope is caused by how much pain they are in and how hopeful they feel. Suppose that the model worked reasonably well in terms of the path coefficients and allocation of effects to direct and indirect causes. Despite the fact that the data are consistent with the hypothesized model, they would also be consistent with alternative (and plausible) models. For example, perhaps patients' poor coping skills "caused" hopelessness, which in turn led these patients to perceive higher levels of pain. This explanation would be difficult to rule out because we do not know whether pain levels preceded or followed coping ability.

In sum, when variables are measured simultaneously, it is often problematic to determine the causal sequence. This does not mean that path analysis cannot be applied to cross-sectional data. Some variables, for example, have implicit temporal information. For example, most demographic variables (age, gender, ethnicity, educational attain-

---

[4]It should be noted that the path coefficients change when the model specification changes, even when the same variables are in the analysis (e.g., $p_{31} \neq p_{13}$). When V_2 and V_3 in Figure 14–3 are interchanged, for example, the path coefficients are $p_{21} = .743$, $p_{32} = .733$, and $p_{31} = .164$.

ment) are temporally prior to other attributes and behaviors. Researchers can also obtain temporal information retrospectively. For example, people can be asked the age at which they began to smoke to rule out the possibility that lung cancer preceded smoking. Finally, and most importantly, a sound theory is an unparalleled resource when developing causal models with cross-sectional data.

We have seen that path models can be evaluated in terms of their consistency with theory and logic, as well as on the basis of reproduced correlations. What about significance testing? An overidentified model can be tested for overall significance, but a just-identified model cannot be tested. Several goodness-of-fit tests have been proposed. The tests are performed by making comparisons between the observed and reproduced correlation matrices. These tests are complex, however, and must generally be computed manually. The interested reader should consult Pedhazur (1982) or other advanced texts.

LINEAR STRUCTURAL RELATIONS ANALYSIS

Path analysis is the most widely used approach to causal modeling used by health care researchers. Strictly speaking, however, its validity depends upon some restrictive assumptions that are often difficult to meet in practice. In addition to the assumptions required for multiple regression, path analysis assumes that (1) the variables in the model are measured without error; (2) the residuals (es) are not intercorrelated; and (3) the causal flow is in one direction—i.e., the model is recursive.

The first assumption is almost never possible to achieve. The greater the unreliability of the instruments used to measure variables in the analysis, the greater is the threat to the validity of a path analysis. The second assumption—that the residuals from different equations are uncorrelated—may also be difficult to achieve; error terms often represent unmeasured sources of systematic individual differences. Finally, it is often theoretically useful to formulate a model involving reciprocal causation, which calls for a nonrecursive model.[5]

A more general and powerful approach that avoids these problems is known as **linear structural relations analysis** (usually abbreviated **LISREL**). LISREL is actually the name of a specific computer program for analyzing covariance structures and for performing structural equations modeling, but the software has come to be almost synonymous with the approach. Some authors prefer to use the generic name of structural equations modeling for this class of techniques. However, inasmuch as path analysis also is based on structural equations, we use the term linear structural relations analysis in this section.

LISREL is an extremely versatile—but extremely complex—analytic tool, and the programs for running these analyses are more difficult than for other multivariate pro-

---

[5]Several extensions of path analysis to accommodate a nopnrecursive model have been proposed, but these approaches have not been widely used by health care researchers or behavioral scientists.

cedures. Therefore, we restrict the discussion here to a rudimentary introduction to LISREL. Readers interested in a more extensive description can consult such references as Kenny (1979), Long (1976), or Sörbom and Jöreskog (1981). Additionally, the computer manuals for LISREL software should be consulted. The software has been continuously updated and is currently in its seventh version (LISREL-7); it is available in mainframe version and also as a separate module that can be run on a personal computer with SPSS/PC (see Jöreskog and Sörbom, 1989).

Basic Concepts of LISREL

LISREL can be used for the analysis of hypothesized causal models under a wide variety of circumstances. Unlike path analysis, LISREL can accommodate measurement errors, correlated errors, correlated residuals, and **nonrecursive models** that allow for reciprocal causation. Another attractive feature of LISREL is that it can be used to analyze causal models involving latent variables. A **latent variable** is an unmeasured variable that corresponds to an abstract construct in which the researcher is interested. For example, *intelligence* can be viewed as a latent variable, while the Stanford-Binet Intelligence Test yields an observed measure of the underlying construct of intelligence. As another example, factor analysis (Chapter 12) yields information about underlying, latent dimensionalities that are not directly measured by the variables in the analysis. In LISREL, latent variables are captured by two or more measured variables—sometimes referred to as the **manifest variables**—that serve as indicators of the underlying construct.

Path analysis, as we have seen, uses least-squares estimation with its associated assumptions and restrictions. LISREL, by contrast, uses maximum likelihood estimation.[6] There are only two noteworthy assumptions for LISREL. First, it is assumed that the matrix of coefficients of the effects of all dependent variables (endogenous on endogenous variables) is nonsingular. Second, it is assumed that latent exogenous variables are uncorrelated with the residuals, or errors, in the equations.

LISREL proceeds in two sequential phases. In the first phase, a measurement model is tested. When there is evidence of an adequate fit of the data to the hypothesized measurement model, the causal model can be tested via structural equation modeling. The causal model is also subjected to a goodness-of-fit test before the overall analysis is considered complete.

The Measurement Model Phase

The **measurement model** stipulates the hypothesized relationships among the latent and manifest variables. In path analysis it is assumed—unrealistically—that underlying constructs on the one hand and the scales or instruments used to measure them on the other are identical. In LISREL, the constructs are treated as unobserved variables measured by two or more fallible indicators. Thus, a major advantage of LISREL is that it

---

[6]Structural equation modeling via maximum likelihood estimation can be performed by other programs in addition to LISREL, such as the EQS program.

enables the researcher to separate latent variables from errors, and to then proceed to study causal relationships among the latent variables. However, the process depends on the judicious selection of indicators. An inadequate selection of measured variables to represent a latent variable will lead to questions about whether or not the theory's constructs are really embedded in the causal model.

During the measurement model phase, LISREL tests three things: (1) causal relationships between the measured variables and latent variables, (2) correlations between pairs of latent variables, and (3) correlations among the errors associated with the measured variables. The measurement model is essentially a factor analytic model that seeks to confirm a hypothesized factor structure. Thus, loadings on the factors (latent variables) provide a method for evaluating relationships between the observed and unobserved variables.

We can illustrate with a simplified example. Figure 14–5 presents a diagram that builds on the example we have been using throughout this chapter. In this diagram, there are two latent variables, depicted by circles by convention: cognitive ability and academic success. Cognitive ability is captured by two indicators: scores on the verbal and quantitative portions of the GRE. According to the model, test scores are *caused by* cognitive ability (and thus the arrows indicating a hypothesized causal path), and are also affected by error (e_1 and e_2). Moreover, it is hypothesized that the error terms are correlated, as indicated by the curved line with double arrows connecting e_1 and e_2. Correlated measurement errors on the GRE might arise, for example, as a result of the stu-

EXAMPLE OF A LATENT MEASUREMENT MODEL

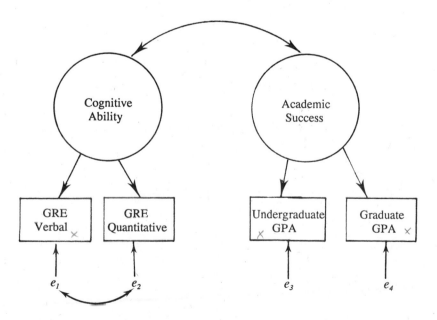

FIGURE 14–5.   EXAMPLE OF A LATENT MEASUREMENT MODEL

dent's test anxiety or level of fatigue—factors that would systematically depress test scores on both portions of the exam. The second latent variable is academic success, which is captured by undergraduate and graduate grades. The error terms associated with these two manifest variables are presumed not to be correlated. Within the measurement model, the two latent variables are hypothesized to be correlated.

After specifying the hypothesized measurement model, the model would be tested against the research data using LISREL.[7] The analysis would provide information on loadings of the observed variables on the latent variables, the correlation between the two latent variables, and the correlation between e_1 and e_2. The analysis would also indicate whether the overall model fit is good, based on a chi-square goodness-of-fit statistic. If the hypothesized model is not a good fit to the study data, the measurement model would need to be respecified and retested.

The Structural Equations Model Phase

Once an adequate measurement model has been found, the second phase of the LISREL analysis can proceed. As in path analysis, the researcher must specify the theoretical causal model to be tested. Both just-identified and overidentified models can be tested with LISREL. **Underidentified models,** which have fewer known parameters than unknown parameters, cannot be estimated.

As an example, we could use LISREL to test a causal model in which we hypothesized that the latent variable cognitive ability caused the latent variable academic success. The model to be tested would look similar to the one shown in Figure 14–5, except that there would be a straight line and an arrow (i.e., a path) from cognitive ability to academic success. There would also be another arrow leading to academic success for a residual term.

In this part of the analysis, LISREL would yield information about the hypothesized causal parameters—i.e., the path coefficients, which are presented as beta weights. The coefficients indicate the expected amount of change in the latent endogenous variable that is caused by a one-unit change in the latent causal variable. The LISREL program provides information on the significance of individual paths via t statistics, thus providing information that might be useful in model trimming.

The residual terms—the amount of unexplained variance for the latent endogenous variables—can also be calculated from the LISREL analysis. The formula for computing the residuals is the same as that in path analysis, i.e., $\sqrt{1 - R^2}$. The LISREL printout provides the value of the squared multiple correlation (R) for each equation predicting an endogenous variable.

The overall fit of the causal model to the research data can be tested by means of several alternative statistics. One statistic is the chi-square goodness-of-fit statistic, which has a low, nonsignificant value when the model fit is good. (As in path analysis, a

---

[7]This first phase of LISREL corresponds to a confirmatory factor analysis (CFA).

just-identified model cannot be tested; the chi-square value is always zero for just-identified models.) One difficulty with the chi-square test is that it is sensitive to sample size. Thus, with a sufficiently large sample size, an overidentified model may be rejected even when the model fit is good. Two alternatives that LISREL offers is the **goodness-of-fit index (GFI)** and the **adjusted goodness-of-fit index (AGFI),** which are independent of sample size. For both of these indexes, a value of .90 or greater indicates a good fit of the model to the data.

Statistical validation is a necessary, but not sufficient means of evaluating the adequacy of the hypothesized causal model. As with path analysis, alternative models tested with LISREL can be consistent with the data. The importance of a sound underlying theory for drawing causal inferences cannot be overemphasized.

COMPUTER EXAMPLE OF PATH ANALYSIS

The data in Table 10–1 on graduate GPA are used here to illustrate computer printouts for path analyses.[8] In this example, the causal model we test is a four-variable mediated-cause model; verbal GRE scores are added to the original model (Figure 14–3) as a second exogenous variable, hypothesized to be a cause of graduate GPA both directly and indirectly through undergraduate GPA. To test this new model, we must run two regressions: one predicting undergraduate grades (z_3) from motivation (z_1) and GRE-Verbal scores (z_2), and the second predicting graduate GPA (z_4) from the three other variables.

Figure 14–6 presents the printout for these analyses.[9] Panel A lists all variables in the analysis, together with the mean and standard deviation for each. As noted beneath the means, there are 20 cases in the analysis. Panel B presents the correlation matrix.

Panel C shows the multiple regression results for the first regression in which undergraduate grades are the dependent variable and motivation and GRE-Verbal scores are the independent variables. The R^2 for this analysis is .55937, and the overall equation is statistically significant ($F = 10.79075$, $p = .0009$). The information needed for the path analysis is at the bottom of the panel, under the heading Variables in the Equation. Here we see that the beta for motivation is .608993 and the beta for the GRE-Verbal scores is .259743. These are, respectively, p_{31} and p_{32} in our path analysis.

Panel D presents the multiple regression results for the prediction of graduate GPA

---

[8]Because of the complexity of LISREL, computer printouts are not presented.

[9]The SPSS/PC commands that generated the printout shown in Figure 14–6 are:

```
REGRESSION VARIABLES=GPA@U GRE@V MOTIV GPA@G
    /DESCRIPTIVES=DEFAULT
    /STATISTICS=DEFAULT
    /DEPENDENT=GPA@U
    /METHOD=ENTER MOTIV GRE@V
    /DEPENDENT=GPA@G
    /METHOD=ENTER MOTIV GRE@V GPA@U.
```

A Listwise Deletion of Missing Data

	Mean	Std Dev	Label
GPA@U	3.305	.296	UNDERGRAD GRADE PT AVERAGE
GRE@V	562.500	57.205	VERBAL GRE SCORE
MOTIV	69.250	10.672	MOTIVATION SCALE SCORE
GPA@G	3.210	.442	GRADUATE GRADE PT AVERAGE

N of Cases =   20

B Correlation:

	GPA@U	GRE@V	MOTIV	GPA@G
GPA@U	1.000	.493	.708	.855
GRE@V	.493	1.000	.383	.727
MOTIV	.708	.383	1.000	.743
GPA@G	.855	.727	.743	1.000

* * * *   M U L T I P L E   R E G R E S S I O N   * * * *

C Equation Number 1   Dependent Variable..   GPA@U   UNDERGRAD GRADE PT AVERAGE

Block Number 1. Method: Enter   MOTIV   GRE@V

Variable(s) Entered on Step Number
   1..   MOTIV   MOTIVATION SCALE SCORE
   2..   GRE@V   VERBAL GRE SCORE

Multiple R	.74791
R Square	.55937
Adjusted R Square	.50754
Standard Error	.20802

Analysis of Variance

	DF	Sum of Squares	Mean Square
Regression	2	.93388	.46694
Residual	17	.73562	.04327

F =   10.79075   Signif F = .0009

------------------ Variables in the Equation ------------------

Variable	B	SE B	Beta	T	Sig T
MOTIV	.016916	.004840	.608993	3.495	.0028
GRE@V	.001346	9.02945E-04	.259743	1.491	.1544
(Constant)	1.376458	.492156		2.797	.0124

End Block Number   1   All requested variables entered.

FIGURE 14–6.   COMPUTER PRINTOUT OF REGRESSIONS FOR A PATH ANALYSIS

```
              * * * *   M U L T I P L E   R E G R E S S I O N   * * * *
D   Equation Number 2    Dependent Variable..   GPA@G   GRADUATE GRADE PT AVERAGE

    Block Number  1.  Method:  Enter     MOTIV    GRE@V    GPA@U


    Variable(s) Entered on Step Number
        1..    MOTIV      MOTIVATION SCALE SCORE
        2..    GRE@V      VERBAL GRE SCORE
        3..    GPA@U      UNDERGRAD GRADE PT AVERAGE


    Multiple R            .94066
    R Square              .88483
    Adjusted R Square     .86324
    Standard Error        .16359

    Analysis of Variance
                          DF       Sum of Squares      Mean Square
    Regression            3             3.28981           1.09660
    Residual              16             .42819            .02676

    F =      40.97604        Signif F =   .0000


    ----------------- Variables in the Equation ------------------

    Variable              B          SE B        Beta        T    Sig T

    MOTIV             .010366      .004990      .250073     2.077   .0542
    GRE@V             .003038   7.55077E-04     .392849     4.023   .0010
    GPA@U             .722009      .190735      .483817     3.785   .0016
    (Constant)      -1.602914      .467684                 -3.427   .0035


    End Block Number   1   All requested variables entered.
```

FIGURE 14–6. (CONTINUED)

on the basis of the three other variables. In this analysis the R^2 is .88483, which is highly significant (F = 40.97604, p = .0000). At the bottom we see that the betas are as follows: motivation (p_{41}) = .250073; GRE-Verbal scores (p_{42}) = .392849; and undergraduate GPA (p_{43}) = .483817.

Figure 14–7 presents the path model with all path coefficients indicated, rounded to three decimal places. As we can see, this is an overidentified model because not all variables are interconnected; V_1 and V_2 do not have a path between them. It would therefore be possible to evaluate the model by examining the extent to which the correlation matrix (panel B of Figure 14–6) could be reproduced from the path coefficients.

Should this model be trimmed? An inspection of the path coefficients reveals that all are fairly substantial. The lowest is for the path between GRE-Verbal scores and undergraduate grades (p_{32} = .260), and this seems large enough to be meaningful. However, returning to Figure 14–6, we find that this path coefficient is *not* statistically significant, a reflection of the small sample size used in this example. This means that p_{32}

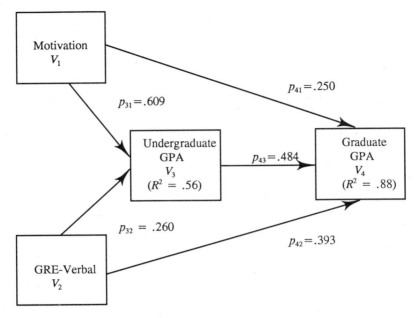

FIGURE 14–7.   FOUR-VARIABLE PATH DIAGRAM FOR COMPUTER PRINTOUT EXAMPLE

is not reliably different from zero, and thus the path could be trimmed from the model on the basis of a statistical criterion.

RESEARCH APPLICATIONS OF CAUSAL MODELS

Causal modeling is an important research tool. This section examines the major applications of causal modeling and discusses methods of effectively displaying causal model information in a research report.

The Uses of Causal Modeling

The primary use of causal modeling is in the testing of theories about causal pathways, and hypotheses relating to those theories. Causal modeling can also be used in an exploratory fashion during the development of theory, but theory development is better suited to a conceptual rather than to an empirical process.

Although causal modeling is most frequently encountered in connection with nonexperimental, correlational research, it can also be applied within experimental research to help unravel underlying causes for observed experimental effects. For example, suppose we wanted to test the effectiveness of an intervention to promote breastfeeding among teenage mothers, using an experimental design in which a sample of pregnant teenagers was randomly assigned to either an experimental group (those exposed to the intervention) or to a control group (those not exposed to it). If the intervention were found to be effective (i.e., a significantly higher percentage of young mothers in the experimental than in the control group breastfed their infants), the researcher might well want to elucidate the causal path through which the intervention had its effect. Was it because of increased knowledge of the benefits of breastfeeding, reduced anxiety about breastfeeding performance, or increased acceptance of breastfeeding via peer group support? If the researcher had included measures of breastfeeding knowledge, breastfeeding anxiety, and peer group support of breastfeeding in the study, the competing hypotheses could be tested via causal modeling. Of course, the analysis of *causes* would still be nonexperimental (i.e., the teenagers were not randomly assigned to different levels of breastfeeding knowledge), but the analysis would be embedded within a rigorous experimental design.

Causal modeling is being used increasingly by health care researchers. Some recent examples of studies that have used causal modeling are summarized in Table 14–3.

The Presentation of Causal Models in Research Reports

Causal model results are complex, and thus the presentation often requires figures, tables, and text if all aspects of the results are to be presented. Supporting tables are

TABLE 14–3. RESEARCH EXAMPLES OF CAUSAL MODELING

Overall Research Question	Theoretical Basis	Analytic Method
What are the direct and indirect effects of child temperament, maternal characteristics, and family circumstances on the maladjustment of school-age children? (McClowry et al., 1994)	Temperament theory	Path analysis
Do cognitive-perceptual and modifying factors such as demographic characteristics affect workers' use of hearing protection in an automotive transmission plant? (Lusk, Ronis, Kerr, & Atwood, 1994)	Pender's Health Promotion Model	Maximum likelihood structural equations model
What is the impact of mother-daughter relationships on the adult daughters' commitment to caregiving of their elderly mothers? (Pohl, Boyd, Liang, & Given, 1995)	Commitment theory; feminist theory	Path analysis
What is the effect of cognitive-perceptual factors, demographic and biologic characteristics, and past exercise behavior on exercise behavior and aerobic fitness in arthritic out-patients? (Neuberger, Kasal, Smith, Hassanein, & DeVíney, 1994)	Pender's Health Promotion Model	Path analysis

not always included in the report, but a figure with the path diagram is essential.

It is often necessary to present two figures with path diagrams—one to lay out the theoretical model and the other to present the estimated parameters. The first figure provides an overview of the model to be tested, and does not contain information about path coefficients—it indicates the construct names, hypothesized paths, and hypothesized (noncausal) correlations. (If LISREL were being used, latent and manifest variables would be indicated.) Often, the researcher marks the paths with pluses and minuses, to indicate the expected direction of the relationship between variables. The initial model is usually shown as the researcher has conceptualized it before any theory trimming, and is usually included in the introduction to the report.

The second path diagram summarizes the results of the final statistical analyses. If paths have been deleted as a result of theory trimming, they typically are omitted in the figure, although the process of deletion and the criteria used to delete paths should be covered in the text. The figure with the final model should include the following information: sample size (usually in a footnote or in the figure title), names of all variables in the analysis,[10] paths in the model, path coefficients, and significance levels for untrimmed models. Researchers often show the value of R^2 in parentheses under each endogenous variable, as we did in Figure 14–7. Residual terms can also be shown, as in Figure 14–3, but are not essential. If goodness-of-fit tests have been performed, this information should be presented at the bottom of the diagram.

Supplementary information can be included in tables, depending upon the nature of the research questions being addressed. For example, a supporting table with full regression results is sometimes included. If the decomposition of the correlation coefficients is an important goal of the research, a table summarizing direct and indirect effects for each predictor should also be presented.

The text should focus on the extent to which there is a good fit between the data and the model—i.e., the extent to which the causal theory (and the measurement model in LISREL) has been supported by the analysis. If the theory was trimmed, a full explanation should be provided regarding the preliminary results and the criteria used to delete paths. If the model fit is poorer than had been anticipated, suggested modifications to the model should be offered.

RESEARCH EXAMPLE

Causal modeling was invented decades ago, but it was not until the last 15 to 20 years that it has been applied with any regularity by health care researchers. This section describes a recent study in which path analysis was used.

Coffman, Levitt, and Brown (1994) used path analysis to test a theoretical model concerning married couples' expectations for mutual support during pregnancy and shortly after childbirth. The

---

[10]In LISREL, the names of the latent variables should always be shown. The manifest variables should be shown if it is possible to do so without resulting in a cluttered presentation.

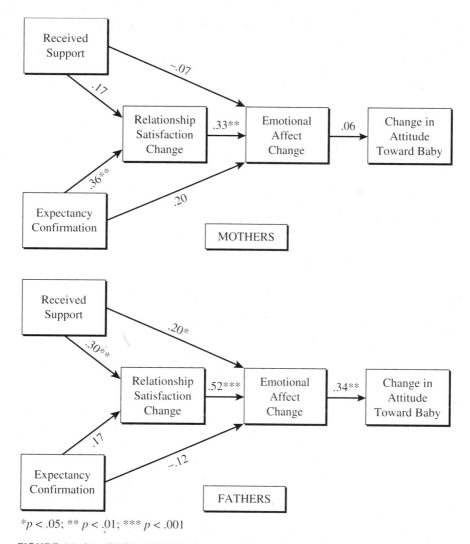

*p < .05; ** p < .01; *** p < .001

FIGURE 14–8.   RESEARCH EXAMPLE OF A PATH ANALYSIS

Originally Figure 1 from Coffman, Levitt, & Brown (1994), entitled Path Model of Interrelations of Support, Expectancy Confirmation, and Outcomes for Mothers and Fathers.

theoretical model stipulated that marital satisfaction depends not only on actual supportiveness but also on the extent to which support is congruent with the person's expectations. Both expectancy confirmation and relationship satisfaction were viewed as determinants of the married partners' emotional well-being, which in turn was hypothesized as a mediator of attitudes toward a newborn. Among the specific hypotheses the researchers tested in their study were the following:

1. Parents who perceive greater confirmation of support expectations postnatally will have more positive outcomes, including better relationship satisfaction, emotional affect, and attitudes toward the baby.
2. Confirmation of support expectations will have an independent effect on relationship satisfaction, over and above the effect of received support.

The researchers conducted a prospective, longitudinal study with a sample of 99 men and 105 women, all of whom were participating in childbirth education classes. Data were gathered prenatally and again 3 to 6 months postnatally. Instruments were administered at both points in time to measure three constructs: emotional affect, attitude toward the baby, and relationship satisfaction. *Changes* on these measures over time were used as the variables in the path analysis. Additionally, two variables were measured postnatally only: level of support received from the spouse and expectancy confirmation (i.e., degree to which support expectations had been met by the partner).

Separate path analyses were run for mothers and fathers. The results are presented in Figure 14–8. (In the report, the path diagram was supported by two tables that completely summarized the two sets of regression results.) As Figure 14–8 shows, the researchers did not do any theory trimming, but rather presented the entire model that they tested. However, they displayed information about the statistical significance of each path coefficient.

The results support the researchers' decision to run separate analyses for men and women because there were important gender differences. Among the women, expectancy confirmation significantly influenced changes in relationship satisfaction, consistent with the theoretical model and both hypotheses. Among the men, by contrast, expectancy confirmation was less important to relationship satisfaction than the *actual* level of support received. For both men and women, changes in satisfaction with the relationship mediated the link between support on the one hand and changes in emotional well-being on the other, consistent with the underlying theory. The mothers' changes in attitude toward the baby were unrelated to emotional affect changes, but among the fathers, improvements in emotional affect resulted in an improved attitude toward the baby.

This study illustrates how longitudinal data can facilitate causal modeling. If the study were cross-sectional and there was a correlation between received support and relationship satisfaction measured contemporaneously, it would be equally plausible to argue that marital satisfaction had an effect on received support (i.e., a strained relationship would result in lower support) as it is to argue that level of support influenced marital satisfaction. By using changes over time, temporal ordering is much more clear-cut.

SUMMARY

Causal modeling involves the development and statistical testing of a hypothesized causal explanation of a phenomenon. **Path analysis,** the most widely used approach to causal modeling, is based on least-squares multiple regression. The causal model being tested should first be specified in a **path diagram** that presents the hypothesized causal linkages among variables. A path diagram shows the expected relationship between the **endogenous variables** (those affected by other variables in the model) and the **exogenous variables** (variables whose determinants are presumed to lie outside the model). Path analysis can be used to test **recursive models** wherein the causal flow is in one direction.

Through a series of multiple regressions, path analysis solves for a set of **structural equations.** The unknown parameters being estimated in path analysis are the **path**

coefficients, which are the beta weights from the regression. Once the path analysis is completed, all correlations can be decomposed to identify **direct effects** of a predictor (effects resulting from a direct path between the predictor and the dependent variable) as well as **indirect effects** (effects resulting through a **mediating variable**). The **tracing rule** can be used to compute indirect effects, as well as **noncausal effects**, such as a spurious relationship between variables.

Identification refers to the existence of sufficient information to estimate the parameters (the path coefficients) of a causal model. A **just-identified model** has an equal number of known and unknown parameters, while an **overidentified model** is one in which there are more known parameters than unknown ones. Just-identified models cannot be tested for overall significance. **Theory trimming** refers to the process of deleting paths from a model on the basis of either statistical criteria or the meaningfulness of a path.

Path analysis has many assumptions and restrictions, and as a result techniques for structural equations modeling using maximum likelihood estimation have been developed, including **linear structural relations analysis** (**LISREL**). LISREL can accommodate measurement errors, **nonrecursive models** that allow for reciprocal causal paths, and correlated errors. LISREL can also analyze causal models involving **latent variables,** which are not directly measured but which are captured by two or more **manifest variables** (i.e., measured variables).

LISREL proceeds in two sequential phases: the measurement model phase and the structural equations modeling phase. The **measurement model** stipulates the hypothesized relationship between latent variables and manifest variables. If the measurement model fits the data, the next phase involves the testing of the hypothesized causal model. LISREL yields several goodness-of-fit indices for testing the overall fit of the model to the data. For both LISREL and path analysis, a sound underlying theory is critical for drawing causal inferences.

EXERCISES

The following exercises cover concepts presented in this chapter. Exercises indicated with a dagger (†) can be checked against answers appearing in Appendix A. Additionally, Chapter 14 of the accompanying *Applications Manual* offers supplementary exercises, including ones that require computer analysis of a data set on diskette.

1. Draw a path diagram depicting a recursive model in which patient satisfaction with nursing care is hypothesized to be caused by both patient characteristics and nurse characteristics. Have you hypothesized a model with independent causes, correlated causes, or mediated causes?

2. Draw a similar path diagram as for Exercise 1, but now use latent variables rather than manifest variables. If appropriate, make the model nonrecursive.

† 3. Write out the structural equations for the model shown in Figure 14–7.

† 4. In Figure 14–1, indicate for each diagram (A, B, and C) whether there would be direct, indirect, and noncausal effects.

† 5. If we wanted to decompose the model shown in Figure 14–7 into various effects, how many correlation coefficients would there be to reproduce? For r_{14}, calculate the direct, indirect, and noncausal effects. How does "all effects" for V_1 through V_4 compare with r_{14}?

† 6. Compute the two residual terms for the path analysis presented in Figure 14–7.

† 7. Are the models in Figure 14–8 just-identified or overidentified?

References

METHODOLOGICAL AND STATISTICAL REFERENCES

American Psychological Association (1983). *Publication manual of the American Psychological Association* (3rd ed.). Washington, DC: Author.

Barnett, V., & Lewis, T. (1985). *Outliers in statistical data* (2nd ed.). New York: John Wiley & Sons.

Becker, H. S. (1970). *Sociological work.* Chicago: Aldine.

Blalock, H. M. (1964). *Causal inferences in nonexperimental research.* Chapel Hill. University of North Carolina.

Cattell, R. B., Balcar, K. R., Horn, J. L., & Nesselroade, J. R. (1969). Factor matching procedures: An improvement of the *s* index with tables. *Educational and Psychological Measurement, 29,* 781–792.

Cohen, J. (1967). An alternative to Marascuilo's large sample multiple comparisons for proportions. *Psychological Bulletin, 67,* 199–201.

Cohen, J. (1977). *Statistical power analysis for the behavioral sciences* (Rev. ed.). New York: Academic Press.

Cohen, J., & Cohen, P. (1975). *Applied multiple regression/correlation analysis for the behavioral sciences.* New York: John Wiley & Sons.

Dixon, W. J., & Massey, F. J. (1969). *Introduction to statistical analysis* (3rd ed.). New York: John Wiley & Sons.

Ferguson, G. A. (1981). *Statistical analysis in psychology and education.* New York: McGraw-Hill.

Ferketich, S., & Verran, J. (1994). An overview of data transformation. *Research in Nursing and Health, 17,* 393–396.

Finn, J. D. (1974). *A general model for multivariate analysis.* New York: Holt, Rinehart and Winston, Inc.

Gibbons, J. D. (1993). *Nonparametric statistics: An introduction.* Thousand Oaks, CA: Sage.

Glass, G. V., McGaw, B., & Smith, M. L. (1981). *Meta-analysis of social research.* Beverly Hills: Sage.

Glass, G., & Stanley, J. C. (1970). *Statistical methods in education and psychology.* Englewood Cliffs, NJ: Prentice-Hall.

Goodman, L. A. (1964). Simultaneous confidence intervals for contrasts among multinomial populations. *Annals of Mathematical Statistics, 35,* 716–725.

Gorsuch, R. L. (1983). *Factor analysis.* Hillsdale, NJ: Erlbaum.

Guilford, J. P. (1964). *Psychometric methods* (2nd ed.). New York: McGraw Hill.

Hays, W. L. (1988). *Statistics for psychologists* (4th ed.). New York: Holt, Rinehart & Winston.

Hedges, L. V., & Olkin, I. (1985). *Statistical methods for meta-analysis.* Orlando: Academic Press.

Jaccard, J., & Becker, M. A. (1990). *Statistics for the behavioral sciences.* Belmont, CA: Wadsworth Publishing Co.

Jöreskog, K. G., & Sörbom, D. (1989). *LISREL 7: A guide to the program and applications* (2nd ed.). Chicago: SPSS, Inc.

Kenny, D. A. (1979). *Correlation and causality.* New York: John Wiley & Sons.

Kirk, R. E. (1968). *Experimental design: Procedures for the behavioral sciences.* Pacific Grove, CA: Brooks/Cole.

Knapp, T. R. (1970). N vs. N − 1. *American Educational Research Journal, 7,* 625–626.

Knapp, T. R. (1994). Regression analyses: What to report. *Nursing Research, 43,* 187–189.

Li, C. C. (1975). *Path analysis: A primer.* Pacific Grove, CA: Boxwood Press.

Little, R. J. A., & Rubin, D. B. (1990). The analysis of social science data with missing values. In J. Fox & J. S. Long (Eds.), *Modern methods of data analysis.* Newbury Park, CA: Sage.

Long, J. S. (1976). Estimation and hypothesis testing in linear models containing measurement error. *Sociological Methods and Research, 5,* 157–206.

Long, J. S. (1983). *Confirmatory factor analysis.* Beverly Hills: Sage.

Marascuilo, L. A., & McSweeney, M. (1977). *Nonparametric and distribution-free methods for the social sciences.* Pacific Grove, CA: Brooks/Cole.

McCall, R. B. (1990). *Fundamental statistics for behavioral sciences* (5th ed.). Fort Worth: Harcourt Brace Jovanovich, Inc.

Miles, M. B., & Huberman, A. M. (1994). *Qualitative data analysis: An expanded sourcebook.* (2nd ed.). Thousand Oaks, CA: Sage.

Norušis, M. J. (1992). *SPSS/PC base system user's guide, version 5.0.* Chicago: SPSS, Inc.

Nunnally, J. (1978). *Psychometric theory.* New York: McGraw-Hill.

Pedhazur, E. J. (1982). *Multiple regression in behavioral research* (2nd ed.). New York: Holt, Rinehart, & Winston.

Polit, D. F., & Hungler, B. P. (1995). *Nursing research: Principles and methods* (5th ed.). Philadelphia: J. B. Lippincott.

Polit, D. F., & Sherman, R. (1990). Statistical power in nursing research. *Nursing Research, 39,* 365–369.

Rummel, R. J. (1970). *Applied factor analysis.* Evanston, IL: Northwestern University Press.

Siegel, S. (1956). *Nonparametric statistics for the behavioral sciences.* New York: McGraw-Hill.

Sörbom, D., & Jöreskog, K.G. (1981). The use of LISREL in sociological model building. In D. J. Jackson and E. F. Borgatta (Eds.), *Factor analysis and measurement in sociological research.* Beverly Hills: Sage.

Tabachnick, B. G. & Fidell, L. S. (1989). *Using multivariate statistics* (2nd ed.). New York; Harper Collins.

Timm, N. H. (1975). *Multivariate analysis with applications in education and psychology.* Monterey, CA: Brooks/Cole.

Welkowitz, J., Ewen, R.B., & Cohen, J. (1991). *Introductory Statistics for the behavorial sciences* (4th ed.). New York: Academic Press.

Winer, B. J. (1971). *Statistical principles in experimental design.* New York: McGraw-Hill.

Wolcott, H. F. (1993). *Transforming qualitative data: Description, analysis, and interpretation.* Thousand Oaks, CA: Sage.

REFERENCES FOR CITED NURSING RESEARCH STUDIES

Affonso, D. D., Mayberry, L. J., Lovett, S. M., & Paul, S. (1994). Cognitive adaptation to stressful events during pregnancy and postpartum: Development and testing of the CASE instrument. *Nursing Research, 43,* 338–343.

Algase, D. L., & Beel-Bates, C. A. (1993). Everyday indicators of impaired cognition: Development of a new screening scale. *Research in Nursing and Health, 16,* 57–66.

Allan, J. D., Mayo, K., & Michel, Y. (1993). Body size values of white and black women. *Research in Nursing and Health, 16,* 323–333.

Archbold, P. G., Stewart, B. J., Miller, L. L., Harvath, T. A., Greenlick, M. R., VanBuren, L., Kirschling, J. M., Valanis, B. G., Brody, K. K., Schook, J. E., & Hagan, J. M. (1995). The PREP system of nursing interventions: A pilot test with families caring for older members. *Research in Nursing and Health, 18,* 3–16.

Beckstrand, J., Ellett, M., Welch, J., Dye, J., Games, C., Henrie, S., & Barlow, R. S. (1990). The distance to the stomach for feeding tube placement in children predicted from regression on height. *Research in Nursing and Health, 13,* 411–420.

Bond, E. F., Heitkemper, M. M., & Jarrett, M. (1994). Intestinal transit and body weight responses to ovarian hormones and dietary fiber in rats. *Nursing Research, 43,* 18–23.

Braden, B. J., & Bergstrom, N. (1994). Predictive validity of the Braden Scale for pressure sore risk in a nursing home population. *Research in Nursing and Health, 17,* 459–470.

Bruce, S. L., & Grove, S. K. (1994). The effect of a coronary artery risk evaluation program on serum lipid values and cardiovascular risk levels. *Applied Nursing Research, 7,* 67–74.

Buchko, B. L., Pugh, L. C., Bishop, B. A., Cochran, J. F., Smith, L. R., & Lerew, D. J. (1994). Comfort measures in breastfeeding primiparous women. *Journal of Obstetric, Gynecologic, and Neonatal Nursing, 23,* 46–52.

Campos, R. G. (1994). Rocking and pacifiers: Two comforting interventions for heelstick pain. *Research in Nursing and Health, 17,* 321–331.

Coffman, S., Levitt, M. J., & Brown, L. (1994). Effects of clarification of support expectations in prenatal couples. *Nursing Research, 43,* 111–116.

Corff, K. E., Seideman, R., Venkataraman, P. S., Lutes, L., & Yates, B. (1995). Facilitated tucking: A non-pharmacologic comfort measure for pain in preterm neonates. *Journal of Obstetric, Gynecologic, and Neonatal Nursing, 24,* 143–147.

Cox, R. P. (1993). The human/animal bond as a correlate of family functioning. *Clinical Nursing Research, 2,* 224–231.

Crumlish, C. M. (1994). Coping and emotional response in cardiac surgery patients. *Western Journal of Nursing Research, 16,* 57–68.

Daly, K., Kleinpell, R.M., Lawinger, S., & Casey, G. (1994). The effect of two nursing interventions on families of ICU patients. *Clinical Nursing Research, 3,* 414–422.

DiIorio, C., vanLier, D., & Manteuffel, B. (1994). Recommendations by clinicians for nausea and vomiting of pregnancy. *Clinical Nursing Research, 3,* 209–227.

Duckett, L., Henly, S. J., & Garvis, M. (1993). Predicting breastfeeding duration during the postpartum hospitalization. *Western Journal of Nursing Research, 15,* 177–198.

Farran, C. J., & Keane-Hagerty, E. (1994). Interventions for caregivers of persons with dementia: Educational support groups and Alzheimer's Association support groups. *Applied Nursing Research, 7,* 112–117.

Glick, O. J., & Swanson, E. A. (1995). Motor performance correlates of functional dependence in long-term care residents. *Nursing Research, 44,* 4–8.

Gray, M., Rayome, R., & Anson, C. (1995). Incontinence and clean intermittent catheterization following spinal cord injury. *Clinical Nursing Research, 4,* 6–21.

Griffith, P., James, B., & Cropp, A. (1994). Evaluation of the safety and efficacy of topical nitroglycerin ointment to facilitate venous cannulation. *Nursing Research, 43,* 203–206.

Gulick, E. E. (1994). Social support among persons with multiple sclerosis. *Research in Nursing and Health, 17,* 195–206.

Hagerty, B. M. K., & Patusky, K. (1995). Developing a measure of sense of belonging. *Nursing Research, 44,* 9–13.

Hahn, E. J. (1995). Predicting Head Start parent involvement in an alcohol and other drug prevention program. *Nursing Research, 44,* 45–51.

Hamilton, G. A., & Seidman, R. N. (1993). A comparison of the recovery period for women and men after an acute myocardial infarction. *Heart and Lung, 22,* 308–315.

Hanneman, S. K. G. (1994). Multidimensional predictors of success or failure with early weaning from mechanical ventilation after cardiac surgery. *Nursing Research, 43,* 4–10.

Haq, M. B. (1993). Understanding older adults' satisfaction with primary health care services at a nursing center. *Applied Nursing Research, 6,* 125–131.

Hays, B. J. (1995). Nursing intensity as a predictor of resource consumption in public health nursing. *Nursing Research, 44,* 106–110.

Heidrich, S. (1994). The self, health, and depression in elderly women. *Western Journal of Nursing Research, 16,* 544–555.

Hilbert, G. A. (1994). Cardiac patients and spouses: Family function and emotions. *Clinical Nursing Research, 3,* 243–252.

Hockenberry-Eaton, M., Kemp, V., & DiIorio, C. (1994). Cancer stressors and protective factors: Predictors of stress experienced during treatment for childhood cancer. *Research in Nursing and Health, 17,* 351–361.

Hofgren, C., Karlson, B. W., & Herlitz, J. (1995). Prodromal symptoms in subsets of patients hospitalized for suspected acute myocardial infarction. *Heart and Lung, 24,* 3–10.

Hurley, A. C., Volicer, B. J., Hanrahan, P.A., Houde, S., & Volicer, L. (1992). Assessment of discomfort in advanced Alzheimer patients. *Research in Nursing and Health, 15,* 369–377.

Kidd, P., & Huddleston, S. (1994). Psychometric properties of the Driving Practices Questionnaire: Assessment of risky driving. *Research in Nursing and Health, 17,* 51–58.

Kocher, K. M., & Thomas, G. W. (1994). Retaining Army nurses: A longitudinal model. *Research in Nursing and Health, 17,* 59–65.

Kollef, M. H. (1995). The identification of ICU-specific outcome predictors: A comparison of medical, surgical, and cardiothoracic ICUs from a single institution. *Heart and Lung, 24,* 60–66.

Koniak-Griffin, D., Ludington-Hoe, S., & Verzemnieks, I. (1995). Longitudinal effects of unimodal and multimodal stimulation on development and interaction of healthy infants. *Research in Nursing and Health, 18,* 27–38.

Lattavo, K., Britt, J., & Dobal, M. (1995). Agreement between measures of pulmonary artery and tympanic temperatures. *Research in Nursing and Health, 18,* 365–370.

Levine, C. D. (1991). Premature rupture of the membranes and sepsis in preterm neonates. *Nursing Research, 40,* 36–41,

Lowe, N. K. (1993). Maternal confidence for labor: Development of the Childbirth Self-Efficacy Inventory. *Research in Nursing and Health, 16,* 141–149.

Lusk, S. L., Ronis, D. L., Kerr, M. J., & Atwood, J. R. (1994). Test of the Health Promotion Model as a causal model of workers' use of hearing protection. *Nursing Research, 43,* 151–157.

Mahon, N. E. (1994). Positive health practices and perceived health status in adolescents. *Clinical Nursing Research, 3,* 86–103.

Martin, L. L. (1994). Validity and reliability of a quality-of-life instrument: The Chronic Respiratory Disease Questionnaire. *Clinical Nursing Research, 3,* 146–156.

McClowry, S. G., Giangrande, S. K., Tommasini, N. R., Clinton, W., Foreman, N. S., Lynch, K., & Ferketich, S. L. (1994). The effect of child temperament, maternal characteristics, and family circumstances on the maladjustment of school-age children. *Research in Nursing and Health, 17,* 25–35.

McCorkle, R., Jepson, C., Malone, D., Lusk, E., Braitman, L., Buhler-Wilkerson, K., & Daly, D. (1994). The impact of posthospital home care on patients with cancer. *Research in Nursing and Health, 17,* 243–251.

McDonald, D. D. (1993). Postoperative narcotic analgesic administration. *Applied Nursing Research, 6,* 106–110.

Meischke, H., Eisenberg, M. S., Schaeffer, S. M., Damon, S. K., Larsen, M. P., & Henwood, D. K. (1995). Utilization of emergency medical services for symptoms of acute myocardial infarction. *Heart and Lung, 24,* 11–18.

Melnyk, B. M. (1994). Coping with unplanned childhood hospitalization: Effects of informational interventions on mothers and children. *Nursing Research, 43,* 50–55.

Metheny, N., Reed, L., Wiersema, L., McSweeney, M., Wehrle, M. A., & Clark, J. (1993). Effectiveness of pH measurements in predicting feeding tube placement: An update. *Nursing Research, 42,* 324–331.

Miaskowski, C., Franck, L. S., Putris, J., & Levine, J. D. (1993). Temporal dissociation of recovery from antinociceptive and motor effects following intrathecal administration of a selective μ-opioid agonist. *Nursing Research, 42,* 344–348.

Mitchell, E. S., Woods, N. F., & Lentz, M. J. (1994). Differentiation of women with three perimenstrual symptom patterns. *Nursing Research, 43,* 25–30.

Neill, K. M. (1993). Ethnic pain styles in acute myocardial infarction. *Western Journal of Nursing Research, 15,* 531–547.

Neuberger, G. B., Kasal, S., Smith, K. V., Hassanein, R., & DeViney, S. (1994). Determinants of exercise and aerobic fitness in outpatients with arthritis. *Nursing Research, 43,* 11–17.

Nyamathi, A. M., Leake, B., Flaskerud, J., Lewis, C., & Bennett, C. (1993). Outcomes of specialized and traditional AIDS counseling programs for impoverished women of color. *Research in Nursing and Health, 16,* 11–21.

O'Brien, M. T. (1993). Multiple sclerosis: The relationship among self-esteem, social support, and coping behavior. *Applied Nursing Research, 6,* 54–63.

Perry, P. A. (1995). Effect of supplemental dietary calcium on the development of DOCA-salt hypertension in weanling rats. *Western Journal of Nursing Research, 17,* 63–75.

Pohl, J. M., Boyd, C., Liang, J., & Given, C. W. (1995). Analysis of the impact of mother-daughter relationships on the commitment to caregiving. *Nursing Research, 44,* 68–75.

Prattke, T. W., & Gass-Sternas, K. A. (1993). Appraisal, coping, and emotional health of infertile couples undergoing donor artificial insemination. *Journal of Obstetric, Gynecologic, and Neonatal Nursing, 22,* 516–527.

Prescott, P. A., Soeken, K. L., & Griggs, M. (1995). Identification and referral of hospitalized patients in need of home health care. *Research in Nursing and Health, 18,* 85–95.

Roberts, S. J., Krouse, H. J., & Michaud, P. (1995). Negotiated and nonnegotiated nurse-patient interactions. *Clinical Nursing Research, 4,* 67–77.

Rudy, S. F., Guckes, A. D., Li, S., McCarthy, G. R., & Brahim, J. S. (1993). Body and orofacial cathexis in edentulous complete-denture-wearing clients. *Clinical Nursing Research, 2,* 296–308.

Schneider, J. K., Hornberger, S., Booker, J., Davis, A., & Kralicek, R. (1993). A medication discharge planning program. *Clinical Nursing Research, 2,* 41–53.

Shelledy, D. C., Rau, J. L., & Thomas-Goodfellow, L. (1995). A comparison of the effects of assist-control, SIMV, and SIMV with pressure support on ventilation, oxygen consumption, and ventilatory equivalent. *Heart and Lung, 24,* 67–75.

Sommers, M. S., Stevenson, J. S., Hamlin, R. L., & Ivey, T. D. (1995). Skin temperature and limb blood flow as predictors of cardiac index. *Clinical Nursing Research, 4,* 22–37.

Tappen, R. M. (1994). The effect of skill training on functional abilities of nursing home residents with dementia. *Research in Nursing and Health, 17,* 159–165.

Topp, R., & Stevenson, J. S. (1994). The effects of attendance and effort on outcomes among older adults in a long-term exercise program. *Research in Nursing and Health, 17,* 15–24.

Tumulty, G., Jernigan, I. E., & Kohut, G. F. (1994). The impact of perceived work environment on job satisfaction of hospital staff nurses. *Applied Nursing Research, 7,* 84–90.

Verdeber, A., Gallagher, K. J., & Severino, R. (1995). The effect of nursing interventions on transcutaneous oxygen and carbon dioxide tensions. *Western Journal of Nursing Research, 17,* 76–90.

Vessey, J. A., Carlson, K. L., & McGill, J. (1994). Use of distraction with children during an acute pain experience. *Nursing Research, 43,* 369–372.

Wallace, D. C., Lockhart, J. G., & Boyle, D. K. (1995). Service use by elders with heart disease. *Research in Nursing and Health, 18,* 293–301.

Wells, N. (1994). Perceived control over pain: Relation to distress and disability. *Research in Nursing and Health, 17,* 295–302.

White, R. E., & Frasure-Smith, N. (1995). Uncertainty and psychologic stress after coronary angioplasty and coronary bypass surgery. *Heart and Lung, 24,* 19–27.

Williams, M. A., Oberst, M. T., & Bjorklund, B. C. (1994). Early outcomes after hip fracture among women discharged home and to nursing homes. *Research in Nursing and Health, 17,* 175–183.

Wineman, N. M., Durand, E. J., & Steiner, R. P. (1994). A comparative analysis of coping behaviors in persons with multiple sclerosis or a spinal cord injury. *Research in Nursing and Health, 17,* 185–194.

Woods, N. F., Lentz, M. J., Mitchell, E. S., & Kogan, H. (1994). Arousal and stress response across the menstrual cycle in women with three perimenstrual symptom patterns. *Research in Nursing and Health, 17,* 99–110.

Workman, M. L. (1995). Comparison of blot-drying versus air-drying of povidone-iodine—cleansed skin. *Applied Nursing Research, 8,* 15–17.

Youngblut, J. M., Loveland-Cherry, C. J., & Horan, M. (1994). Maternal employment effects on families and preterm infants at 18 months. *Nursing Research, 43,* 331–337.

Ziemer, M. M., & Pigeon, J. G. (1993). Skin changes and pain in the nipple during the first week of lactation. *Journal of Obstetric, Gynecologic, and Neonatal Nursing, 22,* 247–256.

Zotti, M. E., & Siegel, E. (1995). Preventing unplanned pregnancies among married couples: Are services for only the wife sufficient? *Research in Nursing and Health, 18,* 133–142.

Glossary

abscissa. The horizontal dimension of a two-dimensional graph; also known as the *X axis*.

absolute frequencies. The count of the number of cases with a given score value.

absolute value. The value of a number regardless of its positive or negative sign (e.g., the absolute value of -10, symbolized $|-10|$, is 10).

adjusted means. The mean values of the dependent variable for different groups, after removing the effects of covariates through multiple regression or ANCOVA.

adjusted R^2. The squared multiple correlation coefficient adjusted for sample size and number of predictors to give a more accurate estimate of relationships in the population; also known as the *shrunken R^2* and sometimes symbolized as $\tilde{R}^2$.

alpha (α). (1) In tests of statistical significance, the level designating the established risk of committing a Type I error; (2) an index used to evaluate internal consistency reliability *(Cronbach's alpha* or *coefficient alpha)*.

alpha factor method. A method of factor analysis that analyzes common factor variance and strives to maximize Cronbach's alpha (internal consistency reliability) for the factors.

alternative hypothesis. In hypothesis testing, a hypothesis different from the one being tested—usually, different from the null hypothesis; often symbolized as H_1.

analysis. A method of organizing data in such a way that research questions can be answered.

analysis of covariance (ANCOVA). A statistical procedure used to test mean group differences on a dependent variable, while controlling for one or more extraneous variables (covariates).

analysis of variance (ANOVA). A statistical procedure for testing mean differences among three or more groups by comparing the variability between groups to the variability within groups.

assumption. In statistical analysis, characteristics of the data presumed to be true for the purpose of the analysis being performed, a violation of which can invalidate the results.

asymmetric distribution. A distribution of values that is skewed, i.e., has two halves that are not mirror images of the each other.

attenuation. The reduction in a correlation coefficient attributable to measurement error.

attrition bias. The bias resulting from the loss of participants during the course of a study, which can alter the composition of the sample initially drawn.

bar graph. A graphical presentation of a frequency distribution for a categorical variable.

Bartlett's test of sphericity. A statistical test used to determine whether dependent variables in MANCOVA or canonical analysis are correlated.

Bartlett's test of Wilks' lambda. In canonical analysis, a significance test used to evaluate whether an R_c (or a set of R_cs) is significantly different from zero.

beta (β). (1) In statistical testing, the probability of committing a Type II error; (2) in multiple regression, a coefficient indicating the relative weight of a standardized independent variable in the regression equation.

between-subjects design. A research design in which there are separate groups of people being compared, calling for a statistical test for independent groups.

bimodal distribution. A distribution of values with two peaks (high frequencies).

binomial distribution. A probability distribution for a dichotomous variable.

bivariate normal distribution. A distribution of two variables (X and Y) such that scores on X are normally distributed for each value of Y, and vice versa.

bivariate statistics. Statistics used to analyze the empirical relationship between two variables.

Bonferroni correction. A correction used to correct the significance level following post hoc tests.

Box M test. A statistical test used to test the homogeneity of a variance-covariance matrix, an assumption underlying several multivariate analyses.

canonical analysis. A multivariate statistical procedure for examining the relationship between two or more independent variables *and* two or more dependent variables.

canonical correlation coefficient (R_c). The index summarizing the correlation between pairs of canonical variates.

canonical variate. In canonical analysis, the composite formed by a linear combination of independent variables or dependent variables.

canonical variate score. In canonical analysis, the score of individual subjects on a canonical variate.

canonical weight. In canonical analysis, the standardized weight associated with each independent and dependent variable.

categorical variable. A variable that has discrete categories, such as a nominal-level variable (e.g., a person's marital status).

causal modeling. The development and statistical testing of hypothesized causal relationships among phenomena.

causal relationship. A relationship between two variables such that one variable (the "cause") determines the presence/absence or value of the other (the "effect").

ceiling effect. The effect of having scores at or near the highest possible value, which can constrain the amount of upward change possible and also tends to reduce variability in a variable.

cell. The intersection of a row and column in a table with two or more dimensions.

central limit theorem. A statistical principle stipulating that (a) the larger the sample, the more closely the sampling distribution of the mean will approach a normal distribution; and (b) the mean of a sampling distribution is equal to the population mean.

central tendency. An index that comes from the center of a distribution of scores, describing what is a "typical" value; the three most common indices of central tendency are the mode, the median, and the mean.

centroid. A group mean on a discriminant score in discriminant analysis.

change score. The score value obtained by subtracting scores on a variable at one point in time from scores on the same variable measured at an earlier point in time.

chi-square goodness-of-fit test. A statistical test used in several contexts to determine the fit of the data to hypothesized population values or a hypothesized model.

chi-square test of independence. A nonparametric test of statistical significance used to assess whether a relationship exists between two categorical variables; symbolized as χ^2.

class interval. A grouping of data on a continuous variable that makes data easier to interpret when displayed in a grouped frequency distribution.

Cochran's *Q*-test. A nonparametric test for population differences in proportions; used when the dependent variable is dichotomous and the design is within subjects.

code. An arbitrary numerical value assigned to a variable according to a set of rules to represent a status on that variable (e.g., for gender, code 1 for males, code 2 for females).

coefficient alpha. See *Cronbach's alpha*.

coefficient of determination. An index indicating the proportion of variance in the dependent variable accounted for or explained by independent variables, more commonly referred to as r^2 or R^2.

common factor variance. A measure of the variance that two or more measures share in common; also referred to as *communality*.

communality. A measure of a variable's shared variance in the context of a factor analysis; also referred to as *common factor variance* and sometimes symbolized as h^2.

confidence interval. The range of values within which a population parameter is estimated to lie; abbreviated *CI*.

confidence level. The estimated probability that a population parameter lies within a given confidence interval.

confidence limits. The upper and lower boundaries of a confidence interval.

confirmatory factor analysis (CFA). A factor analysis, based on maximum likelihood estimation, designed to confirm a hypothesized measurement model.

construct validity. The degree to which an instrument measures the construct under investigation.

contingency table. A two-dimensional table that displays a crosstabulation of the frequencies of two categorical variables.

continuous variable. A variable that can take on an infinite range of values between two points on a continuum (e.g., height).

control. The process of holding constant possible influences on the dependent variable under investigation.

control group. Subjects in an experiment who do not receive the experimental treatment and whose performance provides a baseline against which the effects of the treatment can be measured.

correlation. A bond between variables, wherein variation in one variable is related to variation in the other.

correlation coefficient. An index that summarizes the magnitude and direction of the relationship between two variables; correlation coefficients typically range from $+1.00$ (for a perfect direct relationship) through 0.00 (for no relationship) to -1.00 (for a perfect negative relationship).

correlation matrix. A two-dimensional display showing the correlation coefficients between all variable pairs.

covariance. A measure of the joint variance of two variables, computed by summing the crossproducts of each variable's deviation scores and dividing by degrees of freedom.

covariate. A variable that is statistically controlled (held constant) in analysis of covariance; the covariate is typically an extraneous, confounding influence on the dependent variable or a pretest measure of the dependent variable.

Cramér's *V*. An index describing the magnitude of relationship between nominal-level data, used when the contingency table to which it is applied is larger than 2×2.

criterion-related validity. The extent to which scores on an instrument are correlated with an external criterion.

critical region. The area in the sampling distribution representing values that are "improbable" if the null hypothesis is true.

Cronbach's alpha. A reliability coefficient that indicates how much the items on a scale are measuring the same underlying dimension—thus a measure of internal consistency; also referred to as *coefficient alpha*.

crossproducts. The multiplication of deviation scores for one variable by the deviation scores for the second; used in the calculation of covariances and correlations.

crosstabulation. The calculation of a two-dimensional frequency distribution for two categorical variables (e.g., gender—male/female—crosstabulated with smoking status—smoker/nonsmoker); the results are typically presented in a contingency table.

cross-validation. The process of verifying the validity of the results of an analysis done with one subset of a sample by replicating the analysis with a second subset from the same sample.

cumulative relative frequency. In a frequency distribution, the percentage of cases with a given score value, combined with percentages for all those values that preceded it.

curvilinear relationship. A relationship between two continuous variables such that, when plotted in a scatterplot, a curve rather than a straight line is formed.

data. The pieces of information obtained in a research investigation.

data analysis. The systematic organization and synthesis of research data, and the testing of hypotheses with those data.

data analysis plan. The overall plan for the analysis of research data that serves as a guide toward the goal of answering the research questions.

data cleaning. The preparation of data for statistical analysis through checks to ensure that the data are accurate and internally consistent.

data matrix. A two-dimensional array of data (subjects $\times$ variables).

data set. The total collection of data on all variables for the entire research sample.

data transformation. An alteration of the raw research data, designed to put them in a form that can be meaningfully analyzed.

default. In statistical computer packages, the standard analysis performed (or criterion used in an analysis), unless a specific alternative request is made to override it.

degrees of freedom (*df*). A concept used in tests of statistical significance, referring to the number of components that are free to vary about a parameter (e.g., by knowing a sample mean, all but one value would be free to vary).

dependent variable. The variable that is hypothesized to depend on or be caused by another variable (the independent variable).

descriptive statistics. Statistics used to describe and summarize data (e.g., mean, standard deviation).

deviation score. A score computed by subtracting an individual score value from the mean of the distribution of scores.

dichotomous variable. A variable having only two values or categories (e.g., gender).

direct effect. In a causal model, the effect of an independent variable on a dependent variable represented by a direct (nonmediated) path between the two variables.

directional hypothesis. A hypothesis that makes a specific prediction about the nature and direction of the relationship between two variables.

discrete variable. A variable that has a finite number of values between any two points.

discriminant analysis. A statistical procedure used to predict group membership or status on a categorical (nominal level) variable on the basis of two or more independent variables.

discriminant function. In discriminant analysis, a linear combination of independent variables formed to maximally separate groups.

discriminant score (*D* score). The predicted value from a discriminant analysis equation, used as a basis for classifying cases into groups.

dummy coding. A method of coding categorical variables into dichotomous variables, using codes of 0 and 1 to represent the presence or absence of an attribute (e.g., female = 1, male = 0).

Duncan's multiple-range test. A post hoc test used following a significant ANOVA to test differences between all possible pairs of means.

Dunn procedure. A procedure involving the post hoc comparison of all possible pairs of groups following a significant overall test (e.g., the Mann-Whitney U test or Friedman test), using a Bonferroni correction to adjust the level of significance.

Durbin-Watson statistic. A statistical test used to detect nonindependence of errors of prediction in a regression analysis.

effect coding. A way of coding categorical variables for multivariate analysis that uses 1, 0, and -1 to designate categories.

effect coefficient. In the decomposition of effects in causal models, the value of direct plus indirect effects of an independent variable on a dependent variable; also referred to as the *total effect*.

effect size. A statistical expression of the magnitude of the relationship between two variables, or the magnitude of the difference between groups, with regard to some attribute of interest.

eigenvalue. The value equal to the sum of the squared weights for a linear composite (e.g., a factor in factor analysis), indicating how much variance in the solution is explained.

endogenous variable. In causal models, a variable whose variation is determined by other variables in the model.

errors of prediction. The differences between the actual values of a dependent variable and the predicted values in a regression analysis; the portion of the dependent variable not explained by the predictor variables; also called the *residuals*.

estimation procedures. The procedures used in inferential statistics to estimate a population parameter on the basis of sample data.

eta squared. A statistic calculated (often in connection with ANOVA) to indicate the proportion of variance in the dependent variable explained by the independent variables, analogous to R^2 in multiple regression; computed by dividing the sum of squares between groups by the total sum of squares.

exogenous variable. In causal models, a variable whose determinants lie outside the model.

experimental group. The subjects who receive the experimental treatment or intervention.

exploratory factor analysis. A factor analysis undertaken to determine the underlying dimensionality of a set of variables.

extraneous variable. A variable that confounds the relationship between the independent and dependent variables and that needs to be controlled either in the research design or through statistical procedures.

F ratio. The statistic obtained in several statistical tests (e.g., ANOVA) in which variation attributable to different sources (e.g., between groups and within groups) is compared.

factor. In factor analysis, a linear combination of variables in a data matrix that captures an underlying dimension or latent variable.

factor analysis. a statistical procedure for reducing a large set of variables into a smaller set of variables (factors) with common characteristics or underlying dimensions.

factor correlation matrix. In factor analysis with oblique rotation, the factor $\times$ factor matrix that indicates the correlations among the factors.

factor extraction. The first phase of a factor analysis, which involves the extraction of as much variance as possible through the successive creation of linear combinations of the variables in the data set.

factor loading. In factor analysis, the b weight associated with a variable on a given factor.

factor matrix. A matrix produced in factor analysis that has variables on one dimension and factors on the other.

factor rotation. The second major phase of factor analysis, during which the reference axes for the factors are moved such that variables more clearly align with a single factor.

factor score. A person's score on a latent variable (factor).

factorial design. An experimental design in which two or more independent variables are simultaneously manipulated, permitting an analysis of the main effects of the independent variables, plus the interaction effects.

Fisher's exact test. A statistical procedure used to test the significance of the difference in proportions; used when the sample size is small or cells in the contingency table have no observations.

Fisher's *LSD* test. A post hoc test, also known as the *protected t-test*, used following a significant ANOVA to test differences between all possible pairs of means; *LSD* is an acronym for least significant difference.

floor effect. The effect of having scores at or near the lowest possible value, which can constrain the amount of downward change possible and can reduce variability in a variable.

frequency distribution. A systematic array of data values (usually from the lowest to the highest), together with a count of the number of times each value was obtained.

frequency polygon. Graphic display of a frequency distribution, in which dots connected by a straight line indicate the number of times a score value occurs.

Friedman test. A nonparametric analog of ANOVA, used when the researcher is working with paired groups or a repeated measures situation.

goodness-of-fit test. See *chi-square goodness-of-fit test.*

grand mean. The overall mean for a set of scores, for all groups.

grouped frequency distribution. A frequency distribution in which score values are clustered into sets (class intervals); used to facilitate interpretation of the distribution when the range of values is wide.

heterogeneity. The degree to which objects are dissimilar with respect to some attribute (i.e., characterized by high variability).

heteroscedasticity. A property describing the variability of two variables (X and Y) such that for different values of X the variability of the Y scores differs; the opposite of homoscedasticity.

hierarchical multiple regression. A multiple regression analysis in which predictor variables are entered into the equation in steps that are prespecified by the analyst.

histogram. A graphic presentation of frequency distribution data, in which bars are used to indicate the number of times the score value occurs.

homogeneity. The degree to which objects are similar (i.e., characterized by low variability).

homogeneity of regression assumption. In ANCOVA and MANCOVA, the assumption that the covariate has the same relationship with the dependent variable in every group being compared.

homogeneity of variance assumption. The assumption in several statistical tests that the variance of the groups being compared is equal in the populations.

homogeneity of the variance-covariance matrix assumption. The multivariate analog of the assumption of homogeneous variances for dependent variables.

homoscedasticity. A property describing the variability of two variables (X and Y) such that for each value of X the variability of the Y scores is about the same and vice versa; the opposite of heteroscedasticity.

Hotelling's trace criterion. A statistical index used in MANOVA and other multivariate tests to test the significance of group differences.

Hotelling's T^2 test. An extension of the *t*-test to multivariate situations (i.e., more than one dependent variable).

hypothesis testing. The application of inferential statistics in which sampling distributions are used to make objective decisions about the acceptance or rejection of hypotheses.

identification. The existence of sufficient information for estimating the parameters in a set of regression equations (e.g., in a causal model).

independent variable. The variable that is the hypothesized cause of or influence on the dependent variable.

indirect effect. In a causal model, the effect of an independent variable on a dependent variable that occurs *through* a mediating variable.

inferential statistics. Statistics that rely on the laws of probability to help researchers draw conclusions about whether relationships and characteristics observed in a sample are likely to occur in the population.

interaction hypothesis. A hypothesis regarding the effect on a dependent variable of two or more independent variables acting in combination (interactively) rather than as unconnected factors.

intercept. The point at which a regression line intercepts (crosses) the Y axis when the value on the X axis is zero.

interrater reliability. A coefficient indicating agreement between raters, i.e., the extent to which the ratings of two independent raters or observers are intercorrelated.

interval estimation. A statistical estimation approach in which the researcher uses sample data to establish a range of values that are likely, within a given level of confidence, to contain the true population parameter.

interval measurement. A level of measurement that involves assigning numbers to indicate both the ordering on an attribute and the distance between different amounts of the attribute.

inverse relationship. A negative relationship between two variables, i.e., a relationship characterized by the tendency of high values on one variable to be associated with low values on the second.

item reversal. In scoring scales, the process of reversing the direction of the scoring on certain items, usually by subtracting the value of the item from 1 + the item's maximum value.

jackknifing. A method for estimating errors or improving estimates, involving an iterative process of eliminating observations one at a time.

just-identified model. A model in which the number of known parameters equals the number of unknown parameters being estimated.

Kendall's tau. A nonparametric statistic used to indicate the magnitude and direction of a relationship between ordinal-level data.

known-groups technique. A technique for estimating the construct validity of an instrument through an analysis of the degree to which the instrument differentiates groups that are predicted to differ on the basis of some theory or known characteristic.

Kruskal-Wallis test. A nonparametric test used to test the difference between three or more independent groups, based on ranked scores.

kurtosis. An aspect of the shape of a frequency distribution, referring to how pointed or flat its peak is.

latent variable. An unmeasured variable that represents an underlying, abstract construct (e.g., in factor analysis and LISREL).

laws of probability. The established laws that stipulate the likelihood that a particular event or relationship will occur.

least-squares criterion. The criterion used to estimate parameters in a model, such that the sum of the squared error terms is minimized; also called *ordinary least-squares (OLS)*.

leptokurtic distribution. A frequency distribution in which the peak is thin and pointed.

level of measurement. A system of classifying measurements according to the nature of the measurement and the type of mathematical operations to which they are amenable; the four levels are nominal, ordinal, interval, and ratio.

level of significance. The probability of making a Type I error, established by the researcher before the statistical analysis (e.g., the .05 level).

likelihood index. An index used to evaluate a logistic regression equation, indicating the probability of the observed results given the parameters estimated from the analysis; typically shown as 2 times the log of the likelihood ($-2LL$).

line graph. A graph used for plotting values over time, in which values for a given value are connected by a line.

linear model. The general equation for a straight line (that is, $Y = a + bX$).

linear relationship. A relation between two continuous variables such that when data values are plotted in a scatterplot, a straight line is formed.

linear structural relations analysis. See *LISREL*.

LISREL. The acronym for linear structural relations analysis, used for testing causal models and performing confirmatory factor analysis via maximum likelihood estimation.

listwise deletion. A method of dealing with missing values in a data set, involving the elimination of cases with missing data.

logistic regression. A multivariate regression procedure that uses maximum likelihood estimation for analyzing relationships between multiple independent variables and categorical dependent variables; also referred to as *logit analysis*.

logit. The natural log of the odds, used as the dependent variable in logistic regression; short for logistic probability unit.

log-linear analysis. A statistical technique for analyzing relationships among three or more categorical variables.

main effect. The simple effect of an independent variable on the dependent variable, uninfluenced by other variables.

Mahalanobis distance (D^2). A statistic that is a generalized measure of the distance between groups; used, for example, in stepwise discriminant analysis as a criterion for entering predictors.

MANCOVA. See *multivariate analysis of covariance*.

manifest variable. An observed, measured variable that serves as an indicator of an underlying construct (i.e., a latent variable).

Mann-Whitney U-test. A nonparametric test used to test the difference between two independent groups, based on ranked scores.

MANOVA. See *multivariate analysis of variance*.

marginal frequencies. Frequency distributions of grouped data in a crosstabulation—so called because they are found in the margins of the table; sometimes called *marginals*.

marker variable. In factor analysis, a variable that is highly correlated with only one factor and that helps to define the underlying dimensionality of the factor.

matrix algebra. A branch of mathematics that deals with rules for adding, subtracting, multiplying, and dividing matrices.

maximum likelihood estimation. An estimation approach in which the estimators are ones that estimate the parameters most likely to have generated the observed measurements.

maximum likelihood factoring method. A method of factor analysis that uses maximum likelihood criteria as the method of estimation.

McNemar test. A nonparametric test for comparing differences in proportions when the values are derived from paired (nonindependent) groups.

mean. A descriptive statistic measuring central tendency, computed by summing all scores and dividing by the number of subjects.

mean square. In an ANOVA context, the term used to designate the variance; often abbreviated *MS*; calculated by dividing a sum of squares by its respective degrees of freedom.

mean substitution. A technique for addressing missing data problems by substituting missing values on a variable with the mean for that variable.

measurement. The assignment of numbers to objects to designate the quantity of an attribute, according to specified rules.

measurement model. In LISREL, the model that stipulates the hypothesized relationships among the manifest and latent variables.

median. A descriptive statistic measuring central tendency, representing the exact middle score or value in a distribution of scores; the value above and below which 50% of the scores lie.

mediating variable. A variable that mediates or acts like a "go-between" in a path linking two other variables.

missing values. Values missing from a data set for some subjects as a result of such factors as subject refusals, researcher error, or skip patterns.

modality. A characteristic of a frequency distribution describing the number of peaks or values with high frequencies.

mode. A descriptive statistic that indicates the score or value that occurs most frequently in a distribution of scores.

model. A symbolic representation of concepts or variables, and interrelationships among them.

multicollinearity. A term that describes a correlation matrix in which two or more independent variables are highly correlated with each other.

multifactor ANOVA. An analysis of variance used to test the relationship between two or more independent variables and a dependent variable simultaneously.

multimodal distribution. A distribution of values with more than one peak (high frequency).

multiple classification analysis. An analysis that yields adjusted group means on a dependent variable after controlling for the effects of covariates.

multiple comparison procedures. Statistical tests, normally applied after preliminary results indicate overall statistically significant group differences, that compare different pairs of groups; also referred to as *post hoc tests*.

multiple correlation coefficient. An index that summarizes the magnitude of the relationship between two or more independent variables and a dependent variable; symbolized as *R*.

multiple regression analysis. A statistical procedure for understanding the effects of two or more independent variables on a dependent variable, using least-squares estimation.

multivariate analysis of covariance (MANCOVA). A statistical procedure used to test the significance of differences between the means of two or more groups on two or more dependent variables, after controlling for one or more covariate.

multivariate analysis of variance (MANOVA). A statistical procedure used to test the significance of differences between the means of two or more groups on two or more dependent variables, considered simultaneously.

multivariate normal distribution. A distribution of several variables such that each variable and all linear combinations of the variables are normally distributed; multivariate normality is assumed for many multivariate statistical tests.

multivariate statistics. Statistical procedures for analyzing the relationships among three or more variables simultaneously.

n. Often used to designate the number of subjects in a subgroup or in a cell of a study (e.g., "each of the four groups had an *n* of 125, for a total *N* of 500").

N. Often used to designate the total number of subjects in a study (e.g., "the total *N* was 500").

negative relationship. A relationship between two variables in which there is a tendency for higher values on one variable to be associated with lower values on the other; also referred to as an *inverse relationship*.

negatively skewed distribution. An asymmetrical distribution of values that has a disproportionately large number of cases with high values—i.e., values falling at the upper end of the distribution; when displayed graphically, the tail points to the left.

net effect. The effect of an independent variable on a dependent variable, after controlling for the effect of one or more covariates through multiple regression or ANCOVA.

nominal measurement. The lowest level of measurement, involving the assignment of characteristics into categories (e.g., females, category 1; males, category 2).

noncausal effect. Covariation between two variables in a causal model that is *not* a causal effect; can be either an unanalyzed effect or a spurious effect.

nondirectional hypothesis. A research hypothesis that does not stipulate in advance the direction and nature of the relationship between variables.

nonparametric statistics. A general class of inferential statistics that does not involve rigorous assumptions about the distribution of the variables; most often used when the data are measured on the nominal or ordinal scales.

nonrecursive model. A causal model that hypothesizes reciprocal effects wherein a variable can be both the cause of and an effect of another variable.

nonsignificant result. The result of a statistical test that indicates that the result could have occurred as a result of chance, given the researcher's level of significance; sometimes abbreviated as *NS* in research journals.

normal distribution. A theoretical distribution that is unimodal, symmetric, and not too peaked or flat; also referred to as a *normal curve* or *bell-shaped curve*.

null hypothesis (H_0). The hypothesis that states there is no relationship between the variables under study; used in connection with tests of statistical significance as the hypothesis to be rejected.

oblique rotation. A rotation of factors in factor analysis such that the reference axes are allowed to move to acute or oblique angles and hence the factors are allowed to be correlated.

odds. The ratio of two probabilities, namely, the probability of an event occurring to the probability that it will not occur.

odds ratio. The ratio of one odds to another odds; used in logistic regression as a measure of association and as an estimate of relative risk.

one-sample *t*-test. The test used to evaluate the probability that the value of the sample mean equals the researcher's hypothesis about the population mean.

one-tailed test. A test of statistical significance in which only values at one extreme (tail) of a distribution are considered in determining significance; used when the researcher has predicted the direction of a relationship (i.e., posits a directional hypothesis).

one-way ANOVA. An analysis of variance used to test the relationship between a single independent variable and a dependent variable.

ordinal measurement. A level of measurement that yields a rank ordering of a variable along a specified dimension.

ordinary least-squares (OLS) regression. Regression analysis that uses the least-squares criterion for estimating the parameters in the regression equation.

ordinate. The vertical dimension of a two-dimensional graph; also known as the *Y axis*.

orthogonal. A term used to describe variables that are uncorrelated.

orthogonal coding. A method of coding categorical variables in a regression analysis to make specific planned comparisons.

orthogonal rotation. A rotation of factors in factor analysis such that the reference axes are kept at right angles, and hence the factors remain uncorrelated.

outliers. Wild codes or numerical values that lie outside the normal range of values.

overidentified model. A model in which the number of known parameters is greater than the number of unknown parameters being estimated.

***p* value.** In statistical testing, the probability that the obtained results are due to chance alone; the probability of committing a Type I error.

pairwise deletion. A method of dealing with missing values in a data set, involving the deletion of cases with missing data on a selective basis (i.e., deletion of a case only when one variable is paired with another variable that has missing data).

parameter. An index describing a characteristic of a population.

parametric statistics. A class of inferential statistics that involves (a) assumptions about the distribution of the variables, (b) the estimation of a parameter, and (c) the use of interval or ratio measures.

partial correlation. The correlation between a dependent variable (Y) and an independent variable (X_1) while controlling for the effect of a third variable (X_2); symbolized as $r_{y1.2}$.

partitioning variance. The process of dividing up the total variance in the dependent variable into its contributing components (e.g., between-group variance versus within-group variance).

pattern matrix. In factor analysis, the matrix that indicates partial regression coefficients between variables and factors; in oblique rotation, the matrix used to interpret the meaning of the factors.

path analysis. A regression-based procedure for testing causal models, typically using nonexperimental data.

path coefficient. The weight representing the impact of one variable on another in a causal model; for the path showing the effect of variable 1 on variable 2, the path coefficient is symbolized p_{21}.

path diagram. A graphic representation of the hypothesized linkages and causal flow among variables in a causal network.

Pearson's r. The most widely used correlation coefficient, designating the magnitude and direction of a relationship between two variables measured on at least an interval scale; also referred to as the *product-moment correlation coefficient.*

percentile. An index indicating the ranking of a score by specifying what percentage of the cases fall below that score.

perfect relationship. A relationship between two variables such that the values of one variable permit perfect prediction of the values of the other; indicated as 1.00 or -1.00.

phi coefficient. An index describing the magnitude of relationship between two dichotomous variables.

pie chart. A graphic presentation that shows frequency distribution information in a circle, with "slices" of the pie representing the proportion for each category or score value; also known as a *circle graph.*

Pillai's trace criterion. A statistical index used in MANOVA and other multivariate tests to test the significance of group differences.

planned comparisons. Comparisons between group means in an ANOVA or regression analysis, for comparisons that are specified at the outset of the research.

platykurtic distribution. A frequency distribution in which the peak is flat.

point biserial correlation coefficient. An index of the magnitude and direction of the relationship between two variables, one of which is continuous and the other of which is dichotomous.

point estimation. A statistical estimation procedure in which the researcher uses information from a sample to estimate a single statistic to best represent the value of the population parameter.

pooled variance estimate. In *t*-tests, the standard formula for estimating the standard error of the difference; used if the assumption of homogeneous variances is tenable or if sample sizes in the two groups are approximately equal.

population. The entire set of individuals (or objects) having some common characteristic(s) (e.g., all AIDS patients in the U.S.).

positive relationship. A relationship between two variables in which there is a tendency for high values on one variable to be associated with high values on the other.

positively skewed distribution. An asymmetrical distribution of values that has a disproportionately large number of low values—i.e., values falling at the lower end of the distribution; when displayed graphically, the tail points to the right.

post hoc test. A test for comparing all possible pairs of groups following a significant test of overall group differences (e.g., a significant ANOVA).

power. The probability of correctly rejecting a false null hypothesis; power equals $1 - \beta$, the risk of a Type II error.

power analysis. A procedure for estimating either (a) the likelihood of committing a Type II error or (b) sample size requirements to reduce the risk of a Type II error.

predictor variable. In correlational and regression analyses, the independent variable; used to predict the value of the dependent variable.

principal components method. A method of factor analysis that analyzes all variance in the observed variables, not just common factor variance.

principal factors method. A method of factor analysis that analyzes only common factor variance, using estimates of the communality on the diagonal of the correlation matrix; sometimes referred to as *principal-axis factoring method.*

prior probability. The establishment of a hypothesized probability distribution; used in discriminant analysis for classification of cases into groups.

probability distribution. A frequency distribution that displays all possible outcomes of some event, together with each of their probabilities; sometimes referred to as a *probability density function* for continuous variables.

probit analysis. A statistical method used to analyze the relationship between multiple independent variables and a dichotomous dependent variable; involves the transformation of the dependent variable to the value of the normal curve below which the observed proportion of the area is found, and maximum likelihood estimation of the parameters.

product-moment correlation coefficient (*r*). The most widely used correlation coefficient, designating the magnitude and direction of the relationship between two variables measured on at least an interval scale; also referred to as *Pearson's r.*

protected *t*-test. A post hoc test used following a significant ANOVA to test differences between all possible pairs of means; also known as *Fisher's LSD test.*

qualitative data. Information that is in narrative (nonnumerical) form.

qualitative variable. A variable measured on the nominal scale—i.e., a variable that conveys no quantitative information.

quantitative analysis. The manipulation of numerical data through statistical procedures for the purpose of describing phenomena or assessing the magnitude and reliability of relationships among them.

quantitative data. Information collected in the course of a study that is in a quantified (numerical) form.

quantitative variable. A variable that conveys information about the amount of an attribute—i.e., a variable measured on the ordinal, interval, or ratio scale.

quasi-statistics. A system of "accounting" that involves frequency counts in qualitative analysis.

r. The symbol typically used to designate a bivariate correlation coefficient, summarizing the magnitude and direction of a relationship between two variables.

r-to-z transformation. A logarithmic transformation of correlation coefficients to z scores that allows the use of the normal distribution for comparing correlation coefficients.

R. The symbol used to designate the multiple correlation coefficient, indicating the magnitude (but not direction) of the relationship between the dependent variable and multiple independent variables, taken together.

R^2. The squared multiple correlation coefficient, indicating the proportion of variance in the dependent variable accounted for or explained by a group of independent variables; also referred to as the *coefficient of determination.*

R statistic. An index used in logistic regression to indicate the partial correlation between the dependent variable and each predictor.

random assignment. The assignment of subjects to treatment conditions in a random manner (i.e., in a manner determined by chance alone); also known as *randomization.*

random sample. A sample selected in such a way that each member of the population has an equal probability of being included.

range. A measure of variability, consisting of the difference between the highest and lowest values in a distribution.

Rao's V. A statistic that measures the distance between groups; used, for example, in stepwise discriminant analysis as a criterion for entering predictors.

ratio measurement. A level of measurement of attributes in which there are equal distances between score units and a true meaningful zero point (e.g., weight).

raw data. The actual numerical values of collected data prior to any transformations.

real limits (of a number). The points indicating half a measurement unit below the number (lower real limit) and half a measurement unit above the number (upper real limit).

rectangular matrix. A matrix of data (variables $\times$ subjects) that contains no missing values for any of the variables.

recursive model. A causal model in which the hypothesized causal flow is unidirectional, without any feedback loops.

redundancy index. An index used in canonical analysis to measure how much variance the canonical variates from the independent variables extract from the dependent variables, and vice versa.

reference group. The omitted category in coding schemes for multivariate analyses, against which the effects for other categories are compared.

regression. A statistical procedure for predicting values of a dependent variable based on the values of one or more independent variables.

regression coefficient. The weight associated with an independent variable when predicting values of the dependent variable in regression analysis; also referrred to as a *b weight* (unstandardized) or *beta weight* (standardized).

regression equation. The equation for the best-fitting straight line to characterize the relationship between independent and dependent variables.

relationship. A bond or association between two or more variables.

relative frequency. The frequency of a given score value given as a percentage (i.e., relative to other score values).

relative risk. The risk of an event occurring given one condition, versus the risk of it occurring given another condition.

reliability. The degree of consistency or dependability with which an instrument measures the attribute it is designed to measure.

reliability coefficient. A quantitative index, usually ranging in value from .00 to 1.00, that provides an estimate of how reliable or consistent an instrument is.

repeated measures ANOVA. A statistical procedure for testing mean differences in a within-subjects design involving three or more conditions/observation periods.

research. Systematic inquiry that uses orderly scientific methods to answer questions or solve problems.

research hypothesis. The researcher's expectation regarding the relationship between variables.

residual correlation matrix. A correlation matrix that shows partial correlations between variables with the effects of factors (from a factor analysis) removed.

residual scatterplot. A scatterplot from a multivariate analysis that plots errors of prediction on one axis and predicted values of the dependent variable on the other.

residuals. In multiple regression and other analyses, the error term or unexplained variance.

results. The answers to research questions, obtained through an analysis of the collected data; in a quantitative study, the information obtained through statistical tests.

robust. A characteristic attributed to a statistic that remains useful and believable even when the underlying assumptions have been violated.

rotated factor matrix. A factor matrix (variables $\times$ factors) after the reference axes have been rotated in factor space.

Roy's greatest characteristic root (gcr) criterion. A statistical index used in MANOVA and other multivariate tests to test the significance of group differences.

salient similarity index. A statistic used to determine the significance of similarity between patterns of loadings in two separate factor analyses.

sample. A subset of a population selected to participate in a research study.

sampling distribution. A theoretical distribution of a statistic using an infinite number of samples as a basis and the values of the statistic computed from these samples as the data points in the distribution.

sampling error. The fluctuation of the value of a statistic from one sample from a population to another sample.

scatterplot. A graph depicting the relationship between two continuous variables.

Scheffé test. A post hoc test used following a significant ANOVA to test differences between all possible pairs of means; a conservative test that tends to err on the side of underestimating significance.

scree test. An approach to determining the appropriate number of factors in a factor analysis that plots eigenvalues against factors; discontinuities in the scree plot suggest where factoring should stop.

selection bias. A threat to the internal validity of the study resulting from preexisting differences between the groups under study.

semipartial correlation. A correlation between two variables (Y and X_1) that partials out a third variable (X_2), but only from one of the variables being correlated; symbolized as $r_{y(2\cdot1)}$.

semiquartile range. An index of variability, equal to the difference between the value of the upper quartile (Q_3) and lower quartile (Q_1), divided by 2.

separate variance estimate. In t-tests, an alternative formula for estimating the standard error of the difference; used if the assumption of homogeneous variances is untenable or if sample sizes in the two groups are unequal.

significance level. The probability that an observed value or relationship could be caused by chance (i.e., as a result of sampling error); significance at the .05 level indicates the probability that the observed values would be found by chance only 5 times out of 100.

simultaneous multiple regression. A multiple regression analysis in which all predictor variables are entered into the equation simultaneously; sometimes referred to as *direct* or *standard multiple regression*.

singularity. A term that describes a correlation matrix in which two or more independent variables are perfectly correlated with each other.

skewed distribution. A distribution of data values that is asymmetric, with the bulk of scores clustering at one end and a tail trailing off at the other end.

slope. The rate at which a line rises across a horizontal distance; the steepness of a regression line, usually symbolized by b in a regression equation.

Spearman's rank-order correlation. A correlation coefficient indicating the magnitude and direction of a relationship between variables measured on the ordinal scale.

standard deviation. A descriptive statistic for measuring the degree of variability in a set of scores.

standard error. The standard deviation of a sampling distribution (e.g., the *SD* of the sampling distribution of means is the standard error of the mean, abbreviated *SEM*).

standard error of estimate. In regression analysis, the standard deviation of the errors from the regression line; used to indicate the accuracy of the predictions from regression.

standard scores. Scores expressed in terms of standard deviations from the mean; raw scores are transformed to scores with a mean of zero and a standard deviation of one; referred to as z scores when the distribution is normal.

statistic. A descriptive index calculated from sample data as an estimate of a population parameter.

statistical analysis. The organization and analysis of quantitative data using statistical procedures.

statistical control. The use of statistical techniques to isolate or nullify variance in the dependent variable that is associated with variables extraneous to the analysis.

statistical inference. The process of inferring attributes about the population based on information from a sample.

statistical significance. A term indicating that the results obtained in an analysis of sample data are unlikely to have been caused by chance, at some specified level of probability.

statistical test. An analytic procedure that allows a researcher to determine the likelihood that obtained results from a sample reflect true population results, according to the laws of probability.

stepdown analysis. A supplementary analysis used following a significant MANOVA to test the importance of the dependent variables in the analysis.

stepwise multiple regression. A multiple regression analysis in which predictor variables are entered into the equation in steps, in the order in which the increment to R is greatest.

structural equations. Equations representing the magnitude and nature of hypothesized relations among sets of variables in a theory.

structural equations model. A model made up of a set of structural equations; designed to describe causal relations among variables.

structure coefficients. The correlation between the original variables in the analysis and scores on linear composites (e.g., canonical variate scores or discriminant scores); also called *loadings*.

structure matrix. The matrix that contains the correlations between variables on the one hand and linear composites (factor scores, canonical variate scores, or discriminant scores) on the other.

sum of squares. The sum of squared deviation scores, often abbreviated *SS*.

suppression. A phenomenon that sometimes occurs in multiple regression when a variable obscures (suppresses) or alters a relationship between other variables because of overlapping variability.

symmetrical distribution. A distribution of values that has two halves that are mirror images of the each other; a distribution that is not skewed.

t **distribution.** A family of theoretical probability distributions used in hypothesis testing that are similar to the normal distribution in that *t* distributions are unimodal, symmetrical, and bell-shaped; also referred to as *Student's t distribution*.

t-**test.** A parametric statistical test; most often used for analyzing the difference between two means (the two-sample *t*-test).

test for dependent groups. The class of statistical tests used for within-subjects (or matched-subjects) designs.

test for independent groups. The class of statistical tests used to compare independent groups, i.e., for between-subjects designs.

test statistic. A statistic computed for the purpose of testing the statistical significance of relationships between variables; the sampling distributions of test statistics are known for circumstances in which the null hypothesis is true.

test-retest reliability. Assessment of the stability of an instrument by correlating the scores obtained on repeated administrations.

theory. An abstract generalization that presents a systematic explanation about the relationships among phenomena.

theory trimming. The process of deleting paths from a causal model on the basis of initial empirical results.

tolerance. A statistical index used to detect multicollinearity among independent variables; computed by regressing each independent variable on other independent variables, and subtracting the resulting R^2 from 1.00.

total effect. In the decomposition of effects in causal models, the sum of direct and indirect effects of an independent variable on a dependent variable; also referred to as the *effect coefficient*.

tracing rule. An algorithm used to decompose correlations in a causal model by tracing the paths in a path diagram according to specified criteria.

Tukey's honestly significant difference (HSD) test. A post hoc test used following a significant ANOVA to test differences between all possible pairs of means.

two-tailed test. A test of statistical significance in which values at both extremes (tails) of a distribution are considered in determining significance; used when the researcher has not predicted the direction of a relationship.

Type I error. An error created by rejecting the null hypothesis when it is true (i.e., the researcher concludes that a relationship exists when in fact it does not).

Type II error. An error created by accepting the null hypothesis when it is false (i.e., the researcher concludes that *no* relationship exists when in fact it does).

underidentified model. A model in which there is a greater number of unknown parameters to be estimated than the number of known parameters.

unimodal distribution. A distribution of values with one peak (high frequency).

univariate statistics. Statistical procedures for analyzing a single variable at a time.

unrotated factor matrix. A factor matrix (variables × factors) produced through factor extraction, prior to having the reference axes rotated in factor space.

validity. The degree to which an instrument measures what it is intended to measure.

validity coefficient. A quantitative index, usually ranging in value from .00 to 1.00, that provides an estimate of how valid an instrument is.

variability. The degree to which values on a set of scores are spread out or dispersed.

variable. An attribute of a person or object that varies (i.e., takes on different values).

variance. A measure of variability or dispersion; equal to the square of the standard deviation.

variance-covariance matrix. A square matrix with the variances of variables on the diagonal and the covariance of pairs of variables on the off-diagonal.

Wald statistic. A statistic used to evaluate the significance of individual predictors in a logistic regression equation.

Wilcoxon signed ranks test. A nonparametric statistical test for comparing two paired groups; based on the relative ranking of values between the pairs.

wild code. A code that is inconsistent with the coding scheme established by the researcher.

Wilks' lambda. An index used in several multivariate analyses to test the significance of group differences; indicates the proportion of variance in the dependent variable *un*accounted for by predictors.

within-subjects design. A research design in which a single group of subjects is compared under different conditions or at different points in time and that calls for statistical tests for dependent groups.

X **axis.** The horizontal dimension of a two-dimensional graph; also known as the *abscissa*.

Y **axis.** The vertical dimension of a two-dimensional graph; also known as the *ordinate*.

Yates' correction. A correction to the chi-square statistic that is used when the expected frequency for any cell of a contingency table is less than 10.

z **score.** A standard score expressed in terms of standard deviations from the mean in a normal distribution.

zero-order correlation. The bivariate correlation between two variables, without controlling or partialling out the effect of other variables.

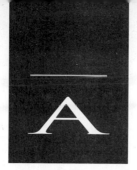

Answers to Selected Exercises

CHAPTER 1

1. a. Constant   b. variable   c. constant   d. variable
2. a. Independent: age; dependent: psychosocial adjustment
   b. Independent: handicap status; dependent: health self-concept
   c. Independent: self versus nurse administration of pain medication; dependent: pain rating
   d. Independent: presence vs. absence of conversing visitors; dependent: intracranial pressure
   e. Independent: type of head covering; dependent: heat loss
3. a. Discrete   b. continuous   c. discrete   d. continuous   e. continuous   f. discrete   g. discrete
4. a. Interval   b. ordinal   c. ratio   d. ordinal (but usually treated as interval)   e. nominal   f. ordinal   g. nominal   h. ratio

CHAPTER 2

1.

Number of Falls	f	%	cum %
0	13	32.5	32.5
1	15	37.5	70.0
2	5	12.5	82.5
3	3	7.5	90.0
4	2	5.0	95.0
5	1	2.5	97.5
6	1	2.5	100.0
	40	100.0	

2. a. 67.5%   b. 1 fall   c. 5 and 6 falls   d. 82.5%
   e. sample size = 40   f. there are no outliers
3. Grouping would result in insufficient detail; with only seven different score values, the values should not be grouped.
5. The distribution is unimodal and positively skewed. The data are not normally distributed.
6. A bar graph; clinical specialty is a nominal-level variable.

CHAPTER 3

1. Mean = 30.37; median = 29.0; mode = 27. The distribution is positively skewed.
2. a. 7.0   b. 7.0   c. 3.83   d. 4.17   e. 5.0
3. d. This distribution has an extreme value (20) that would result in a distorted view of a "typical" value if the mean were used.
4. Mean = 140.0; range = 60; SD = 20.0 Var = 400.0
5.

Original	Z Score	Transformed
130	−0.5	450
120	−1.0	400
110	−1.5	350
150	+0.5	550
160	+1.0	600
140	0.0	500
120	−1.0	400
160	+1.0	600
170	+1.5	650
140	0.0	500

CHAPTER 4

1.

	Experimental	Control	Total
Complied	9	5	14
	64.3% (R)	35.7% (R)	
	60.0% (C)	33.3% (C)	
Did Not Comply	6	10	16
	37.5% (R)	62.5% (R)	
	40.0% (C)	66.7% (C)	
Total	15	15	30

2. Teenaged mothers: M = 102.5; older mothers: M = 106.7; overall sample: M = 104.6
4. r = .91, strong positive correlation

CHAPTER 5

1. $p = .25$ ($1 \div 4$ suits); $p = .0009765$ ($.25^5$)
3. $z = -0.5; +1.5; -2.0; +3.0$
4. $p = .023$ ($z = -2.00$)
5. An *SEM* of 0.0 implies that all the sample means are equal to the population mean—there is no variability in any of the sample means as estimates of the population mean. This, in turn, implies the absence of variability of scores in the population, because under any other circumstance sampling error would result in some sample means being different from the population mean.
6. Mean = 5.0; $SD = 1.211$; $SEM = 0.303$
7. The estimate for sample B is likely to be more accurate than that for sample A because the standard error of the mean will be smaller as a result of the fact that the sample size is larger.
8. 95% $CI = 7.155 \leq \mu \leq 8.445$; 99% $CI = 6.942 \leq \mu \leq 8.658$
9. $t = 1.768$; tabled value is about 2.01 for $df = 49$, so the result is not statistically significant ($p > .05$).
10. Tabled value for a one-tailed test with $\alpha = .05$ and $df = 49$ is about 1.68, so the obtained result ($t = 1.768$) *is* statistically significant at the .05 level.

CHAPTER 6

1. a. Inappropriate—there are three groups, not two
   b. Inappropriate—the dependent groups *t*-test should be used because the subjects are paired
   c. Appropriate
   d. Inappropriate—the DV is measured on the nominal scale
   e. Inappropriate—the dependent groups *t*-test should be used because it is the same subjects in both groups.
2. a. Appropriate, assuming the same subjects are used in both conditions
   b. Appropriate
   c. Inappropriate—there are three time periods, not two
   d. Inappropriate—the groups are independent (unless the data were collected longitudinally from the same subjects over a lengthy time period).
   e. Inappropriate—the DV is measured on the nominal scale.
3. $t = 3.54$, $df = 48$, statistically significant at $\alpha = .05$
4. $r_{pb} = .21$, a modest relationship
6. $\gamma = .91$, $\delta = 3.21$, $1 - \beta = .89$, $\beta = .11$
7. a. No   b. yes   c. yes   d. yes
8. a. About 2.02   b. about 2.39   c. 2.878   d. about 1.66   e. 2.807
9. $\delta = 1.50$, $1 - \beta = .32$; n needed for power = .80 is about 62 per group
10. $t = 4.58$, $df = 9$, statistically significant at $\alpha = .05$

CHAPTER 7

1. a. Appropriate—-one-way ANOVA
   b. Appropriate—-two-way (multifactor) ANOVA
   c. Inappropriate—-there are only two groups
   d. Appropriate—-mixed design ANOVA: between subjects on treatment factor, within subjects for time of measurement
   e. Inappropriate—-dependent variable is nominal-level
   f. Appropriate—repeated measures ANOVA
2. The group means are: nonsmokers = 21.0; smokers = 26.0; quitters = 35.0; $SS_B = 503.33$, $SS_W = 222.00$; $df_B = 2$, $df_W = 12$; $MS_B = 251.67$, $MS_W = 18.50$; $F = 13.60$, significant at the .05 level.
3. $t_{1-2} = -1.84$; $t_{1-3} = -5.15$; $t_{2-3} = -3.31$; $LSD = 5.93$. Quitters are significantly different from both nonsmokers and smokers. Smokers are *not* significantly different from nonsmokers.
4. $Eta^2 = .69$; estimated power is greater than .99. Thus, there is a strong relationship between smoking status and somatic complaints; the risk of a Type II error is negligible.
6. a. Not significant   b. not significant   c. significant   d. significant   e. not significant
7. $MS_A = 74.50$; $MS_B = 37.00$; $MS_{AB} = 54.00$; $MS_W = 13.49$; $F_A = 5.52$; $F_B = 2.74$; $F_{AB} = 4.00$. With $df = 1$ and 76 for all three tests, the tabled value of F is 3.96. Thus, the F tests for gender (Factor A) differences and for the interaction (AB) are both significant, but the F test for differences by exercise status is not.
9. $df_{site} = 2$; $df_{error} = 28$; $MS_{site} = 8.996.50$; $MS_{error} = 1,726.75$; the computed value of F for within subjects is 5.21. With $df = 2$ and 28, the tabled value of F at $\alpha = .05$ is 3.34. Thus, we reject the null hypothesis that the three site means are equal.
10. a. .75   b. .45   c. .70   d. .68   e. .92

CHAPTER 8

1. $\chi^2 = 16.66$, $df = 2$. The tabled value of χ^2 at $\alpha = .05$ is 5.99, so the results are statistically significant. Group B's high rate of obtaining a flu shot is substantially higher than expected; the value of $(O - E)^2/E$ for that cell was 7.50.
2. Cramér's $V = .24$. If the value of V were .20, power would be between .85 and .90 (i.e., for a sample size between 273 and 316). Since V is larger than .20, power in this case exceeds .90.
4. a. No   b. yes   c. no   d. yes
5. Approximately 200 subjects
6. 1. c   2. d   3. b   4. a
7. a. Mann-Whitney U-test   b. repeated measures ANOVA   c. Cochran's Q test   d. chi-square test of independence   e. Kruskal-Wallis test   f. McNemar's test
8. a. Fisher's exact test   b. regular chi-square test   c. chi-square test with Yates' continuity correction.

9. $U_{men} = 18$, $U_{women} = 31$, not statistically significant
10. Wilcoxon signed-ranks test, $z = 2.29$, $p < .05$

CHAPTER 9

1. a. No b. no c. yes d. yes e. no
2. a. .58 b. .11 c. .83 d. .02
3. a. .81 b. .36 c. .54 d. .26
4. a. r likely would get smaller b. r likely would get larger c. r likely would get larger
5. $a = 9.8$; $Y' = 9.8 - .10X$
6. a. 4.6 b. 3.0 c. 7.5 d. 8.8
7. Yes: $z_{obs} = 1.97$, which is greater than the critical value of 1.96
8. $\delta = 1.55$; power $(1 - \beta)$ is about .34; risk of Type II error (β) is about .66
9. About 243 subjects for $\delta = 2.8$
10. $r_S = .54$, not significant

CHAPTER 10

1. 2.91 (18); 3.16 (19); 3.60 (20)
2. a. $F (5,114) = 25.73, p < .05$ b. $F (5,24) = 5.41, p < .05$ c. $F (4,59) = 5.74, p < .05$ d. $F (4,59)= 2.40, p > .05$ *(NS)*
3. a and c
4. a. Lowest $R^2 = .29$ b. VARA c. cannot be determined
6. Male smokers = 1, female smokers = 0, male nonsmokers = 0, female nonsmokers = 0
7. a. .51 b. .23 c. .14 d. .27
8. a. The increment = .03 b. the increment is the squared semipartial correlation coefficient, $r^2_{y(3.12)}$; $F (1,46) = 2.34, p > .05$ *(NS)*.
9. a. FULLTIME (1,0), PARTTIME (1,0) b. PREMENO (1,0), PERIMENO (1,0), MENOPAUS (1,0) c. HOSPITAL (1,0)
11. a. $N = 79$ b. $N = 234$ c. $N = 66$ d. $N = 35$

CHAPTER 11

1. a. Canonical analysis b. two-way MANCOVA c. repeated measures ANCOVA d. MANOVA
3.

	Unadjusted Mean	Adjusted Mean
1 No insurance	17.961	16.631
2 Private insurance	24.331	25.491
3 Medicaid	18.871	18.051

4. Data that are suitable for a MANOVA *could* also be analyzed by canonical analysis. The group variable would need to be dummy coded, so that one set of variables in the canonical analysis would consist of two dummy variables and the other set would consist of the four dependent variables.
5. .005
6. Four

CHAPTER 12

1. I = 1.38 (13.8%); II = 1.22 (12.2%); III = 1.21 (12.1%); total = 38.1%
2. 1 = .39; 2 = .41; 3 = .59; 4 = .44; 5 = .58; 6 = .29; 7 = .25; 8 = .35; 9 = .27; 10 = .25
3. $Y' = .10$; $X' = .60$; test G is likely to be a quantitative aptitude test
4. Subject 1: Factor I = 347.0, Factor II = 300.0; Subject 2: Factor I = 265.8, Factor II = 264.2
5. 58.6%, 49.1%

CHAPTER 13

1. No. 16: .82; No. 17: −1.53; No. 18: −1.83; No. 19: −.87; No. 20: .70
2. Predicted classification—Finished: Nos. 16 and 20; Did not finish, Nos. 17, 18, and 19; 100% of these five cases were correctly classified.
3. a. Two functions   b. two functions   c. one function
4. a. $D = 8.29 + 1.32(\text{PARTNR}) - .74(\text{BCBASE}) - .60(\text{DIPLOMA}) + .51(\text{WELFARE}) + .32(\text{ASPIREHI}) + .64 \ (\text{PREGCNT}) + .02(\text{BASECESD}) - .52(\text{BASEAGE})$

   b. $\log\left[\dfrac{\text{Prob (repeat)}}{\text{Prob (no repeat)}}\right] =$

   $3.91 + .59(\text{PARTNR}) - .33(\text{BCBASE}) - .27(\text{DIPLOMA}) + .23(\text{WELFARE}) + .14(\text{ASPIREHI}) + .28(\text{PREGCNT}) + .01(\text{BASECESD}) - .23(\text{BASEAGE})$
5. Smokers odds   = $.37 \div .63 = .587$

   Nonsmokers odds = $.11 \div .89 = .124$

   Odds ratio   = $.587 \div .124 = 4.73$

CHAPTER 14

3. $z_1 = e_1$

   $z_2 = e_2$

   $z_3 = p_{31}z_1 + p_{32}z_2 + e_3$

   $z_4 = p_{41}z_1 + p_{42}z_2 + p_{43}z_3 + e_4$
4. A—direct only;   B—direct and noncausal (unanalyzed);   C—direct, indirect, and noncausal (spurious)

5. Six correlations: r_{12}, r_{13}, r_{14}, r_{23}, r_{24}, r_{34}. Decomposition of r_{14} (.743): Direct = p_{41} = .250; indirect = $p_{31}p_{43}$ = .295; total causal = .545; noncausal = $p_{41}p_{31}p_{43}$ = .074; all effects = .619. (The model does not exactly reproduce r_{14} because it does not account for the relationship between V_1 and V_2; i.e., the model assumes these two variables are uncorrelated, but r_{12} = .383.)

6. e_3 = .664; e_4 = .339

7. Overidentified (e.g., there is no path between Received Support and Expectancy Confirmation)

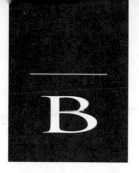

Theoretical Probability Distribution Tables

TABLE B-1. AREAS OF THE NORMAL DISTRIBUTION FOR SELECTED z SCORES

Column (1): z Score (or $-z$)

Column (2):   Probability of a value $\geq z$

or

Probability of a value $\leq -z$

Column (3):   Probability of a value ≥ 0 and $\leq z$

or

Probability of a value $\geq -z$ and ≤ 0

(1) z	(2) $\geq z$	(3) ≥ 0 and $\leq z$	(1) z	(2) $\geq z$	(3) ≥ 0 and $\leq z$
0.00	.500	.000	1.10	.136	.364
0.05	.480	.020	1.20	.115	.385
0.10	.460	.040	1.30	.097	.403
0.15	.440	.060	1.40	.081	.419
0.20	.421	.079	1.50	.067	.433
0.25	.401	.099	1.60	.055	.445
0.30	.382	.118	1.70	.045	.455
0.35	.363	.137	1.80	.036	.464
0.40	.345	.155	1.90	.029	.471
0.45	.326	.174	2.00	.023	.477
0.50	.309	.192	2.10	.018	.482
0.55	.291	.209	2.20	.014	.486
0.60	.274	.226	2.30	.011	.489
0.65	.258	.242	2.40	.008	.492
0.70	.242	.258	2.50	.006	.494
0.75	.227	.273	2.60	.005	.495
0.80	.212	.288	2.70	.004	.496
0.85	.198	.302	2.80	.003	.497
0.90	.184	.316	2.90	.002	.498
0.95	.171	.329	3.00	.001	.499
1.00	.159	.341			

TABLE B–2. CRITICAL VALUES OF *t*

df	Test 2-Tailed α:	Level of Significance .10	.05	.02	.01	.001
1		6.31	12.71	31.82	63.66	636.62
2		2.92	4.30	6.97	9.93	31.60
3		2.35	3.18	4.54	5.84	12.94
4		2.13	2.78	3.75	4.60	8.61
5		2.02	2.57	3.37	4.03	6.86
6		1.94	2.45	3.14	3.71	5.96
7		1.90	2.37	3.00	3.45	5.41
8		1.86	2.31	2.90	3.36	5.04
9		1.83	2.26	2.82	3.25	4.78
10		1.81	2.23	2.76	3.17	4.58
11		1.80	2.20	2.72	3.11	4.44
12		1.78	2.18	2.68	3.06	4.32
13		1.77	2.16	2.65	3.01	4.22
14		1.76	2.15	2.62	2.98	4.14
15		1.75	2.13	2.60	2.95	4.07
16		1.75	2.12	2.58	2.92	4.02
17		1.74	2.11	2.57	2.90	3.97
18		1.73	2.10	2.55	2.88	3.92
19		1.73	2.09	2.54	2.86	3.88
20		1.73	2.09	2.53	2.85	3.85
21		1.72	2.08	2.52	2.83	3.82
22		1.72	2.07	2.51	2.82	3.79
23		1.71	2.07	2.50	2.81	3.77
24		1.71	2.06	2.49	2.80	3.75
25		1.71	2.06	2.49	2.79	3.73
26		1.71	2.06	2.48	2.78	3.71
27		1.71	2.05	2.47	2.77	3.69
28		1.70	2.05	2.47	2.76	3.67
29		1.70	2.05	2.46	2.76	3.66
30		1.70	2.04	2.46	2.75	3.65
40		1.68	2.02	2.42	2.70	3.55
60		1.67	2.00	2.39	2.66	3.46
120		1.66	1.98	2.36	2.62	3.73
∞		1.65	1.96	2.33	2.58	3.29
df	1-Tailed α:	.05	.025	.01	.005	.0005

TABLE B–3. CRITICAL VALUES OF F: $\alpha = .05$

$\dfrac{df_B}{df_W}$	1	2	3	4	5	6	8	12	24	∞
1	161.4	199.5	215.7	224.6	230.2	234.0	238.9	243.9	249.0	254.3
2	18.51	19.00	19.16	19.25	19.30	19.33	19.37	19.41	19.45	19.50
3	10.13	9.55	9.28	9.12	9.01	8.94	8.84	8.74	8.64	8.53
4	7.71	6.94	6.59	6.39	6.26	6.16	6.04	5.91	5.77	5.63
5	6.61	5.79	5.41	5.19	5.05	4.95	4.82	4.68	4.53	4.26
6	5.99	5.14	4.76	4.53	4.39	4.28	4.15	4.00	3.84	3.67
7	5.59	4.74	4.35	4.12	3.97	3.87	3.73	3.57	3.41	3.23
8	5.32	4.46	4.07	3.84	3.69	3.58	3.44	3.28	3.12	2.93
9	5.12	4.26	3.86	3.63	3.48	3.37	3.23	3.07	2.90	2.71
10	4.96	4.10	3.71	3.48	3.33	3.22	3.07	2.91	2.74	2.54
11	4.84	3.98	3.59	3.36	3.20	3.09	2.95	2.79	2.61	2.40
12	4.75	3.88	3.49	3.26	3.11	3.00	2.85	2.69	2.50	2.30
13	4.67	3.80	3.41	3.18	3.02	2.92	2.77	2.60	2.42	2.21
14	4.60	3.74	3.34	3.11	2.96	2.85	2.70	2.53	2.35	2.13
15	4.54	3.68	3.29	3.06	2.90	2.79	2.64	2.48	2.29	2.07
16	4.49	3.63	3.24	3.01	2.85	2.74	2.59	2.42	2.24	2.01
17	4.45	3.59	3.20	2.96	2.81	2.70	2.55	2.38	2.19	1.96
18	4.41	3.55	3.16	2.93	2.77	2.66	2.51	2.34	2.15	1.92
19	4.38	3.52	3.13	2.90	2.74	2.63	2.48	2.31	2.11	1.88
20	4.35	3.49	3.10	2.87	2.71	2.60	2.45	2.28	2.08	1.84
21	4.32	3.47	3.07	2.84	2.68	2.57	2.42	2.25	2.05	1.81
22	4.30	3.44	3.05	2.82	2.66	2.55	2.40	2.23	2.03	1.78
23	4.28	3.42	3.03	2.80	2.64	2.53	2.38	2.20	2.00	1.76
24	4.26	3.40	3.01	2.78	2.62	2.51	2.36	2.18	1.98	1.73
25	4.24	3.38	2.99	2.76	2.60	2.49	2.34	2.16	1.96	1.71
26	4.22	3.37	2.98	2.74	2.59	2.47	2.32	2.15	1.95	1.69
27	4.21	3.35	2.96	2.73	2.57	2.46	2.30	2.13	1.93	1.67
28	4.20	3.34	2.95	2.71	2.56	2.44	2.29	2.12	1.91	1.65
29	4.18	3.33	2.93	2.70	2.54	2.43	2.28	2.10	1.90	1.64
30	4.17	3.32	2.92	2.69	2.53	2.42	2.27	2.09	1.89	1.62
40	4.08	3.23	2.84	2.61	2.45	2.34	2.18	2.00	1.79	1.51
60	4.00	3.15	2.76	2.52	2.37	2.25	2.10	1.92	1.70	1.39
120	3.92	3.07	2.68	2.45	2.29	2.17	2.02	1.83	1.61	1.25
∞	3.84	2.99	2.60	2.37	2.21	2.09	1.94	1.75	1.52	1.00

TABLE B–3. (CONTINUED) CRITICAL VALUES OF F: $\alpha = .01$

$\dfrac{df_B}{df_W}$	1	2	3	4	5	6	8	12	24	∞
1	4052	4999	5403	5625	5764	5859	5981	6106	6234	6366
2	98.49	99.00	99.17	99.25	99.30	99.33	99.36	99.42	99.46	99.50
3	34.12	30.81	29.46	28.71	28.24	27.91	27.49	27.05	26.60	26.12
4	21.20	18.00	16.69	15.98	15.52	15.21	14.80	14.37	13.93	13.46
5	16.26	13.27	12.06	11.39	10.97	10.67	10.29	9.89	9.47	9.02
6	13.74	10.92	9.78	9.15	8.75	8.47	8.10	7.72	7.31	6.88
7	12.25	9.55	8.45	7.85	7.46	7.19	6.84	6.47	6.07	5.65
8	11.26	8.65	7.59	7.01	6.63	6.37	6.03	5.67	5.28	4.86
9	10.56	8.02	6.99	6.42	6.06	5.80	5.47	5.11	4.73	4.31
10	10.04	7.56	6.55	5.99	5.64	5.39	5.06	4.71	4.33	3.91
11	9.65	7.20	6.22	5.67	5.32	5.07	4.74	4.40	4.02	3.60
12	9.33	6.93	5.95	5.41	5.06	4.82	4.50	4.16	3.78	3.36
13	9.07	6.70	5.74	5.20	4.86	4.62	4.30	3.96	3.59	3.16
14	8.86	6.51	5.56	5.03	4.69	4.46	4.14	3.80	3.43	3.00
15	8.68	6.36	5.42	4.89	4.56	4.32	4.00	3.67	3.29	2.87
16	8.53	6.23	5.29	4.77	4.44	4.20	3.89	3.55	3.18	2.75
17	8.40	6.11	5.18	4.67	4.34	4.10	3.79	3.45	3.08	2.65
18	8.28	6.01	5.09	4.58	4.25	4.01	3.71	3.37	3.00	2.57
19	8.18	5.93	5.01	4.50	4.17	3.94	3.63	3.30	2.92	2.49
20	8.10	5.85	4.94	4.43	4.10	3.87	3.56	3.23	2.86	2.42
21	8.02	5.78	4.87	4.37	4.04	3.81	3.51	3.17	2.80	2.36
22	7.94	5.72	4.82	4.31	3.99	3.76	3.45	3.12	2.75	2.31
23	7.88	5.66	4.76	4.26	3.94	3.71	3.41	3.07	2.70	2.26
24	7.82	5.61	4.72	4.22	3.90	3.67	3.36	3.03	2.66	2.21
25	7.77	5.57	4.68	4.18	3.86	3.63	3.32	2.99	2.62	2.17
26	7.72	5.53	4.64	4.14	3.82	3.59	3.29	2.96	2.58	2.13
27	7.68	5.49	4.60	4.11	3.78	3.56	3.26	2.93	2.55	2.10
28	7.64	5.45	4.57	4.07	3.75	3.53	3.23	2.90	2.52	2.06
29	7.60	5.42	4.54	4.04	3.73	3.50	3.20	2.87	2.49	2.03
30	7.56	5.39	4.51	4.02	3.70	3.47	3.17	2.84	2.47	2.01
40	7.31	5.18	4.31	3.83	3.51	3.29	2.99	2.66	2.29	1.80
60	7.08	4.98	4.13	3.65	3.34	3.12	2.82	2.50	2.12	1.60
120	6.85	4.79	3.95	3.48	3.17	2.96	2.66	2.34	1.95	1.38
∞	6.64	4.60	3.78	3.32	3.02	2.80	2.51	2.18	1.79	1.00

(Continued)

TABLE B–3. (CONTINUED) CRITICAL VALUES OF F: $\alpha = .001$

$\dfrac{df_B}{df_W}$	1	2	3	4	5	6	8	12	24	∞
1	405284	500000	540379	562500	576405	585937	598144	610667	623497	636619
2	998.5	999.0	999.2	999.2	999.3	999.3	999.4	999.4	999.5	999.5
3	167.5	148.5	141.1	137.1	134.6	132.8	130.6	128.3	125.9	123.5
4	74.14	61.25	56.18	53.44	51.71	50.53	49.00	47.41	45.77	44.05
5	47.04	36.61	33.20	31.09	29.75	28.84	27.64	26.42	25.14	23.78
6	35.51	27.00	23.70	21.90	20.81	20.03	19.03	17.99	16.89	15.75
7	29.22	21.69	18.77	17.19	16.21	15.52	14.63	13.71	12.73	11.69
8	25.42	18.49	15.83	14.39	13.49	12.86	12.04	11.19	10.30	9.34
9	22.86	16.39	13.90	12.56	11.71	11.13	10.37	9.57	8.72	7.81
10	21.04	14.91	12.55	11.28	10.48	9.92	9.20	8.45	7.64	6.76
11	19.69	13.81	11.56	10.35	9.58	9.05	8.35	7.63	6.85	6.00
12	18.64	12.97	10.80	9.63	8.89	8.38	7.71	7.00	6.25	5.42
13	17.81	12.31	10.21	9.07	8.35	7.86	7.21	6.52	5.78	4.97
14	17.14	11.78	9.73	8.62	7.92	7.43	6.80	6.13	5.41	4.60
15	16.59	11.34	9.34	8.25	7.57	7.09	6.47	5.81	5.10	4.31
16	16.12	10.97	9.00	7.94	7.27	6.81	6.19	5.55	4.85	4.06
17	15.72	10.66	8.73	7.68	7.02	6.56	5.96	5.32	4.63	3.85
18	15.38	10.39	8.49	7.46	6.81	6.35	5.76	5.13	4.45	3.67
19	15.08	10.16	8.28	7.26	6.61	6.18	5.59	4.97	4.29	3.52
20	14.82	9.95	8.10	7.10	6.46	6.02	5.44	4.82	4.15	3.38
21	14.59	9.77	7.94	6.95	6.32	5.88	5.31	4.70	4.03	3.26
22	14.38	9.61	7.80	6.81	6.19	5.76	5.19	4.58	3.92	3.15
23	14.19	9.47	7.67	6.69	6.08	5.65	5.09	4.48	3.82	3.05
24	14.03	9.34	7.55	6.59	5.98	5.55	4.99	4.39	3.74	2.97
25	13.88	9.22	7.45	6.49	5.88	5.46	4.91	4.31	3.66	2.89
26	13.74	9.12	7.36	6.41	5.80	5.38	4.83	4.24	3.59	2.82
27	13.61	9.02	7.27	6.33	5.73	5.31	4.76	4.17	3.52	2.75
28	13.50	8.93	7.19	6.25	5.66	5.24	4.69	4.11	3.46	2.70
29	13.39	8.85	7.12	6.19	5.59	5.18	4.64	4.05	3.41	2.64
30	13.29	8.77	7.05	6.12	5.53	5.12	4.58	4.00	3.36	2.59
40	12.61	8.25	6.60	5.70	5.13	4.73	4.21	3.64	3.01	2.23
60	11.97	7.76	6.17	5.31	4.76	4.37	3.87	3.31	2.69	1.90
120	11.38	7.31	5.79	4.95	4.42	4.04	3.55	3.02	2.40	1.56
∞	10.83	6.91	5.42	4.62	4.10	3.74	3.27	2.74	2.13	1.00

TABLE B–4. CRITICAL VALUES OF χ^2

df	Level of Significance				
	.10	.05	.02	.01	.001
1	2.71	3.84	5.41	6.63	10.83
2	4.61	5.99	7.82	9.21	13.82
3	6.25	7.82	9.84	11.34	16.27
4	7.78	9.49	11.67	13.28	18.46
5	9.24	11.07	13.39	15.09	20.52
6	10.64	12.59	15.03	16.81	22.46
7	12.02	14.07	16.62	18.48	24.32
8	13.36	15.51	18.17	20.09	26.12
9	14.68	16.92	19.68	21.67	27.88
10	15.99	18.31	21.16	23.21	29.59
11	17.28	19.68	22.62	24.72	31.26
12	18.55	21.03	24.05	26.22	32.91
13	19.81	22.36	25.47	27.69	34.53
14	21.06	23.68	26.87	29.14	36.12
15	22.31	25.00	28.26	30.58	37.70
16	23.54	26.30	29.63	32.00	39.25
17	24.77	27.59	31.00	33.41	40.79
18	25.99	28.87	32.35	34.81	42.31
19	27.20	30.14	33.69	36.19	43.82
20	28.41	31.41	35.02	37.57	45.32
21	29.62	32.67	36.34	38.93	46.80
22	30.81	33.92	37.66	40.29	48.27
23	32.01	35.17	38.97	41.64	49.73
24	33.20	36.42	40.27	42.98	51.18
25	34.38	37.65	41.57	44.31	52.62
26	35.56	38.89	42.86	45.64	54.05
27	36.74	40.11	44.14	46.96	55.48
28	37.92	41.34	45.42	48.28	56.89
29	39.09	42.56	46.69	49.59	58.30
30	40.26	43.77	47.96	50.89	59.70

TABLE B–5. CRITICAL VALUES OF THE U STATISTIC FOR $\alpha = .05$ (TWO-TAILED TEST)

$n_2\downarrow$ \ $n_1\rightarrow$	1	2	3	4	5	6	7	8	9	10	11	12	13	14	15	16	17	18	19	20
1	—a	—	—	—	—	—	—	—	—	—	—	—	—	—	—	—	—	—	—	—
2	—	—	—	—	—	—	—	0	0	0	0	1	1	1	1	1	2	2	2	2
3	—	—	—	—	0	1	1	2	2	3	3	4	4	5	5	6	6	7	7	8
4	—	—	—	0	1	2	3	4	4	5	6	7	8	9	10	11	11	12	13	13
5	—	—	0	1	2	3	5	6	7	8	9	11	12	13	14	15	17	18	19	20
6	—	—	1	2	3	5	6	8	10	11	13	14	16	17	19	21	22	24	25	27
7	—	—	1	3	5	6	8	10	12	14	16	18	20	22	24	26	28	30	32	34
8	—	0	2	4	6	8	10	13	15	17	19	22	24	26	29	31	34	36	38	41
9	—	0	2	4	7	10	12	15	17	20	23	26	28	31	34	37	39	42	45	48
10	—	0	3	5	8	11	14	17	20	23	26	29	33	36	39	42	45	48	52	55
11	—	0	3	6	9	13	16	19	23	26	30	33	37	40	44	47	51	55	58	62
12	—	1	4	7	11	14	18	22	26	29	33	37	41	45	49	53	57	61	65	69
13	—	1	4	8	12	16	20	24	28	33	37	41	45	50	54	59	63	67	72	76
14	—	1	5	9	13	17	22	26	31	36	40	45	50	55	59	64	67	74	78	83
15	—	1	5	10	14	19	24	29	34	39	44	49	54	59	64	70	75	80	85	90
16	—	1	6	11	15	21	26	31	37	42	47	53	59	64	70	75	81	86	92	98
17	—	2	6	11	17	22	28	34	39	45	51	57	63	67	75	81	87	93	99	105
18	—	2	7	12	18	24	30	36	42	48	55	61	67	74	80	86	93	99	106	112
19	—	2	7	13	19	25	32	38	45	52	58	65	72	78	85	92	99	106	113	119
20	—	2	8	13	20	27	34	41	48	55	62	69	76	83	90	98	105	112	119	127

Note: To be statistically significant, the calculated U must be *equal to or less than* the tabled value.
aA dash indicates that no decision is possible for the specified ns.

TABLE B–6. CRITICAL VALUES OF r

Test	Level of Significance				
df 2-Tailed α: (1)	.10 (2)	.05 (3)	.02 (4)	.01 (5)	.001 (6)
1	.988	.997	.9995	.9999	1.00
2	.900	.950	.980	.990	.999
3	.805	.878	.934	.959	.991
4	.729	.811	.882	.917	.974
5	.669	.754	.833	.874	.951
6	.622	.707	.789	.834	.925
7	.582	.666	.750	.798	.898
8	.549	.632	.716	.765	.872
9	.521	.602	.685	.735	.847
10	.497	.576	.658	.708	.823
11	.476	.553	.634	.684	.801
12	.458	.532	.612	.661	.780
13	.441	.514	.592	.641	.760
14	.426	.497	.574	.623	.742
15	.412	.482	.558	.606	.725
16	.400	.468	.542	.590	.708
17	.389	.456	.528	.575	.693
18	.378	.444	.516	.561	.679
19	.369	.433	.503	.549	.665
20	.360	.423	.492	.537	.652
25	.323	.381	.445	.487	.597
30	.296	.349	.409	.449	.554
35	.275	.325	.381	.418	.519
40	.257	.304	.358	.393	.490
45	.243	.288	.338	.372	.465
50	.231	.273	.322	.354	.443
60	.211	.250	.295	.325	.408
70	.195	.232	.274	.302	.380
80	.183	.217	.256	.283	.357
90	.173	.205	.242	.267	.338
100	.164	.195	.230	.254	.321
125	.147	.174	.206	.228	.288
150	.134	.159	.189	.208	.264
200	.116	.138	.164	.181	.235
300	.095	.113	.134	.148	.188
500	.074	.088	.104	.115	.148
1000	.052	.062	.073	.081	.104
2000	.037	.044	.056	.058	.074
df 1-Tailed α:	.05	.025	.01	.005	.0005

These are the critical values for the test that $\rho = 0$

TABLE B–7. TRANSFORMATION OF r TO z_r

r	z_r	r	z_r	r	z_r	r	z_r	r	z_r
.000	.000	.200	.203	.400	.424	.600	.693	.800	1.1099
.005	.005	.205	.208	.405	.430	.605	.701	.805	1.113
.010	.010	.210	.213	.410	.436	.610	.709	.810	1.127
.015	.015	.215	.218	.415	.442	.615	.717	.815	1.142
.020	.020	.220	.224	.420	.448	.620	.725	.820	1.157
.025	.025	.225	.229	.425	.454	.625	.733	.825	1.172
.030	.030	.230	.234	.430	.460	.630	.741	.830	1.188
.035	.035	.235	.239	.435	.466	.635	.750	.835	1.204
.040	.040	.240	.245	.440	.472	.640	.758	.840	1.221
.045	.045	.245	.250	.445	.478	.645	.767	.845	1.238
.050	.050	.250	.255	.450	.485	.650	.775	.850	1.256
.055	.055	.255	.261	.455	.491	.655	.784	.855	1.274
.060	.060	.260	.266	.460	.497	.660	.793	.860	1.293
.065	.065	.265	.271	.465	.504	.665	.802	.865	1.313
.070	.070	.270	.277	.470	.510	.670	.811	.870	1.333
.075	.075	.275	.282	.475	.517	.675	.820	.875	1.354
.080	.080	.280	.288	.480	.523	.680	.829	.880	1.376
.085	.085	.285	.293	.485	.530	.685	.838	.885	1.398
.090	.090	.290	.299	.490	.536	.690	.848	.890	1.422
.095	.095	.295	.304	.495	.543	.695	.858	.895	1.447
.100	.100	.300	.310	.500	.549	.700	.867	.900	1.472
.105	.105	.305	.315	.505	.556	.705	.877	.905	1.499
.110	.110	.310	.321	.510	.563	.710	.887	.910	1.528
.115	.116	.315	.326	.515	.570	.715	.897	.915	1.557
.120	.121	.320	.332	.520	.576	.720	.908	.920	1.589
.125	.126	.325	.337	.525	.583	.725	.918	.925	1.623
.130	.131	.330	.343	.530	.590	.730	.929	.930	1.658
.135	.136	.335	.348	.535	.597	.735	.940	.935	1.697
.140	.141	.340	.354	.540	.604	.740	.950	.940	1.738
.145	.146	.345	.360	.545	.611	.745	.962	.945	1.783
.150	.151	.350	.365	.550	.618	.750	.973	.950	1.832
.155	.156	.355	.371	.555	.626	.755	.984	.955	1.886
.160	.161	.360	.377	.560	.633	.760	.996	.960	1.946
.165	.167	.365	.383	.565	.640	.765	1.008	.965	2.014
.170	.172	.370	.388	.570	.648	.770	1.020	.970	2.092
.175	.177	.375	.394	.575	.655	.775	1.033	.975	2.185
.180	.182	.380	.400	.580	.662	.780	1.045	.980	2.298
.185	.187	.385	.406	.585	.670	.785	1.058	.985	2.443
.190	.192	.390	.412	.590	.678	.790	1.071	.990	2.647
.195	.198	.395	.418	.595	.685	.795	1.085	.995	2.994

TABLE B–8. CRITICAL VALUES FOR SPEARMAN'S RHO (r_s)

Test N 2-Tailed α:	Level of Significance			
	.10	.05	.02	.01
(1)	(2)	(3)	(4)	(5)
5	.900	1.000	1.000	—
6	.829	.886	.943	1.000
7	.714	.786	.893	.929
8	.643	.738	.833	.881
9	.600	.683	.783	.833
10	.564	.648	.746	.794
12	.506	.591	.712	.777
14	.456	.544	.645	.715
16	.425	.506 —	.601	.665
18	.399	.475	.564	.625
20	.377	.450	.534	.591
22	.359	.428	.508	.562
24	.343	.409	.485	.537
25	.337	.398	.465	.510
26	.329	.392	.456	.515
28	.317	.377	.448	.496
30	.306	.363	.432	.467
N 1-Tailed α:	.05	.025	.01	.005

These are the critical values for the test that $\rho_S = 0$; note that column 1 specifies the number of pairs of scores (N), not degrees of freedom. The critical values are both + and − for two-tailed tests.

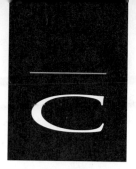

Tables for Power Analyses

TABLE C–1. TABLE OF POWER $(1 - \beta)$ AS A FUNCTION OF δ AND α

(1) δ	(2) .10	(3) .05	(4) .02	(5) .01	(1) δ	(2) .10	(3) .05	(4) .02	(5) .01
0.0	.10	.05	.02	.01	2.5	.80	.71	.57	.47
0.1	.10	.05	.02	.01	2.6	.83	.74	.61	.51
0.2	.11	.05	.02	.01	2.7	.85	.77	.65	.55
0.3	.12	.06	.03	.01	2.8	.88	.80	.68	.59
0.4	.13	.07	.03	.01	2.9	.90	.83	.72	.63
0.5	.14	.08	.03	.02	3.0	.91	.85	.75	.66
0.6	.16	.09	.04	.02	3.1	.93	.87	.78	.70
0.7	.18	.11	.05	.03	3.2	.94	.89	.81	.73
0.8	.21	.13	.06	.04	3.3	.96	.91	.83	.77
0.9	.23	.15	.08	.05	3.4	.96	.93	.86	.80
1.0	.26	.17	.09	.06	3.5	.97	.94	.88	.82
1.1	.30	.20	.11	.07	3.6	.97	.96	.92	.87
1.2	.33	.22	.13	.08	3.7	.98	.96	.93	.89
1.3	.37	.26	.15	.10	3.8	.98	.97	.93	.89
1.4	.40	.29	.18	.12	3.9	.99	.97	.94	.91
1.5	.44	.32	.20	.14	4.0	.99	.98	.95	.92
1.6	.48	.36	.23	.16	4.1	.99	.98	.96	.94
1.7	.52	.40	.27	.19	4.2	.99	.99	.97	.95
1.8	.56	.44	.30	.22	4.3	.99+	.99	.98	.96
1.9	.60	.48	.33	.25	4.4	.99+	.99	.98	.97
2.0	.64	.52	.37	.28	4.5	.99+	.99	.99	.97
2.1	.68	.56	.41	.32	4.6	.99+	.99+	.99	.98
2.2	.71	.59	.45	.35	4.7	.99+	.99+	.99	.98
2.3	.74	.63	.49	.39	4.8	.99+	.99+	.99	.99
2.4	.77	.67	.53	.43	4.9	.99+	.99+	.99	.99
δ	.05	.025	.01	.005	δ	.05	.025	.01	.005

Top headers: Two-tailed significance (α) (both sides).
Bottom headers: One-tailed significance (α) (both sides).

To find power for two-tailed significance tests, find appropriate α in top row and read down; to find power for one-tailed significance tests, find appropriate α in bottom row and read up.

TABLE C–2. POWER TABLES FOR ANOVA

A. Number of Groups = 4, α = .05[a]

Power	.01	.03	.05	.07	.10	.15	.20	.25	.30	.40	.50	.60	.70	.80
							Population Eta^2							
.10	21	7	5	4	3	2	2	2	—	—	—	—	—	—
.50	144	48	28	20	14	9	7	5	4	3	2	2	2	—
.70	219	72	43	30	21	13	10	8	6	4	3	2	2	2
.80	272	90	53	37	26	17	12	9	7	5	4	3	2	2
.90	351	115	68	48	33	21	15	12	9	6	5	3	3	2
.95	426	140	83	58	40	25	18	14	11	7	5	4	3	2
.99	583	191	113	79	54	34	24	19	15	10	7	5	4	2

B. Number of Groups = 5, α = .05

Power	.01	.03	.05	.07	.10	.15	.20	.25	.30	.40	.50	.60	.70	.80
							Population Eta^2							
.10	19	7	5	3	3	2	2	2	—	—	—	—	—	—
.50	128	43	25	18	13	8	6	5	4	3	2	2	2	—
.70	193	64	38	27	18	12	9	7	6	4	3	2	2	2
.80	238	78	46	33	23	15	10	8	7	5	3	3	2	2
.90	306	101	59	42	29	18	13	10	8	6	4	3	2	2
.95	369	121	72	50	34	22	16	12	10	7	5	3	3	2
.99	501	164	97	68	46	30	21	16	13	9	6	4	3	2

C. Number of Groups = 6, α = .05

Power	.01	.03	.05	.07	.10	.15	.20	.25	.30	.40	.50	.60	.70	.80
							Population Eta^2							
.10	18	7	4	3	3	2	—	—	—	—	—	—	—	—
.50	117	39	23	17	12	8	6	5	4	3	2	2	2	—
.70	174	57	34	24	17	11	8	6	5	4	3	2	2	2
.80	213	70	42	29	20	13	9	7	6	4	3	2	2	2
.90	273	90	53	37	26	17	12	9	7	5	4	3	2	2
.95	328	108	64	45	31	20	14	11	9	6	4	3	3	2
.99	442	145	86	60	41	26	19	14	11	8	5	4	3	2

NOTE: Entries in body of table are for n, the number of subjects *per group*.
[a] The power table for 3 groups with α =.05 is presented in Table 7-7.

(Continued)

TABLE C–2. (CONTINUED) POWER TABLES FOR ANOVA

D. Number of Groups = 3, α = .01

Power	.01	.03	.05	.07	.10	.15	Population Eta^2 .20	.25	.30	.40	.50	.60	.70	.80
.10	77	26	16	11	8	5	5	3	3	2	2	2	—	—
.50	272	89	53	37	26	16	13	9	7	5	4	3	2	2
.70	383	126	74	52	36	23	17	13	10	7	5	4	3	2
.80	459	151	89	62	43	27	20	15	12	8	6	4	3	2
.90	576	189	111	78	53	34	25	18	15	10	7	5	3	2
.95	683	224	132	93	63	40	29	22	17	11	8	6	4	3
.99	906	297	175	122	83	53	38	28	22	15	10	7	5	3

E. Number of Groups = 4, α = .01

Power	.01	.03	.05	.07	.10	.15	Population Eta^2 .20	.25	.30	.40	.50	.60	.70	.80
.10	70	23	14	10	7	5	4	3	3	2	2	—	—	—
.50	232	76	45	32	22	14	11	8	6	4	3	3	2	2
.70	323	106	63	44	30	19	14	11	9	6	4	3	2	2
.80	384	126	75	52	36	23	17	13	10	7	5	4	3	2
.90	478	157	93	65	44	28	21	15	12	8	6	4	3	2
.95	563	184	109	76	52	33	24	18	14	10	7	5	3	2
.99	740	242	143	100	68	43	31	23	18	12	8	6	4	3

F. Number of Groups = 5, α = .01

Power	.01	.03	.05	.07	.10	.15	Population Eta^2 .20	.25	.30	.40	.50	.60	.70	.80
.10	64	21	13	9	7	5	4	3	3	2	2	—	—	—
.50	204	67	40	28	19	13	10	7	6	4	3	3	2	2
.70	280	92	55	38	26	17	13	9	8	6	4	3	2	2
.80	333	109	65	46	31	20	15	11	9	6	4	3	2	2
.90	412	135	80	56	38	25	18	13	11	7	5	4	3	2
.95	483	158	94	66	45	29	21	16	12	8	6	4	3	2
.99	631	207	122	86	58	37	27	20	16	11	7	5	4	3

TABLE C–2. (CONTINUED) POWER TABLES FOR ANOVA

G. Number of Groups = 6, α = .01

	Population Eta²													
Power	.01	.03	.05	.07	.10	.15	.20	.25	.30	.40	.50	.60	.70	.80
.10	59	20	12	9	6	4	4	3	2	2	2	—	—	—
.50	183	61	36	25	18	11	9	7	5	4	3	2	2	2
.70	251	83	49	35	24	15	11	9	7	5	4	3	2	2
.80	296	97	58	41	28	18	13	10	8	5	4	3	2	2
.90	365	120	71	50	34	22	16	12	10	7	5	3	3	2
.95	426	140	83	58	40	25	18	14	11	7	5	4	3	2
.99	554	182	107	75	51	33	24	18	14	9	7	5	3	2

NOTE: Entries in body of table are for *n*, the number of subjects *per group*.

TABLE C–3. POWER TABLES FOR THE CHI-SQUARE TEST FOR $\alpha = .05$

FOR A 2 × 2 TABLE:

Power	Population Value of Cramér's Statistic								
	.10	.20	.30	.40	.50	.60	.70	.80	.90
.25	165	41	18	10	7	5	3	3	2
.50	384	96	43	24	15	11	8	6	5
.60	490	122	54	31	20	14	10	8	6
.70	617	154	69	39	25	17	13	10	8
.75	694	175	77	43	28	19	14	11	9
.80	785	196	87	49	31	22	16	12	10
.85	898	224	100	56	36	25	18	14	11
.90	1,051	263	117	66	42	29	21	16	13
.95	1,300	325	144	81	52	36	27	20	16
.99	1,837	459	204	115	73	51	37	29	23

FOR A 2 × 3 TABLE:

Power	Population Value of Cramér's Statistic								
	.10	.20	.30	.40	.50	.60	.70	.80	.90
.25	226	56	25	14	9	6	5	4	3
.50	496	124	55	31	20	14	10	8	6
.60	621	155	69	39	25	17	13	10	8
.70	770	193	86	48	31	21	16	12	10
.75	859	215	95	54	34	24	18	13	11
.80	964	241	107	60	39	27	20	15	12
.85	1,092	273	121	68	44	30	22	17	13
.90	1,265	316	141	79	51	35	26	20	16
.95	1,544	386	172	97	62	43	32	24	19
.99	2,140	535	238	134	86	59	44	33	26

TABLE C–3. (CONTINUED) POWER TABLES FOR THE CHI-SQUARE TEST FOR $\alpha = .05$

FOR A 2 × 4 TABLE:

Power	Population Value of Cramér's Statistic								
	.10	.20	.30	.40	.50	.60	.70	.80	.90
.25	258	65	29	16	10	7	5	4	3
.50	576	144	64	36	23	16	12	9	7
.60	715	179	79	45	29	20	15	11	9
.70	879	220	98	55	35	24	18	14	11
.75	976	244	108	61	39	27	20	15	12
.80	1,090	273	121	68	44	30	22	17	13
.85	1,230	308	137	77	49	34	25	19	15
.90	1,417	354	157	89	57	39	29	22	17
.95	1,717	429	191	107	69	48	35	27	21
.99	2,352	588	261	147	94	65	48	37	29

FOR A 3 × 3 TABLE:

Power	Population Value of Cramér's Statistic								
	.10	.20	.30	.40	.50	.60	.70	.80	.90
.25	154	39	17	10	6	4	3	2	2
.50	321	80	36	20	13	9	7	5	4
.60	396	99	44	25	16	11	8	6	5
.70	484	121	54	30	19	13	10	8	6
.75	536	134	60	34	21	15	11	8	7
.80	597	149	66	37	24	17	12	9	7
.85	671	168	75	42	27	19	14	10	8
.90	770	193	86	48	31	21	16	12	10
.95	929	232	103	58	37	26	19	15	11
.99	1,262	316	140	79	50	35	26	20	16

TABLE C–3. (CONTINUED) POWER TABLES FOR THE CHI-SQUARE TEST FOR $\alpha = .05$

FOR A 3 × 4 TABLE:

Power	Population Value of Cramér's Statistic								
	.10	.20	.30	.40	.50	.60	.70	.80	.90
.25	185	46	21	12	7	5	4	3	2
.50	375	94	42	23	15	10	8	6	5
.60	460	115	51	29	18	13	9	7	6
.70	557	139	62	35	22	15	11	9	7
.75	615	154	68	38	25	17	13	10	8
.80	681	170	76	43	27	19	14	11	8
.85	763	191	85	48	31	21	16	12	9
.90	871	218	97	54	35	24	18	14	11
.95	1,043	261	116	65	42	29	21	16	13
.99	1,403	351	156	88	56	39	29	22	17

FOR A 4 × 4 TABLE:

Power	Population Value of Cramér's Statistic								
	.10	.20	.30	.40	.50	.60	.70	.80	.90
.25	148	37	16	9	6	4	3	2	2
.50	294	73	33	18	12	8	6	5	4
.60	357	89	40	22	14	10	7	6	4
.70	430	107	48	27	17	12	9	7	5
.75	472	118	52	30	19	13	10	7	6
.80	522	130	58	33	21	14	11	8	6
.85	582	145	65	36	23	16	12	9	7
.90	661	165	73	41	26	18	13	10	8
.95	786	197	87	49	31	22	16	12	10
.99	1,046	262	116	65	42	29	21	16	13

Name Index

Subject Index

MULTIVARIATE STATISTICAL ANALYSES

Name	Purpose	Measurement Level*			Number of:		
		IV	DV	Cov	IVs	DVs	Cov
Multiple correlation/ regression	To test the relationship between 2+ IVs and 1 DV; to predict a DV from 2+ IVs	N,I,R	I,R	—	2+	1	—
Analysis of covariance (ANCOVA)	To test the difference between the means of 2+ groups, while controlling for 1+ covariate	N	I,R	N,I,R	1+	1	1+
Multivariate analysis of variance (MANOVA)	To test the difference between the means of 2+ groups for 2+ DVs simultaneously	N	I,R	—	1+	2+	—
Multivariate analysis of covariance (MANCOVA)	To test the difference between the means of 2+ groups for 2+ DVs simultaneously, while controlling for 1+ covariate	N	I,R	N,I,R	1+	2+	1+
Canonical analysis	To test the relationship between 2 sets of variables (variables on the right, variables on the left)	N,I,R	N,I,R	—	2+	2+	—
Factor analylis	To determine the dimensionality/ structure of a set of variables	—	—	—	—	—	—
Discriminant analysis	To test the relationship between 2+ IVs and 1 DV; to predict group membership; to classify cases into groups	N,I,R	N	—	2+	1	—
Logistic regression regression	To test the relationship between 2+ IVs and 1 DV; to predict the probability of an event; to estimate relative risk	N,I,R	N	—	2+	1	—

*Measurement level of the independent variable (IV), dependent variable, (DV), and covariates (Cov): N = nominal, I= interval, R = ratio